1.99

369 0289830

Aberdeen Mackenzie Library
MacRobert

2012
YEAR BOOK OF
NEONATAL AND
PERINATAL MEDICINE®

# The 2012 Year Book Series

Year Book of Anesthesiology and Pain Management™: Drs Chestnut, Abram, Black, Gravlee, Lien, Mathru, and Roizen

Year Book of Cardiology®: Drs Gersh, Cheitlin, Elliott, Gold, Graham, and Thourani

Year Book of Critical Care Medicine®: Drs Dries, Zanotti-Cavazzoni, Latenser, Martinez, Rincon, and Zwank

Year Book of Dermatology and Dermatologic Surgery™: Dr Del Rosso

Year Book of Diagnostic Radiology®: Drs Elster, Abbara, Oestreich, Offiah, Rosado de Christenson, Stephens, and Strickland

Year Book of Emergency Medicine®: Drs Hamilton, Bruno, Handly, Minczak, Mullin, Quintana, and Ramoska

Year Book of Endocrinology®: Drs Schott, Apovian, Clarke, Eugster, Meikle, Oetgen, Ovalle, Schteingart, and Toth

Year Book of Hand and Upper Limb Surgery®: Drs Yao, Adams, Isaacs, Lee, and Rizzo

Year Book of Medicine®: Drs Barker, Garrick, Gersh, Khardori, LeRoith, Panush, Talley, and Thigpen

Year Book of Neonatal and Perinatal Medicine®: Drs Fanaroff, Benitz, Donn, Neu, Papile, and Van Marter

Year Book of Neurology and Neurosurgery®: Drs Klimo, Minagar, Gandhi, House, Kevill, Liu, Mazia, Panagariya, Ragel, Riesenburger, Robottom, Schwendimann, Shafazand, Uhm, and Yang

Year Book of Obstetrics, Gynecology, and Women's Health®: Drs Dungan and Shulman

Year Book of Oncology®: Drs Arceci, Bauer, Chiorean, Gordon, Lawton, Murphy, Thigpen, and Tsao

Year Book of Ophthalmology®: Drs Rapuano, Cohen, Flanders, Hammersmith, Milman, Myers, Nagra, Nelson, Penne, Pyfer, Sergott, Shields, Talekar, and Vander

Year Book of Orthopedics®: Drs Morrey, Huddleston, Rose, Swiontkowski, and Trigg

Year Book of Otolaryngology-Head and Neck Surgery®: Drs Sindwani, Balough, Franco, Gapany, and Mitchell

Year Book of Pathology and Laboratory Medicine®: Drs Raab and Bissell

Year Book of Pediatrics®: Dr Stockman

Year Book of Plastic and Aesthetic Surgery™: Drs Miller, Gosman, Gurtner, Gutowski, Ruberg, Salisbury, and Smith

**Year Book of Psychiatry and Applied Mental Health®:** Drs Talbott, Ballenger, Buckley, Frances, Krupnick, and Mack

**Year Book of Pulmonary Disease®:** Drs Barker, Jones, Maurer, Spradley, Tanoue, and Willsie

**Year Book of Sports Medicine®:** Drs Shephard, Cantu, Feldman, Galea, Jankowski, Janssen, Lebrun, and Nieman

**Year Book of Surgery®:** Drs Copeland, Behrns, Daly, Eberlein, Fahey, Huber, Klodell, Mozingo, and Pruett

**Year Book of Urology®:** Drs Andriole and Coplen

**Year Book of Vascular Surgery®:** Drs Moneta, Gillespie, Starnes, and Watkins

Alistair Mackenzie Library
Wishaw General Hospital
50 Netherton Street
Wishaw
ML2 0DP

MUSEUM

2012

# The Year Book of
# NEONATAL AND
# PERINATAL
# MEDICINE®

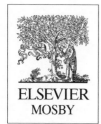

ELSEVIER
MOSBY

ALISTAIR MACKENZIE LIBRARY
Barcode: ~~26905~~
Class no:

ALISTAIR MACKENZIE LIBRARY
Barcode: 36902898 30
Class no: WS 420 FAN

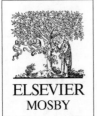

# ELSEVIER
## MOSBY

*Vice President, Continuity:* Kimberly Murphy
*Editor:* Kerry Holland
*Production Supervisor, Electronic Year Books:* Donna M. Skelton
*Electronic Article Manager:* Emily Ogle
*Illustrations and Permissions Coordinator:* Dawn Vohsen

**2012 EDITION**
**Copyright 2012, Mosby, Inc. All rights reserved.**

No part of this publication may be reproduced, stored in a retrieval system, or transmitted, in any form or by any means, electronic, mechanical, photocopying, recording, or otherwise, without prior written permission from the publisher.

Permission to photocopy or reproduce solely for internal or personal use is permitted for libraries or other users registered with the Copyright Clearance Center, provided that the base fee of $35.00 per chapter is paid directly to the Copyright Clearance Center, 21 Congress Street, Salem, MA 01970. This consent does not extend to other kinds of copying, such as copying for general distribution, for advertising or promotional purposes, for creating new collected works, or for resale.

Composition by TNQ Books and Journals Pvt Ltd, India

Editorial Office:
Elsevier
Suite 1800
1600 John F. Kennedy Blvd.
Philadelphia, PA 19106-3399

International Standard Serial Number: 8756-5005
International Standard Book Number: 978-0-323-09108-4

Printed and bound by CPI Group (UK) Ltd, Croydon, CR0 4YY

Transferred to digital print 2012

# Editorial Board

## Avroy A. Fanaroff, MD, FRCPE, FRCP&CH

*Eliza Henry Barnes Chair of Neonatology, Rainbow Babies & Children's Hospital; Professor, Department of Pediatrics and Reproductive Biology, Case Western Reserve University School of Medicine, Cleveland, Ohio*

## William E. Benitz, MD

*Philip Sunshine Professor of Neonatology, Stanford University School of Medicine, Palo Alto, California*

## Steven M. Donn, MD

*Professor of Pediatrics, Division of Neonatal-Perinatal Medicine, University of Michigan Health System, C.S. Mott Children's Hospital, Ann Arbor, Michigan*

## Josef Neu, MD

*Professor of Pediatrics, University of Florida College of Medicine, Gainesville, Florida*

## Lu-Ann Papile, MD

*Professor of Pediatrics, Baylor College of Medicine, Houston, Texas*

## Linda J. Van Marter, MD, MPH

*Director of Clinical Research, Associate Professor of Pediatrics, Harvard Medical School, Boston, Massachusetts*

# Contributing Editors

## Jill E. Baley, MD
*Professor of Pediatrics, Case Western Reserve University School of Medicine; Medical Director, Neonatal Transitional Unit, Rainbow Babies & Children's Hospital, Cleveland, Ohio*

## John Donald E. Barks, MD
*Professor of Pediatrics, Director, Neonatal-Perinatal Medicine, C.S. Mott Children's Hospital, University of Michigan Health System, Ann Arbor, Michigan*

## Rachel L. Chapman, MD
*Clinical Associate Professor of Pediatrics, University of Michigan School of Medicine, C.S. Mott Children's Hospital, Ann Arbor, Michigan*

## Ritu Chitkara, MD
*Attending Neonatologist, Department of Pediatrics, Cedars-Sinai Medical Center; Clinical Instructor, Department of Pediatrics, David Geffen School of Medicine at UCLA, Los Angeles, CA*

## Helen Christou, MD
*Assistant Professor of Pediatrics, Harvard Medical School; Associate Director, Harvard Perinatal-Neonatal Fellowship program; Brigham and Women's Hospital and Boston Children's Hospital, Boston Massachusetts*

## Nicholas Evans, DM, MRCPCH
*Clinical Associate Professor, Department of Neonatal Medicne, Royal Prince Alfred Hospital, and University of Sydney, Sydney, Australia*

## Jonathan M. Fanaroff, MD, JD
*Associate Professor of Pediatrics, Case Western Reserve University School of Medicine; Director, Rainbow Center for Pediatric Ethics; Co-Director, Neonatal Intensive Care Unit, Rainbow Babies & Children's Hospital, Cleveland, Ohio*

## Jay P. Goldsmith, MD
*Clinical Professor, Department of Pediatrics, Tulane University, New Orleans, Louisiana*

## Samir Gupta, DM, MRCP, MD, FRCPCH, FRCPI
*Senior Lecturer, University of Durham; Consultant Neonatologist and Co-Director Research and Development, North Tees Hospital, Stockton, United Kingdom*

## Jonathan Hellmann, MBBCh, FCP(SA), FRCPC, MHSc
*Professor of Paediatrics, University of Toronto; Staff Neonatologist, The Hospital for Sick Children, Toronto, Ontario, Canada*

## Naomi Laventhal, MD
*Clinical Lecturer of Pediatrics and Communicable Diseases, Division of Neonatal-Perinatal Medicine, University of Michigan Health System, C.S. Mott Children's Hospital, Ann Arbor, Michigan*

## Richard J. Martin, MD
*Professor, Pediatrics, Case Western Reserve University; Drusinksy-Fanaroff Chair in Neonatology, Rainbow Babies & Children's Hospital, Cleveland, Ohio*

## Fernando Moya, MD
*Director of Neonatology, Betty Cameron Women & Children's Hospital; Clinical Professor of Pediatrics, University of North Carolina; and President and CEO, Coastal Carolina Neonatology, PLLC, Wilmington, North Carolina*

## Karen M. Puopolo, MD, PhD
*Assistant Professor of Pediatrics, Harvard Medical School; Division of Newborn Medicine, Brigham and Women's Hospital, Boston, Massachusetts*

## Robert E. Schumacher, MD
*Professor, Department of Pediatrics, University of Michigan Health System, Ann Arbor, Michigan*

## Renée A. Shellhaas, MD, MS
*Clinical Assistant Professor, Department of Pediatrics and Communicable Diseases, Division of Pediatric Neurology, Department of Pediatrics, University of Michigan, Ann Arbor, Michigan*

## Eileen K. Stork, MD
*Professor of Pediatrics, Director, Neonatal and ECMO Program, Rainbow Babies & Children's Hospital, Cleveland, Ohio*

## Rebecca J. Vartanian, MD
*Clinical Lecturer, Division of Neonatal-Perinatal Medicine, C.S. Mott Children's Hospital, University of Michigan Health System, Ann Arbor, Michigan*

## Deanne Wilson-Costello, MD
*Professor of Pediatrics, Co-Director of High Risk Follow-up, Rainbox Babies & Children's Hospital, Cleveland, Ohio*

## Fiona E. Wood, MBBS (Lond), MRCPCH
*Clinical Research Fellow in Neonatology, James Cook University Hospital, South Tees Hospitals NHS Foundation Trust, Middlesbrough; Honorary Clinical Teaching Associate, University of Newcastle-upon-Tyne, Tyne and Wear, United Kingdom*

# Table of Contents

# Journals Represented

Journals represented in this YEAR BOOK are listed below.

Acta Obstetricia et Gynecologica Scandinavica
Acta Paediatrica
Advances in Neonatal Care
American Journal of Clinical Nutrition
American Journal of Obstetrics and Gynecology
American Journal of Perinatology
American Journal of Respiratory and Critical Care Medicine
Annals of Neurology
Annals of Thoracic Surgery
Archives of Disease in Childhood Education and Practice Edition
Archives of Disease in Childhood Fetal and Neonatal Edition
Archives of Facial Plastic Surgery
Archives of General Psychiatry
Archives of Pediatrics & Adolescent Medicine
Australia & New Zealand Journal of Obstetrics & Gynaecology
British Medical Journal
Childs Nervous System
Circulation
Clinical Chemistry
Clinical Infectious Diseases
Drugs
Early Human Development
European Journal of Obstetrics & Gynecology and Reproductive Biology
European Journal of Paediatric Neurology
Human Reproduction
Intensive Care Medicine
Israel Medical Association Journal
Journal of Allergy and Clinical Immunology
Journal of Child Neurology
Journal of Clinical Nursing
Journal of Molecular Diagnostics
Journal of Nursing Scholarship
Journal of Pediatric Gastroenterology and Nutrition
Journal of Pediatric Surgery
Journal of Pediatrics
Journal of Perinatology
Journal of the American Academy of Dermatology
Journal of the American College of Cardiology
Journal of the American Medical Association
Journal of the American Society of Echocardiography
Journal of Thoracic and Cardiovascular Surgery
Journal of Ultrasound in Medicine
Lancet
Neurology
New England Journal of Medicine
Obstetrics & Gynecology
Ophthalmology

Pediatric Cardiology
Pediatric Infectious Disease Journal
Pediatric Neurology
Pediatric Research
Pediatrics
Proceedings of the National Academy of Sciences of the United States of America
Public Library of Science One
Science Translational Medicine
Seminars in Fetal & Neonatal Medicine
Southern Medical Journal
Ultrasound in Obstetrics & Gynecology

## STANDARD ABBREVIATIONS

The following terms are abbreviated in this edition: acquired immunodeficiency syndrome (AIDS), cardiopulmonary resuscitation (CPR), central nervous system (CNS), cerebrospinal fluid (CSF), computed tomography (CT), deoxyribonucleic acid (DNA), electrocardiography (ECG), health maintenance organization (HMO), human immunodeficiency virus (HIV), intensive care unit (ICU), intramuscular (IM), intravenous (IV), magnetic resonance (MR) imaging (MRI), ribonucleic acid (RNA), and ultrasound (US).

## NOTE

The YEAR BOOK OF NEONATAL AND PERINATAL MEDICINE® is a literature survey service providing abstracts of articles published in the professional literature. Every effort is made to assure the accuracy of the information presented in these pages. Neither the editors nor the publisher of the YEAR BOOK OF NEONATAL AND PERINATAL MEDICINE® can be responsible for errors in the original materials. The editors' comments are their own opinions. Mention of specific products within this publication does not constitute endorsement.

To facilitate the use of the YEAR BOOK OF NEONATAL AND PERINATAL MEDICINE® as a reference tool, all illustrations and tables included in this publication are now identified as they appear in the original article. This change is meant to help the reader recognize that any illustration or table appearing in the YEAR BOOK OF NEONATAL AND PERINATAL MEDICINE® may be only one of many in the original article. For this reason, figure and table numbers will often appear to be out of sequence within the YEAR BOOK OF NEONATAL AND PERINATAL MEDICINE®.

# Introduction

After a seemingly very short year, the 2012 YEAR BOOK OF NEONATAL AND PERINATAL MEDICINE is complete, and work is already underway on the 2013 edition. The literature related to the fetus and newborn has expanded exponentially, yet there have not been any major therapeutic breakthroughs published in the past year. Rather, there has been consolidation of the evidence and a more intense focus on patient safety, avoidance of medical errors, and an awareness of the importance of the Statewide Quality Improvement Collaborative. Some highlights from this issue include the evidence supporting the use of antenatal corticosteroids as early as 23 weeks' gestation; the dangers of fetal exposure to environmental teratogens; the changing patterns of labor over the past 50 years; the effectiveness of an alcohol-free mouthwash in reducing premature birth in a high-risk population; and a more precise definition of oligohydramnios—beneficial in predicting adverse neonatal outcomes. We are reminded of the dangers of prolonged and unnecessary antibiotic administration in the neonatal period, the remarkable success in preventing early onset Group B streptococcal infections, and the need to find adjunctive therapies for use with hypothermia to improve the outcomes for severely asphyxiated term neonates. The shift to gentler ventilation and alternative methods of administering surfactant is also addressed. Further benefits from delayed clamping of the umbilical cord and the feeding of human milk are documented, and the use of nonspecific intravenous immunoglobulin for the treatment of neonatal sepsis is put to rest.

Neonatal—perinatal medicine has come a long way. The outlook for intact survival of preterm and malformed infants continues to improve. However, we are still mired in the era of evidence-based medicine, awaiting further application of the human genome to move to individualized medicine.

The YEAR BOOK provides interpretation and perspectives on a broad range of publications in the field of neonatal—perinatal medicine over the past year. We are grateful to our colleagues who continue to provide their expert comments on various articles. Our goal is to be informative, provocative, and at times even humorous, but our main objective is for the information to be educational, thought provoking, and stimulating for the reader. We thank Kerry Holland, our editor, for her considerable help and thank the Elsevier YEAR BOOK team for their continued professionalism and support.

Avroy A. Fanaroff, MD, FRCPE, FRCP&CH

William E. Benitz, MD

Steven M. Donn, MD

Josef Neu, MD

Lu-Ann Papile, MD

Linda Van Marter, MD, MPH

# 1 The Fetus

**Fetal Laboratory Medicine: On the Frontier of Maternal–Fetal Medicine**
Geaghan SM (Stanford Univ School of Medicine, Palo Alto, CA)
*Clin Chem* 58:337-352, 2012

*Background.*—Emerging antenatal interventions and care delivery to the fetus require diagnostic support, including laboratory technologies, appropriate methodologies, establishment of special algorithms, and interpretative guidelines for clinical decision-making.

*Content.*—Fetal diagnostic and therapeutic interventions vary in invasiveness and are associated with a spectrum of risks and benefits. Fetal laboratory assessments are well served by miniaturized diagnostic methods for blood analysis. Expedited turnaround times are mandatory to support invasive interventions such as cordocentesis and intrauterine transfusions. Health-associated reference intervals are required for fetal test interpretation. Fetal blood sampling by cordocentesis carries substantial risk and is therefore performed only when fetal health is impaired, or at risk. When the suspected pathology is not confirmed, however, normative fetal data can be collected. Strategies for assurance of sample integrity from cordocenteses and confirmation of fetal origin are described. After birth, definitive assessment of prenatal environmental and/or drug exposures to the fetus can be retrospectively assessed by analysis of meconium, hair, and other alternative matrices. A rapidly advancing technology for fetal assessment is the use of fetal laboratory diagnostic techniques that use cell-free fetal DNA collected from maternal plasma, and genetic analysis based on molecular counting techniques.

*Summary.*—Developmental changes in fetal biochemical and hematologic parameters in health and disease are continually delineated by analysis of our collective outcome-based experience. Noninvasive technologies for fetal evaluation are realizing the promise of lower risk yet robust diagnostics; examples include sampling and analysis of free fetal DNA from maternal blood, and analysis of fetal products accessible at maternal sites. Application of diagnostic technologies for nonmedical purposes (e.g., sex selection) underscores the importance of ethical guidelines for new technology implementation (Tables 1, 2 and 4).

▶ It is unusual to select a review article that does not summarize a number of randomized trials but is descriptive. Nonetheless, I found this article to be dense with information and very well referenced. It is also a comprehensive review of the past, current, and perhaps future state of fetal evaluation. It traverses the

TABLE 1.—Fetal Therapeutic Interventions (In Order of Increasing Invasiveness) and Clinical Indications[ab]

| Antenatal Intervention | Clinical Indication(s) |
|---|---|
| Delivery of therapeutic drugs, antibiotics, or steroids to fetus by maternal administration | Thyroid hormone in cases of maternal thyroid dysfunction; antibiotics for intrauterine infection; and steroid administration for accelerated lung maturation and to reduce the incidence of respiratory distress and neonatal mortality in the setting of premature births, or for confirmed congenital adrenal hyperplasia |
| Intrauterine transfusion | Fetal anemia (e.g., Rh isoimmunization) |
| Surgery on fetal membranes | Amniotic band syndrome (release) |
| Placental surgery | For placental chorangioma, to prevent cardiac failure and hydrops |
| Laser ablation or photocoagulation of placental vasculature | IUGR or twin—twin transfusion syndrome due to placental vascular anastamoses between monochorionic twins |
| Urinary obstruction decompression by vesicoamniotic catheter placement/shunting | Congenital hydronephrosis (urinary obstruction), with adequate renal function and pulmonary immaturity such that delivery must be delayed |
| Fetoscopy (direct endoscopic visualization) | Percutaneous tracheal occlusion procedure for lung growth promotion in congenital diaphragmatic hernia; tissue biopsies; vascular access; diagnosis and treatment of urinary tract obstruction (see below); surgeries on placenta, membranes, cord |
| Open fetal surgery | Meningomyelocele repair; congenital diaphragmatic hernia repair; thoracic space-occupying lesion removal; cardiac malformation repair; lower urinary tract obstruction decompression; sacrococcygeal teratoma resection |

*Editor's Note*: Please refer to original journal article for full references.
[a]Harrison et al. (1), Crombleholme et al. (2), Deprest et al. (3), Adzick et al. (4), Quintero et al. (5), Leviton et al. (6).
[b]Adapted with permission from Geaghan (95).

high-risk invasive fetal diagnostic tests and comprehensively deals with the new diagnostics, emphasizing the need for rapid turnover of samples and exquisite quality control. The tables summarize the various fields and highlight the important stages in the emergence of this new field called *fetology*.

Tables 1, 2, and 4 provide normal hematologic parameters for the fetus. The parameters for fetal diagnosis and antenatal interventions are transforming rapidly. Noninvasive technologies for fetal evaluation have rapidly emerged with sampling and analysis of free fetal DNA from maternal blood and analysis of fetal products accessible at maternal sites. For interventions to be practical and effective requires robust diagnostics with the establishment of specific algorithms and guidelines for clinical decision making. As these tests become more widely used and reliable, the benefit to risk of fetal intervention will shift dramatically in favor of benefits. After birth, definitive assessment of prenatal environmental or drug exposures to the fetus can be assessed retrospectively by analysis of meconium, hair, and other biologic specimens. Geagham indicates that a major concern is that gender determination from DNA detected in maternal cell free plasma will be used for gender selection; hence, ethical guidelines need to accompany the generalized implementation of this technology.

"Cell-free fetal DNA comprises only 3—6% of the total circulating cell-free DNA, therefore diagnoses are primarily limited to those caused by paternally inherited sequences as well as conditions that can be inferred by the unique gene expression

**TABLE 2.**—Antenatal Diagnostic Laboratory Technologies: Clinical Applications, Associated Risks and Benefits[a,b]

| Diagnostic Test | Clinical Application | Risks | Benefits |
|---|---|---|---|
| Amniocentesis | Detection of aneuploidy or amniocytes for molecular genetic analysis on fetal cells; determination of amniotic fluid OD 450 in Rh incompatibility (infrequent due to use of MCA-PSA); lamellar body count | Amniotic fluid leakage 1%–2%; spontaneous loss rate 0.7% if performed at 14 weeks or later | Reassurance or allows for genetic counseling, OD 450 guides interventions; lamellar body count indicates fetal lung maturity |
| Chorionic villus sampling | Detection of aneuploidy or molecular genetic analysis on fetal cells | If performed at an experienced center after 9 weeks, loss rate approaches that of midtrimester amniocentesis | Reassurance if normal, if abnormal, allows for genetic counseling |
| Cordocentesis: fetal hormones | Testing for congenital adrenal hyperplasia by CYP21 genotyping and assessment of antenatal steroid therapy by following marker 17-hydroxyprogesterone | <2% Fetal loss related to procedure; 9.38% fetal bradycardia | Reduce risk of gender misassignment; possible reduction of gender confusion; may prevent need for corrective genital surgery for ambiguous genitalia |
| Cordocentesis: blood gases | Fetal academia | Same as above | Correlates with reduced development quotient; indicator for emergent delivery |
| Cordocentesis: coagulation testing and platelet counts | Diagnosis and management of hereditary and acquired immune bleeding disorders | Same as above | Planning for minimizing birth trauma (caesarean section); in utero transfusions |
| Maternal site sampling for fetal products | Detection of fetal fibronectin for risk of premature labor; IL-6 and CRP in cervicovaginal fluid; use of $\alpha$-microglobulin-1 test in cervicovaginal fluid | None | fFN: negative predictive value for labor, may reduce admissions; IL-6 and CRP proposed for detection of chorioamnionitis; $\alpha$-microglobulin-1 for detection of premature rupture of membranes |
| Meconium analysis; fetal or segmental maternal hair analysis | Detection of drugs of abuse and alcohol (fatty acid ethyl esters) exposures; environmental exposures | Maternal sanctions, legal and social | Allows for child protection, maternal rehabilitation; allows for removal of environmental risk and ongoing risk surveillance |
| Fetal urine analysis by percutaneous catheter | Assess need to decompress urinary obstruction: if Na <100 mEq/L Cl <90 mEq/L; osmolarity <210 mosmol | Shunt can dislodge, obstruct, migrate | Avert renal damage; possibly promote lung growth |

*Editor's Note:* Please refer to original journal article for full references.

[a]Harrison et al. (1), Crombleholme et al. (2), Deprest et al. (3), Leviton et al. (6), Soothill et al. (30), Ghizzoni et al. (37), Sulcova et al. (38), Daffos et al. (43), Bevis et al. (46), Liley (47), Queenan et al. (48), Mari et al. (49), Gareri et al. (51), Gourley et al. (52), Verma et al. (53), Koren et al (54), Chan et al. (55), Cernichiari et al. (56), Loew et al. (61), Swamy et al. (62), Wei et al. (63), Ashwood et al. (64), Cousins et al. (65), American College of Obstetricians and Gynecologists (68), Borgida et al. (69), Botto et al. (70), Brambati and Tului (71).

[b]Adapted with permission from Geaghan (95).

TABLE 4.—Hematologic Parameters in Healthy Fetuses by Gestational Age[a][b]

| Gestational Age | Sample No. | Hemoglobin, g/dL | Red Blood Cells, ×10⁶/μL | Hematocrit, % | MCV, fL | Total WBC Count, ×10³/μL | Corrected WBC Count, ×10³/μL | Platelets, ×10³/μL |
|---|---|---|---|---|---|---|---|---|
| 15[c] | 6 | 10.9 (0.7) | 2.43 (0.26) | 34.6 (3.6) | 143 (8) | 1.6 (0.7) | — | 190 (31) |
| 16[c] | 5 | 12.5 (0.8) | 2.68 (0.21) | 38.1 (0.21) | 143 (12) | 2.4 (1.7) | — | 208 (57) |
| 17[c] | 16 | 12.4 (0.9) | 2.74 (0.23) | 37.4 (0.28) | 137 (8) | 2.0 (0.8) | — | 202 (25) |
| 18–21[d] | 760 | 11.69 (1.27) | 2.85 (0.36) | 37.3 (4.32) | 131.1 (11.0) | 4.68 (2.96) | 2.57 (0.42) | 234 (57) |
| 22–25[d] | 1200 | 12.20 (1.6) | 3.09 (0.34) | 38.59 (3.94) | 125.1 (7.8) | 4.72 (2.82) | 3.73 (2.17) | 247 (59) |
| 26–29[d] | 460 | 12.91 (1.38) | 3.46 (0.41) | 40.88 (4.4) | 118.5 (8.0) | 5.16 (2.53) | 4.08 (0.84) | 242 (69) |
| >30[d] | 440 | 13.64 (2.21) | 3.82 (0.64) | 43.55 (7.2) | 114.4 (9.3) | 7.71 (4.99) | 6.4 (2.99) | 232 (87) |

*Editor's Note:* Please refer to original journal article for full references.

[a]Hematologic measurements by a Coulter S-plus II instrument on 2860 fetal blood samplings for prenatal diagnostic purposes. Data expressed as mean (SD). Total WBC count includes NRBCs. Corrected WBC count includes WBCs only, after subtracting NRBCs, based on a 100-cell count manual differential.

[b]Adapted with permission from Geaghan (95).

[c]Data from Millar et al. (41).

[d]Data from Forestier et al. (42).

patterns in the fetus and placenta. Broadly, the potential applications of this technology fall into two categories: first, high genetic risk families with inheritable monogenic diseases, including sex determination in cases at risk of X-linked diseases and detection of specific paternally inherited single gene disorders; and second, routine antenatal care offered to all pregnant women, including prenatal screening/diagnosis for aneuploidy, particularly Down syndrome (DS), but also trisomies 13 and 18, and diagnosis of Rhesus factor status in RhD negative women. Already sex determination and Rhesus factor diagnosis are nearing translation into clinical practice for high-risk individuals."[1]

Indeed, Ashoor et al[2] obtained spectacular results in differentiating between trisomy 21, trisomy 18, and normal fetuses at 11 to 13 weeks' gestation. The sensitivity for detecting trisomy 21 was 100% (50 of 50 cases), the sensitivity for trisomy 18 was 98% (49 of 50 cases), and the specificity was 100% (297 of 297 cases). In this study, chromosome-selective sequencing of cell-free DNA separated all cases of trisomy 21 and 98% of trisomy 18 from euploid pregnancies.

As the field of fetal surgery advances, new techniques will allow additional congenital defects to be treated, and an expanded portfolio of minimally invasive technologies will no doubt be developed.

**A. A. Fanaroff, MBBCh, FRCPE**

*References*

1. Wright CF, Burton H. The use of cell-free fetal nucleic acids in maternal blood for non-invasive prenatal diagnosis. *Hum Reprod Update.* 2009;15:139-151.
2. Ashoor G, Syngelaki A, Wagner M, Birdir C, Nicolaides KH. Chromosome-selective sequencing of maternal plasma cell-free DNA for first-trimester detection of trisomy 21 and trisomy 18. *Am J Obstet Gynecol.* 2012;206:322.e1-322.e5.

---

**Reproductive Technologies and the Risk of Birth Defects**
Davies MJ, Moore VM, Willson KJ, et al (Robinson Institute, Adelaide, South Australia, Australia; et al)
*N Engl J Med* 366:1803-1813, 2012

---

*Background.*—The extent to which birth defects after infertility treatment may be explained by underlying parental factors is uncertain.

*Methods.*—We linked a census of treatment with assisted reproductive technology in South Australia to a registry of births and terminations with a gestation period of at least 20 weeks or a birth weight of at least 400 g and registries of birth defects (including cerebral palsy and terminations for defects at any gestational period). We compared risks of birth defects (diagnosed before a child's fifth birthday) among pregnancies in women who received treatment with assisted reproductive technology, spontaneous pregnancies (i.e., without assisted conception) in women who had a previous birth with assisted conception, pregnancies in women with a record of infertility but no treatment with assisted reproductive technology, and pregnancies in women with no record of infertility.

*Results.*—Of the 308,974 births, 6163 resulted from assisted conception. The unadjusted odds ratio for any birth defect in pregnancies involving assisted conception (513 defects, 8.3%) as compared with pregnancies not involving assisted conception (17,546 defects, 5.8%) was 1.47 (95% confidence interval [CI], 1.33 to 1.62); the multivariate-adjusted odds ratio was 1.28 (95% CI, 1.16 to 1.41). The corresponding odds ratios with in vitro fertilization (IVF) (165 birth defects, 7.2%) were 1.26 (95% CI, 1.07 to 1.48) and 1.07 (95% CI, 0.90 to 1.26), and the odds ratios with intracytoplasmic sperm injection (ICSI) (139 defects, 9.9%) were 1.77 (95% CI, 1.47 to 2.12) and 1.57 (95% CI, 1.30 to 1.90). A history of infertility, either with or without assisted conception, was also significantly associated with birth defects.

*Conclusions.*—The increased risk of birth defects associated with IVF was no longer significant after adjustment for parental factors. The risk of birth defects associated with ICSI remained increased after multivariate adjustment, although the possibility of residual confounding cannot be excluded. (Funded by the National Health and Medical Research Council and the Australian Research Council.)

▶ Reproductive technologies (RT) often result in multiple gestations and associated increased risk of prematurity. This is the most recent in a series of reports noting that the risks of RT do not end with prematurity; there also are increased risks of congenital anomalies among infants born following RT-assisted conception. This study of more than 6000 infants born in the context of RT, in comparison with a group of more than 300 000 infants born following spontaneous conception, revealed an approximately 50% increase in risk of any birth defect being observed (unadjusted odds ratio [OR] 1.47; 95% confidence interval [CI], 133, 1.62). The risk appeared to be greatest among infants for whom the RT used was intracytoplasmic sperm injection (ICSI) (OR 1.77; 95% CI, 1.47, 2.12). There were no detected associations with any specific syndrome or chromosomal abnormality. The study populations differed in a number of potential risk factors for birth defects, including maternal age, maternal smoking, singleton versus multiple gestation, and maternal diseases in pregnancy, in each case, with the RT mothers, on average, being more likely to be designated high risk. After adjustment for risk factors, RT overall continued to be associated with any birth defect (OR 1.30; 95% CI, 1.16, 1.45) and some specific classes of defects, but not multiple defects. The elevated risk of birth defects also was noted in risk-adjusted analyses of several specific methods, with the notable exclusion of in vitro fertilization. Another aspect worth considering is that most of the analyses included cerebral palsy (CP) within the birth defect designation. This is a decision with which some investigators might differ, since postnatal factors also might contribute to CP, a diagnosis generally considered valid only when the child is at or beyond 2 years of age. This study underscores the importance of ongoing studies of the growing yet incompletely understood population of children born following RT.

**L. J. Van Marter, MD, MPH**

**Placental pathology in asphyxiated newborns meeting the criteria for therapeutic hypothermia**
Wintermark P, Boyd T, Gregas MC, et al (Children's Hosp Boston, MA)
*Am J Obstet Gynecol* 203:579.e1-579.e9, 2010

*Objective.*—We sought to describe placental findings in asphyxiated term newborns meeting therapeutic hypothermia criteria and to assess whether histopathologic correlation exists between these placental lesions and the severity of later brain injury.

*Study Design.*—We conducted a prospective cohort study of the placentas of asphyxiated newborns, in whom later brain injury was defined by magnetic resonance imaging.

*Results.*—A total of 23 newborns were enrolled. Eighty-seven percent of their placentas had an abnormality on the fetal side of the placenta, including umbilical cord lesions (39%), chorioamnionitis (35%) with fetal vasculitis (22%), chorionic plate meconium (30%), and fetal thrombotic vasculopathy (26%). A total of 48% displayed placental growth restriction. Chorioamnionitis with fetal vasculitis and chorionic plate meconium were significantly associated with brain injury ($P=.03$). Placental growth restriction appears to significantly offer protection against the development of these injuries ($P=.03$).

*Conclusion.*—Therapeutic hypothermia may not be effective in asphyxiated newborns whose placentas show evidence of chorioamnionitis with fetal vasculitis and chorionic plate meconium.

▶ This small cohort study attempted to associate placental histopathology with response to therapeutic hypothermia in 23 infants who met criteria for induced hypothermia. Severity of brain injury was assessed by magnetic resonance imaging (MRI). The authors concluded that therapeutic hypothermia is less effective in babies whose placental histopathology showed evidence of chorioamnionitis with fetal vasculitis or those with evidence of meconium staining of the chorionic plate. Growth restriction of the placenta appeared to have a neuroprotective benefit.

I took away 2 points from this study: First, placental histopathology is an important and integral part of the examination of the encephalopathic neonate. Second, the conclusions reached by the investigators are undersupported by their study design and data. Only 7 of the 23 (30%) patients had cortical gray matter or basal ganglia injury on MRI. An additional 4 had other cerebral lesions usually attributable to hypoxia-ischemia (such as thalamic infarction, periventricular white matter injury, and venous sinus thrombosis). The study design introduces a large potential for selection bias. Given the small number of patients, the best we can do is generate hypotheses for future study.

However, the article is a must-read for neonatologists and obstetricians. If nothing else, perhaps the fabulous color photomicrographs will serve as a strong visual cue to remind us to send the placenta for detailed examination when we deal with a depressed newborn. "Don't make mirth of the afterbirth"—Jack Rudolph.

**S. M. Donn, MD**

## Accuracy of imaging parameters in the prediction of lethal pulmonary hypoplasia secondary to mid-trimester prelabor rupture of fetal membranes: a systematic review and meta-analysis

van Teeffelen ASP, van der Heijden J, Oei SG, et al (Máxima Med Ctr Veldhoven, The Netherlands; VieCuri Med Ctr Venlo, The Netherlands; et al)
*Ultrasound Obstet Gynecol* 39:495-499, 2012

In women who have suffered mid-trimester prelabor rupture of membranes (PPROM), prediction of pulmonary hypoplasia is important for optimal management. We performed a systematic review to assess the capacity of imaging parameters to predict pulmonary hypoplasia. We searched for published articles that reported on biometric parameters and allowed the construction of a 2 × 2 table, comparing at least one of these parameters with the occurrence of pulmonary hypoplasia. The selected studies were scored on methodological quality and we calculated sensitivity and specificity of the tests in the prediction of pulmonary hypoplasia and lethal pulmonary hypoplasia. Overall performance was assessed by summary receiver–operating characteristics (sROC) analyses that were performed with bivariate meta-analysis. We detected 13 studies that reported on the prediction of lethal pulmonary hypoplasia. The quality of the included studies was poor to mediocre. The estimated sROC curves for the chest circumference/abdominal circumference ratio and other parameters showed limited accuracy in the prediction of pulmonary hypoplasia. In women with mid-trimester PPROM, the available evidence indicates limited accuracy of biometric parameters in the prediction of pulmonary hypoplasia.

▶ Over the past 30 years, medicine has made great strides, especially with new imaging techniques. Dazzling MRI, CT scans, and various forms of ultrasound aid clinicians on a daily basis. In neonatal-perinatal medicine, exquisite and accurate imaging not only localizes birth defects but also plays a vital role in the overall patient evaluation and serves as a wonderful guide for counseling families. Pulmonary hypoplasia (PH), a complication midtrimester rupture of the membranes and loss of amniotic fluid, has been elusive to diagnose. Vergani[1] reviewed the literature pertaining to tests for diagnosis of PH and concluded that 2-dimensional biometric parameters were not accurate enough to be applied in clinical practice, but the lung-to-head ratio was a reasonable predictor of PH in fetuses with congenital diaphragmatic hernia (CDH). Vergani's summary noted that a reliable, reproducible, well-defined test to predict pulmonary hypoplasia has not yet emerged. This is disappointing news, as prediction of PH after midtrimester preterm prelabor rupture of membranes (PPROM) is important for optimal management.

Ruano et al[2] prospectively and comprehensively evaluated 108 fetuses at a single center with isolated CDH (82 left-sided and 26 right-sided). The following parameters were taken into consideration: gestational age at diagnosis, side of the diaphragmatic defect, presence of polyhydramnios, presence of liver herniated into the fetal thorax (liver-up), lung-to-head ratio (LHR) and observed/expected LHR (o/e-LHR), observed/expected contralateral and total fetal lung volume (o/e-Cont FLV and o/e-Tot FLV) ratios, ultrasonographic fetal lung volume/fetal weight ratio (US-FLW), observed/expected contralateral and main pulmonary artery diameter (o/e-Cont PA and o/e-MPA) ratios, and the contralateral vascularization index (Cont-VI). The outcomes were neonatal death and severe postnatal pulmonary arterial hypertension (PAH). The diagnosis of PAH was present in 63 of 70 deaths. Only 5 subjects with severe PAH survived. LHR, o/e-LHR, liver-up, o/e-Cont FLV, o/e-Tot FLV, US-FLW, o/e-ContPA, o/e-MPA, and Cont-VI were associated with both neonatal death and severe postnatal PAH ($P < .001$), but not gestational age at diagnosis, presence of polyhydramnios, or side of lesion. From the authors' experience, evaluating total lung volumes was more accurate than measuring only the contralateral lung size. Also evaluation of pulmonary vascularization (Cont-VI) is the most accurate predictor of neonatal outcome.

In 2010 van Teeffelen et al[3] in a literature search found 28 studies that reported on the prediction of PH, but prediction of lethal PH could be analyzed separately in 21 of these studies. They were of the opinion that the quality of the included studies was poor. The estimated summary receiver operator curves (sROC) showed that gestational age at PPROM performed significantly better than the latency time between PPROM and delivery or the amount of amniotic fluid.

In this article, the Dutch group again tackled the problem with a literature review, attempting to predict lethal PH secondary to midtrimester PPROM. They point out that the literature is flawed since all the accounts are single-center studies. Because second-trimester PPROM is a rare condition (0.7% of pregnancies), it is unlikely that a single-center study would reach sufficient power. Indeed all publications had relatively few subjects. Another major flaw is the fact that the technique to diagnose PH in autopsy varies widely. The 3 standard criteria used to define PH are lung weight/body weight ratio, radial alveolar count, and amount of DNA detected in lung tissue (lung DNA, in milligrams, to body weight, in grams, ratio). These are laborious techniques, each with its own set of problems. Although the lung weight/body weight ratio is decreased in pulmonary hypoplasia, tissue edema could increase the ratio, confusing the diagnosis. Radial alveolar counts are difficult to interpret in the preterm lung before the development of alveoli. The numbers in a fixed expanded lung differ from those in a fixed collapsed lung. The lung DNA/body weight ratio is confounded by the presence of increased pulmonary interstitial inflammatory cells.

The prediction of the lethal PH is pivotal to improve counseling and neonatal management. We can state with confidence that PPROM in midtrimester may be associated with PH. It is also true to state that PH carries a high mortality and morbidity. Regrettably, in women with midtrimester PPROM, the available evidence indicates limited accuracy of biometric parameters in the prediction of PH. There is currently no single test that can predict postnatal lung function. Combinations of clinical, ultrasound, and MRI parameters may provide the best approach for these complex patients.

**A. A. Fanaroff, MBBCh, FRCPE**

*References*

1. Vergani P. Prenatal diagnosis of pulmonary hypoplasia. *Curr Opin Obstet Gynecol.* 2012;24:89-94.

2. Ruano R, Takashi E, da Silva MM, Campos JA, Tannuri U, Zugaib M. Prediction and probability of neonatal outcome in isolated congenital diaphragmatic hernia using multiple ultrasound parameters. *Ultrasound Obstet Gynecol.* 2012;39:42-49.
3. van Teeffelen AS, van der Ham DP, Oei SG, Porath MM, Willekes C, Mol BW. The accuracy of clinical parameters in the prediction of perinatal pulmonary hypoplasia secondary to midtrimester prelabour rupture of fetal membranes: a meta-analysis. *Eur J Obstet Gynecol Reprod Biol.* 2010;148:3-12.

## Outcome of fetal exomphalos diagnosed at 11–14 weeks of gestation

Khalil A, Arnaoutoglou C, Pacilli M, et al (Univ College London Hosps NHS Foundation Trust, UK; Great Ormond Street Hosp for Children NHS Trust, London, UK)
*Ultrasound Obstet Gynecol* 39:401-406, 2012

*Objective.*—To determine whether sonographic findings in cases of exomphalos detected at the 11–14-week scan can be used to guide pregnancy management.

*Methods.*—Retrospective study of cases of exomphalos identified from the Fetal Medicine Unit database, University College London Hospitals between January 1998 and January 2010. Pregnancy and neonatal data were ascertained from maternal and neonatal records. Fetal exomphalos was categorized into three groups: exomphalos associated with other major structural malformation(s), isolated exomphalos with increased nuchal translucency (NT) and isolated exomphalos with normal NT.

*Results.*—A total of 98 cases of exomphalos were identified, of which 45 (45.9%) were associated with other major structural malformation(s), identified antenatally. Isolated exomphalos was found with increased NT in 22 cases (22.4%) and with normal NT in 31 cases (31.6%). Of 80 (81.6%) fetuses that were karyotyped, 43 (53.8%) had a chromosomal abnormality; the most common aneuploidy was trisomy 18 ($n = 31$; 72.1%). Where exomphalos was associated with other major structural abnormalities, or was isolated with increased NT, the incidence of aneuploidy was high, at 78.9% and 72.2%, respectively. Cases of isolated exomphalos with normal NT were all euploid. In 21 cases (21.4%), exomphalos resolved later in pregnancy and none had apparent abnormalities at birth; isolated exomphalos persisted in only three neonates (3.1%).

*Conclusions.*—The finding of a major structural abnormality or of increased NT in association with exomphalos in the first trimester implies a high risk of aneuploidy. Parents can be reassured that fetuses with isolated exomphalos and normal NT are likely to be euploid.

▶ The first trimester scan performed at 11 to 14 weeks of gestation aims to establish viability, confirm gestational age, and screen for fetal chromosomal abnormalities and provides an opportunity to look for structural malformations. The group at University College Hospital have been pioneers in this field, and their data base has provided valuable information and guidance over the years for perinatologists. There is and always will be strength in numbers. Although it took more than a decade to accumulate a series of almost 100 cases of omphalocele detected in the first trimester at this large center, the wait was worthwhile, as the data revealed are extremely informative. The presence of an isolated omphalocele without increased nuchal translucency is reassuring. Indeed, in this series, 58% of these have resolved by 16 weeks' gestation, and there are no residual signs when the infants are delivered. On the other hand, the combination of an omphalocele with increased nuchal translucency is ominous. This combination indicates a high prevalence of other malformations and an abnormal karyotype (close to 80%) to boot.

Gastroschisis and omphalocele are often discussed together because they are both congenital abdominal wall defects, yet they are very different. Their anatomy, embryology, and clinical problems are worlds apart, and they should not really be mentioned in the same sentence. Whereas omphalocele is often accompanied by other major anatomic defects and abnormal karyotype, increasing evidence suggests gastroschisis results from environmental teratogens.

Prior studies had indicated that the incidence of omphalocele is 1 in 3000 at birth[1] but 1 in 380 at 11 to 13 weeks' gestation.[2] In addition, some spontaneous resolution insight into the changing numbers is available from the 11-year experience reported from the same University College Hospital by Lakasing et al.[3] In total, 445 cases of exomphalos were identified. In 250 (56%) cases, the fetal karyotype was abnormal, and 99% were terminated. Of 135 cases with normal karyotype, 74 (54%) fetuses had other structural anomalies; 82 (61%) pregnancies resulted in termination of pregnancy (TOP) or fetal death, 42 (31%) resulted in live births, and 11 (8%) were lost to follow-up. Of the remaining pregnancies in which karyotype was refused, 38 (63%) fetuses had other structural anomalies, 41 (69%) pregnancies resulted in TOP or fetal death, 11 (18%) resulted in live births, and 8 (13%) were lost to follow-up. Of the 55 live births, 11 died preoperatively, and 44 had surgery. There were no postoperative deaths. Hence, less than 10% of the antenatal diagnostic workup reached operative repair.

The higher prevalence of exomphalos (omphalocele) in the first trimester may be explained by the strong association of fetal exomphalos with chromosomal abnormalities and other structural anomalies, with the inherent risk of spontaneous fetal loss or termination of pregnancy. The ability to detect those fetuses at minimum risk by detecting normal nuchal translucency is valuable information for the clinician.

**A. A. Fanaroff, MBBCh, FRCPE**

*References*

1. Mann S, Blinman TA, Douglas Wilson R. Prenatal and postnatal management of omphalocele. *Prenat Diagn.* 2008;28:626-632.
2. Kagan KO, Staboulidou I, Syngelaki A, Cruz J, Nicolaides KH. The 11–13-week scan: diagnosis and outcome of holoprosencephaly, exomphalos and megacystis. *Ultrasound Obstet Gynecol.* 2010;36:10-14.
3. Lakasing L, Cicero S, Davenport M, Patel S, Nicolaides KH. Current outcome of antenatally diagnosed exomphalos: an 11 year review. *J Pediatr Surg.* 2006;41:1403-1406.

## Antenatal Corticosteroids Promote Survival of Extremely Preterm Infants Born at 22 to 23 Weeks of Gestation

Mori R, on behalf of the Neonatal Research Network Japan (The Univ of Tokyo, Japan; et al)

*J Pediatr* 159:110-114, 2011

*Objective.*—To evaluate the effectiveness of antenatal corticosteroid (ACS) to improve neonatal outcomes for infants born at <24 weeks of gestation.

*Study Design.*—We performed a retrospective analysis of 11 607 infants born at 22 to 33 weeks of gestation between 2003 and 2007 from the Neonatal Research Network of Japan. We evaluated the gestational age effects of ACS administered to mothers with threatened preterm birth on several factors related to neonatal morbidity and mortality.

*Results.*—By logistic regression analysis, ACS exposure decreased respiratory distress syndrome and severe intraventricular hemorrhage in infants born between 24 and 29 weeks of gestation. Cox regression analysis revealed that ACS exposure was associated with a significant decrease in mortality of preterm infants born at 22 or 23 weeks of gestation (adjusted hazard ratio, 0.72; 95% CI, 0.53 to 0.97; $P = .03$). This effect was also observed at 24 to 25 and 26 to 27 weeks of gestation and in the overall study population.

*Conclusions.*—ACS exposure improved survival of extremely preterm infants. ACS treatment should be considered for threatened preterm birth at 22 to 23 weeks of gestation.

▶ While the 1994 National Institutes of Health Consensus Development Conference yielded a belated consensus regarding the efficacy of and necessity for antenatal steroid therapy (ANS) in the treatment of women with anticipated preterm birth, the margins of gestational age at which benefits can be expected remained imprecise. Given evidence that ANS reduces the incidence of respiratory distress syndrome (RDS) and mortality in infants born at 29 to 34 weeks' gestation as well as severity of RDS and rates of intraventricular hemorrhage (IVH) and mortality in infants born between 24 and 28 weeks' gestation, that conference produced recommendations for ANS use for all fetuses threatened with premature birth at gestational ages between 24 and 34 weeks' gestation but provided no guidance for management at earlier gestations. The use of antenatal steroids at early gestations has remained controversial, with a recent systematic review[1] concluding that there was no evidence to support or refute the efficacy of ANS before 26 weeks' gestation, but the original recommendation survives in the 2011 update to the American College of Obstetricians and Gynecologists recommendations.[2] This report from the Neonatal Research Network of Japan and a similar one from the National Institute of Child Health and Human Development Neonatal Research Network[3] provide data to fill that void. The Japanese authors found that ANS was associated with increased survival to hospital discharge in infants born at 22 to 23 weeks' (hazard ratio [HR], 0.72; 95% confidence interval [CI], 0.53-0.97), 24 to 25 weeks' (HR, 0.65; 95% CI, 0.50-0.86), and 26 to

27 weeks' (HR, 0.64; 95% CI, 0.45-0.91) gestation but (curiously and likely as a result of the current low mortality rates for these infants) not in those born at 28 to 33 weeks' gestation. ANS reduced RDS and severe IVH in infants born between 24 and 29 weeks' but not in those born at 22 to 23 weeks' gestation. American data are similar: ANS was associated with lower rates of death before discharge or before follow-up at 18 to 22 months of age, grade 3 to 4 IVH or PVL, and death or neurodevelopmental impairment at 18- to 22-month follow-up and with increased rates of bronchopulmonary dysplasia for infants born at 23 to 25 weeks' gestation; the point estimates for these outcomes for infants born at 22 weeks were concordant with those for older infants, but confidence intervals all included 1. Together these analyses suggest that the lower gestational threshold for ANS should be reduced to 23 weeks. More evidence will be needed to ascertain or refute benefit at 22 weeks.

**W. E. Benitz, MD**

*References*

1. Onland W, de Laat MW, Mol BW, Offringa M. Effects of antenatal corticosteroids given prior to 26 weeks' gestation: a systematic review of randomized controlled trials. *Am J Perinatol.* 2011;28:33-44.
2. ACOG Committee on Obstetric Practice. ACOG Committee Opinion No. 475: antenatal corticosteroid therapy for fetal maturation. *Obstet Gynecol.* 2011; 117:422-424.
3. Carlo WA, McDonald SA, Fanaroff AA, et al. Association of antenatal corticosteroids with mortality and neurodevelopmental outcomes among infants born at 22 to 25 weeks' gestation. *JAMA.* 2011;306:2348-2358.

## Association of Antenatal Corticosteroids With Mortality and Neurodevelopmental Outcomes Among Infants Born at 22 to 25 Weeks' Gestation

Carlo WA, for the Eunice Kennedy Shriver National Institute of Child Health and Human Development Neonatal Research Network (Univ of Alabama, Birmingham; et al)
*JAMA* 306:2348-2358, 2011

*Context.*—Current guidelines, initially published in 1995, recommend antenatal corticosteroids for mothers with preterm labor from 24 to 34 weeks' gestational age, but not before 24 weeks due to lack of data. However, many infants born before 24 weeks' gestation are provided intensive care.

*Objective.*—To determine if use of antenatal corticosteroids is associated with improvement in major outcomes for infants born at 22 and 23 weeks' gestation.

*Design, Setting, and Participants.*—Cohort study of data collected prospectively on inborn infants with a birth weight between 401 g and 1000 g (N = 10 541) born at 22 to 25 weeks' gestation between January 1, 1993, and December 31, 2009, at 23 academic perinatal centers in the United States. Certified examiners unaware of exposure to antenatal corticosteroids performed follow-up examinations on 4924 (86.5%) of the infants born between 1993 and 2008 who survived to 18 to 22 months. Logistic regression models generated adjusted odds ratios (AORs), controlling for maternal and neonatal variables.

*Main Outcome Measures.*—Mortality and neurodevelopmental impairment at 18 to 22 months' corrected age.

*Results.*—Death or neurodevelopmental impairment at 18 to 22 months was significantly lower for infants who had been exposed to antenatal corticosteroids and were born at 23 weeks' gestation (83.4% with exposure to antenatal corticosteroids vs 90.5% without exposure; AOR, 0.58 [95% CI, 0.42-0.80]), at 24 weeks' gestation (68.4% with exposure to antenatal corticosteroids vs 80.3% without exposure; AOR, 0.62 [95% CI, 0.49-0.78]), and at 25 weeks' gestation (52.7% with exposure to antenatal corticosteroids vs 67.9% without exposure; AOR, 0.61 [95% CI, 0.50-0.74]) but not in those infants born at 22 weeks' gestation (90.2% with exposure to antenatal corticosteroids vs 93.1% without exposure; AOR, 0.80 [95% CI, 0.29-2.21]). If the mothers had received antenatal corticosteroids, the following events occurred significantly less in infants born at 23, 24, and 25 weeks' gestation: death by 18 to 22 months; hospital death; death, intraventricular hemorrhage, or periventricular leukomalacia; and death or necrotizing enterocolitis. For infants born at 22 weeks' gestation, the only outcome that occurred significantly less was death or necrotizing enterocolitis (73.5% with exposure to antenatal corticosteroids vs 84.5% without exposure; AOR, 0.54 [95% CI, 0.30-0.97]).

*Conclusion.*—Among infants born at 23 to 25 weeks' gestation, antenatal exposure to corticosteroids compared with nonexposure was associated with a lower rate of death or neurodevelopmental impairment at 18 to 22 months (Tables 2 and 3).

▶ Despite strong evidence dating back to the 1970s that antenatal corticosteroids (ANS) reduced morbidity and mortality in preterm infants, it was only after the National Institute of Child Health and Human Development (NICHD) Consensus conference in 1994 that ANS became the standard of care for women delivering between 24 and 34 weeks' gestation. Key questions today are whether ANS are beneficial for late preterm deliveries (34–36 weeks, 6 days) and for infants delivering at 22 and 23 weeks' gestation. The available data are derived from post-hoc evaluation of network databases with all the inherent problems of bias. The untreated pregnancies tend to be very abnormal or present late so that there is insufficient time for administration even of an incomplete course of ANS. Carlo et al report that the combined outcome of mortality and neurodevelopmental impairment is reduced in infants exposed to antenatal corticosteroids starting from 23 weeks' gestation. Overall mortality rate was reduced from 56% to 35.5% for the whole cohort and at 23 weeks' gestation from 73% for infants not receiving ANS to 58% for those exposed to ANS (Table 2). Mortality or mental development index ≤70 decreased from 90% at 23 weeks to 83% (Table 3). Subgroup analyses indicated that exposure to antenatal corticosteroids was associated with lower hospital mortality, lower mortality

TABLE 2.—Hospital Outcomes of Infants at 22 to 25 Weeks' Gestation by Exposure to Antenatal Corticosteroids (ANS)[a]

| | Gestational Age | | | | | | | | | |
| | 22 wk | | 23 wk | | 24 wk | | 25 wk | | Total | |
| | ANS | No ANS | ANS | No ANS | ANS | No ANS | ANS | No ANS | ANS | No ANS |
|---|---|---|---|---|---|---|---|---|---|---|
| **Death** | | | | | | | | | | |
| No./total (%) | 86/118 (72.9) | 233/283 (82.3) | 667/1147 (58.2) | 606/831 (72.9) | 1177/2976 (39.6) | 415/814 (51.0) | 834/3555 (23.5) | 276/804 (34.3) | 2764/7796 (35.5) | 1530/2732 (56.0) |
| OR (95% CI)[b] | 0.61 (0.34-1.07)[c] | | 0.49 (0.39-0.61) | | 0.64 (0.54-0.76) | | 0.57 (0.48-0.69) | | 0.58 (0.52-0.65) | |
| **Death, BPD, or both** | | | | | | | | | | |
| No./total (%) | 107/118 (90.7) | 259/278 (93.2)[d] | 972/1131 (85.9) | 751/813 (92.4) | 2340/2928 (79.9) | 615/787 (78.1) | 2287/3463 (66.0) | 508/768 (66.2) | 5706/7640 (74.7) | 2133/2646 (80.6) |
| OR (95% CI)[b] | 0.73 (0.33-1.59)[d] | | 0.63 (0.45-0.90) | | 1.18 (0.95-1.47) | | 0.97 (0.80-1.18) | | 0.97 (0.85-1.10) | |
| **BPD** | | | | | | | | | | |
| No./total (%) | 20/31 (64.5) | 26/45 (57.8) | 305/464 (65.7) | 145/207 (70.1) | 1161/1749 (66.4) | 200/372 (53.8) | 1448/2624 (55.2) | 231/491 (47.1) | 2934/4868 (60.3) | 602/1115 (54.0) |
| OR (95% CI)[b] | 1.33 (0.51-3.45)[d] | | 0.83 (0.57-1.21)[c] | | 1.69 (1.30-2.20) | | 1.33 (1.06-1.67) | | 1.43 (1.23-1.67) | |
| **Death, IVH grade 3-4, PVL, or all 3** | | | | | | | | | | |
| No./total (%) | 93/116 (80.2) | 242/280 (86.4) | 794/1139 (69.7) | 686/825 (83.2) | 1538/2944 (52.2) | 514/803 (64.0) | 1284/3482 (36.9) | 406/773 (52.5) | 3709/7681 (48.3) | 1848/2681 (68.9) |
| OR (95% CI)[b] | 0.65 (0.35-1.23)[c] | | 0.44 (0.34-0.57) | | 0.65 (0.55-0.78) | | 0.52 (0.44-0.62) | | 0.55 (0.50-0.62) | |
| **IVH grade 3-4, PVL, or both** | | | | | | | | | | |
| No./total (%) | 7/30 (23.3) | 9/47 (19.2) | 127/472 (26.9) | 80/219 (36.5) | 361/1767 (20.4) | 99/388 (25.5) | 448/2646 (16.9) | 130/497 (26.2) | 943/4915 (19.2) | 318/1151 (27.6) |
| OR (95% CI)[b] | 0.94 (0.20-4.49)[c] | | 0.59 (0.40-0.87) | | 0.81 (0.61-1.08) | | 0.56 (0.44-0.72) | | 0.67 (0.57-0.79) | |
| **Death, NEC, or both** | | | | | | | | | | |
| No./total (%) | 86/117 (73.5) | 239/283 (84.5) | 722/1145 (63.1) | 640/831 (77.0) | 1356/2974 (45.6) | 453/813 (55.7) | 1100/3552 (31.0) | 309/804 (38.4) | 3264/7788 (41.9) | 1641/2731 (60.0) |
| OR (95% CI)[b] | 0.54 (0.30-0.97)[c] | | 0.47 (0.37-0.59) | | 0.65 (0.55-0.78) | | 0.72 (0.60-0.85) | | 0.62 (0.56-0.69) | |
| **NEC** | | | | | | | | | | |
| No./total (%) | 0/31 (0) | 6/50 (12.0) | 55/478 (11.5) | 34/225 (15.1) | 179/1797 (10.0) | 38/398 (9.6) | 265/2717 (9.8) | 32/527 (6.1) | 499/5023 (9.9) | 110/1200 (9.2) |
| OR (95% CI)[b] | NA | | 0.67 (0.41-1.08)[c] | | 0.85 (0.57-1.26) | | 1.76 (1.18-2.65) | | 1.01 (0.80-1.28) | |

*Abbreviations:* BPD, bronchopulmonary dysplasia; IVH, intraventricular hemorrhage; NA, not able to calculate; NEC, necrotizing enterocolitis; OR, odds ratio; PVL, periventricular leukomalacia.
[a]Cohort includes inborn infants born from 1993 through 2009 with birth weights between 401 g and 1000 g. Outcomes not corrected for mortality are only given for the survivors.
[b]Calculated from logistic regression and adjusted for maternal age, maternal marital status, maternal race, diabetes, maternal hypertension or preeclampsia, and maternal rupture of membranes more than 24 hours antepartum and estimated within each week of gestational age. The no ANS group was used as the referent category.
[c]Model does not include perinatal center (the statistical model did not converge with center included).
[d]Because of convergence problems due to low outcome prevalence, this model adjusts only for sex.

TABLE 3.—Outcomes by 18 to 22 Months' Corrected Age for Infants Born at 22 to 25 Weeks' Gestation From 1993 Through 2008 by Exposure to Antenatal Corticosteroids (ANS)[a]

| | Gestational Age | | | | | | | | Total | |
| | 22 wk | | 23 wk | | 24 wk | | 25 wk | | | |
| | ANS | No ANS | ANS | No ANS | ANS | No ANS | ANS | No ANS | ANS | No ANS |
|---|---|---|---|---|---|---|---|---|---|---|
| **Death by follow up** | | | | | | | | | | |
| No./total (%) | 85/116 (73.3) | 220/267 (82.4)[c] | 634/1072 (59.1) | 585/796 (73.5) | 1141/2768 (41.2) | 411/786 (52.3) | 824/3294 (25.0) | 287/779 (36.8) | 2684/7250 (37.0) | 1503/2628 (57.2) |
| OR (95% CI)[b] | 0.60 (0.34-1.07)[c] | | 0.50 (0.40-0.63) | | 0.66 (0.55-0.79) | | 0.56 (0.47-0.68) | | 0.59 (0.53-0.65) | |
| **Death or NDI** | | | | | | | | | | |
| No./total (%) | 101/112 (90.2) | 243/261 (93.1)[c] | 838/1005 (83.4) | 676/747 (90.5) | 1711/2502 (68.4) | 559/696 (80.3) | 1510/2865 (52.7) | 451/664 (67.9) | 4160/6484 (64.2) | 1929/2368 (81.5) |
| OR (95% CI)[b] | 0.80 (0.29-2.21)[c] | | 0.58 (0.42-0.80) | | 0.62 (0.49-0.78) | | 0.61 (0.50-0.74) | | 0.60 (0.53-0.69) | |
| **NDI** | | | | | | | | | | |
| No./total (%) | 16/27 (59.3) | 23/41 (56.1) | 204/371 (55.0) | 91/162 (56.2) | 570/1361 (41.9) | 148/285 (51.9) | 686/2041 (33.6) | 164/377 (43.5) | 1476/3800 (38.8) | 426/865 (49.2) |
| OR (95% CI)[b] | 1.14 (0.39-3.28)[d] | | 1.11 (0.72-1.71) | | 0.80 (0.60-1.08) | | 0.81 (0.62-1.04) | | 0.83 (0.70-0.99) | |
| **MDI <70** | | | | | | | | | | |
| No./total (%) | 14/21 (66.7) | 16/32 (50.0) | 159/295 (53.9) | 67/134 (50.0) | 425/1008 (42.2) | 118/257 (45.9) | 527/1543 (34.2) | 127/330 (38.5) | 1125/2867 (39.2) | 328/753 (43.6) |
| OR (95% CI)+ | 2.16 (0.36-13.1)[c] | | 1.27 (0.79-2.03) | | 0.85 (0.62-1.16) | | 0.91 (0.69-1.20) | | 0.93 (0.78-1.12) | |
| **PDI <70** | | | | | | | | | | |
| No./total (%) | 10/21 (47.6) | 13/34 (38.2)[d] | 111/293 (37.9) | 55/136 (40.4) | 307/996 (30.8) | 87/254 (34.3) | 348/1533 (22.7) | 91/327 (27.8) | 776/2843 (27.3) | 246/751 (32.8) |
| OR (95% CI)[b] | 1.47 (0.48-4.50)[d] | | 0.93 (0.58-1.50) | | 0.69 (0.49-0.95) | | 0.82 (0.60-1.11) | | 0.79 (0.65-0.96) | |
| **Bayley III cognitive score <70[e]** | | | | | | | | | | |
| No./total (%) | 1/6 (16.7) | 1/8 (12.5) | 10/74 (13.5) | 8/26 (30.8)[f] | 45/346 (13.0) | 6/26 (23.1)[c] | 45/503 (8.9) | 6/48 (12.5) | 101/929 (10.9) | 21/108 (19.4) |
| OR (95% CI)[b] | 1.28 (0.06-27.50)[d] | | 0.31 (0.09-0.998)[f] | | 0.57 (0.17-1.91)[c] | | 0.88 (0.34-2.24)[c] | | 0.63 (0.34-1.17) | |
| **Moderate to severe cerebral palsy** | | | | | | | | | | |
| No./total (%) | 4/28 (14.3) | 7/44 (15.9) | 43/380 (11.3) | 31/167 (18.6)[c] | 140/1432 (9.8) | 36/295 (12.2)[g] | 154/2132 (7.2) | 33/385 (8.6) | 341/3972 (8.6) | 107/891 (12.0) |
| OR (95% CI)[b] | 0.88 (0.23-3.34)[d] | | 0.50 (0.30-0.85)[c] | | 0.71 (0.47-1.08)[g] | | 0.97 (0.62-1.50) | | 0.76 (0.59-0.98) | |
| **Blindness** | | | | | | | | | | |
| No./total (%) | 0/28 (0) | 2/44 (4.5) | 7/379 (1.8) | 8/170 (4.7) | 34/1436 (2.4) | 6/304 (2.0) | 18/2133 (0.8) | 7/393 (1.8) | 59/3976 (1.5) | 23/911 (2.5) |
| OR (95% CI)[b] | NA | | 0.31 (0.10-0.93)[c] | | 1.17 (0.48-2.83)[f] | | 0.46 (0.19-1.10)[d] | | 0.61 (0.36-.03)[c] | |

| Deafness | | | | | | | | | |
|---|---|---|---|---|---|---|---|---|---|
| No./total (%) | 0/28 (0) | 2/42 (4.8) | 11/376 (2.9) | 12/169 (7.1) | 45/1433 (3.1) | 11/305 (3.6) | 50/2127 (2.4) | 10/391 (2.6) | 106/3964 (2.7) | 35/907 (3.9) |
| OR (95% CI)[b] | | NA | 0.39 (0.17-0.93)[f] | | 0.93 (0.45-1.90)[c] | | 0.91 (0.46-1.81)[d] | | 0.76 (0.50-.16)[c] |

*Abbreviations:* MDI, Mental Developmental Index; NA, not able to calculate; NDI, neurodevelopmental impairment; OR, odds ratio; PDI, Psychomotor Developmental Index.

[a]Outcomes not corrected for mortality are only given for the survivors. The follow-up cohort includes inborn infants born from 1993 through 2008 with birth weights between 401 g and 1000 g, and born at gestational age of 22 through 25 weeks. Infants who died within 12 hours without delivery room resuscitation are excluded.

[b]Estimated within each week of gestational age. The no ANS group was used as the referent category.

[c]Model does not include perinatal center (the statistical model did not converge with center included).

[d]Because of convergence problems due to low outcome prevalence, this model adjusts only for sex.

[e]Bayley II is used for infants born between 1993 and 2005; Bayley III is used for infants born after 2005. For all death or NDI and NDI-only models, a cohort effect was included in the model to indicate Bayley II vs Bayley III.

[f]Because of convergence problems due to low outcome prevalence, this model adjusts only for sex and race.

[g]Because of convergence problems due to low outcome prevalence, this model adjusts only for sex, race, and perinatal center.

at 18 to 22 months, and lower mortality or neurodevelopmental impairment at 18 to 22 months in singleton and multiple births, partial and full antenatal corticosteroid treatment groups, betamethasone and dexamethasone treatment groups, and infants of mothers with and without diabetes. Outcomes may be better with ANS, but there is still a disturbingly high number of bad outcomes.

What about the data from Japan where the best outcomes for extremely low gestational aged infants have been published.[1] Mori et al[2] report for the Japanese Neonatal Research Network that only 42% of 11 600 infants born between 22 and 33 weeks' gestation were exposed to antenatal corticosteroids. (This contrasts with more than 80% in the NICHD Neonatal Research Network.) Although antenatal steroid (ANS) treatment was effective in decreasing RDS, surfactant use, and duration of $O_2$ use in preterm infants born between 24 and 29 weeks of gestation, it was not as effective in the 22- to 23-week group. Furthermore, ANS treatment was extremely effective at decreasing both IVH and severe IVH in preterm infants at the gestational age of 24 to 29 weeks but not in infants born at less than 24 weeks of gestation. Although there was no RDS or IVH benefit at 22 to 23 weeks' gestation, survival was increased with maternal corticosteroid treatment. These data represent the largest cohorts of extremely immature babies, but outcomes are not based on randomized treatment assignments. However, they are the best information that we are likely to have regarding the efficacy of ANS for very early—gestation infants. Given the available evidence, ANS treatment should be considered for threatened preterm birth at 23 weeks of gestation and perhaps even 22 weeks' gestation.

**A. A. Fanaroff, MBBCh, FRCPE**

*References*

1. Itabashi K, Horiuchi T, Kusuda S, et al. Mortality rates for extremely low birth weight infants born in Japan in 2005. *Pediatrics*. 2009;123:445-450.
2. Mori R, Kusuda S, Fujimara M. Antenatal corticosteroids promote survival of extremely preterm infants born at 22 to 23 weeks of gestation. *J Pediatr*. 2011;159: 110-114.

**Association of Antenatal Corticosteroids With Mortality and Neurodevelopmental Outcomes Among Infants Born at 22 to 25 Weeks' Gestation**

Carlo WA, for the Eunice Kennedy Shriver National Institute of Child Health and Human Development Neonatal Research Network (Univ of Alabama, Birmingham; et al)

*JAMA* 306:2348-2358, 2011

*Context.*—Current guidelines, initially published in 1995, recommend antenatal corticosteroids for mothers with preterm labor from 24 to 34 weeks' gestational age, but not before 24 weeks due to lack of data. However, many infants born before 24 weeks' gestation are provided intensive care.

*Objective.*—To determine if use of antenatal corticosteroids is associated with improvement in major outcomes for infants born at 22 and 23 weeks' gestation.

*Design, Setting, and Participants.*—Cohort study of data collected prospectively on inborn infants with a birth weight between 401 g and 1000 g (N = 10 541) born at 22 to 25 weeks' gestation between January 1, 1993, and December 31, 2009, at 23 academic perinatal centers in the United States. Certified examiners unaware of exposure to antenatal corticosteroids performed follow-up examinations on 4924 (86.5%) of the infants born between 1993 and 2008 who survived to 18 to 22 months. Logistic regression models generated adjusted odds ratios (AORs), controlling for maternal and neonatal variables.

*Main Outcome Measures.*—Mortality and neurodevelopmental impairment at 18 to 22 months' corrected age.

*Results.*—Death or neurodevelopmental impairment at 18 to 22 months was significantly lower for infants who had been exposed to antenatal corticosteroids and were born at 23 weeks' gestation (83.4% with exposure to antenatal corticosteroids vs 90.5% without exposure; AOR, 0.58 [95% CI, 0.42-0.80]), at 24 weeks' gestation (68.4% with exposure to antenatal corticosteroids vs 80.3% without exposure; AOR, 0.62 [95% CI, 0.49-0.78]), and at 25 weeks' gestation (52.7% with exposure to antenatal corticosteroids vs 67.9% without exposure; AOR, 0.61 [95% CI, 0.50-0.74]) but not in those infants born at 22 weeks' gestation (90.2% with exposure to antenatal corticosteroids vs 93.1% without exposure; AOR, 0.80 [95% CI, 0.29-2.21]). If the mothers had received antenatal corticosteroids, the following events occurred significantly less in infants born at 23, 24, and 25 weeks' gestation: death by 18 to 22 months; hospital death; death, intraventricular hemorrhage, or periventricular leukomalacia; and death or necrotizing enterocolitis. For infants born at 22 weeks' gestation, the only outcome that occurred significantly less was death or necrotizing enterocolitis (73.5% with exposure to antenatal corticosteroids vs 84.5% without exposure; AOR, 0.54 [95% CI, 0.30-0.97]).

*Conclusion.*—Among infants born at 23 to 25 weeks' gestation, antenatal exposure to corticosteroids compared with nonexposure was associated with a lower rate of death or neurodevelopmental impairment at 18 to 22 months.

▶ Current guidelines recommend use of antenatal corticosteroids (ANS) in women with threatened preterm birth between 24 and 34 weeks of gestation but provide no guidance for management of threatened delivery at earlier gestations. This silence does not reflect evidence that ANS are ineffective before 24 weeks of gestation but rather a lack of evidence for efficacy in these circumstances. (The evidence for benefit between 24 and 26 weeks is also sparse.) This report from the NICHD Neonatal Research Network and a similar one from its Japanese counterpart[1] begin to address this uncertainty. Both studies provide logistic regression analyses of retrospective data for more than 10 000 extremely low birth weight infants, demonstrating strong associations of ANS with improved outcomes among infants born at 23 weeks of gestation or later. The US results differ from those from Japan primarily in inclusion of data on neurodevelopmental and sensorineural outcomes at 18 to 22 months of age and in analysis of effects of several potential confounders. For infants born at 23 to 25 weeks of gestation, ANS were associated with significantly lower mortality, less intraventricular hemorrhage or periventricular leukomalacia, or either of those outcomes. The combined outcome of death or bronchopulmonary dysplasia was less frequent with ANS among infants born at 23 weeks of gestation but not among more mature infants for whom rates of BPD were significantly greater with ANS (likely reflecting their higher survival rates). As detailed in the abstract, ANS were associated with lower rates of death or neurodevelopment impairment (NDI) after 23 weeks of gestation; although the reduction in NDI was significant for the full cohort, it was not significant for each individual week of gestation, and the point estimate was less than 1 only for infants at 24 or 25 weeks of gestation. Notably, however, rates of Bayley III cognitive scores < 70, moderate to severe cerebral palsy, blindness, and deafness were all lower in ANS-exposed infants born at 23 weeks but not in other age strata. Beneficial effects of ANS were apparent in infants in both the presence and absence of several comorbidities (multiple gestation, maternal diabetes, prolonged rupture of membranes, chorioamnionitis, antepartum hemorrhage, cesarean birth) and were independent of sex or race; only maternal hypertension and intrauterine growth restriction were associated with nonsignificant effects. These results provide substantial support for routine use of antenatal steroids for women expected to deliver at 23 weeks.

**W. E. Benitz, MD**

*Reference*

1. Mori R, Kusuda S, Fujimura M. Antenatal corticosteroids promote survival of extremely preterm infants born at 22 to 23 weeks of gestation. *J Pediatr.* 2011;159: 110-114.

---

**Magnesium sulfate therapy for the prevention of cerebral palsy in preterm infants: a decision-analytic and economic analysis**

Cahill AG, Odibo AO, Stout MJ, et al (Depts of Obstetrics and Gynecology at Washington Univ in St Louis School of Medicine, MO; et al)
*Am J Obstet Gynecol* 205:542.e1-542.e7, 2011

*Objective.*—We sought to estimate the cost-effectiveness of magnesium neuroprophylaxis for all women at risk for preterm birth <32 weeks.

*Study Design.*—A decision analytic and cost-effectiveness model was designed to compare use of magnesium for neuroprophylaxis vs no treatment for women at risk for preterm birth <32 weeks due to preterm premature rupture of membranes or preterm labor from 24-32 weeks. Outcomes included neonatal death and moderate-severe cerebral palsy. Effectiveness was reported in quality-adjusted life years.

*Results.*—Magnesium for neuroprophylaxis led to lower costs ($1739 vs $1917) and better outcomes (56.684 vs 56.678 quality-adjusted life years). However, sensitivity analysis revealed the model to be sensitive to estimates of effect of magnesium on risk of moderate or severe cerebral palsy as well as neonatal death.

*Conclusion.*—Based on currently published evidence for efficacy, magnesium for neuroprophylaxis in women at risk to deliver preterm is cost-effective.

▶ After 10 years of effort and at a cost of $25 million, the National Institutes of Health Maternal Fetal Medicine Units Network BEAM trial completed enrollment and follow-up of 2241 women at imminent risk for delivery between 24 and 31 weeks of gestation.[1] Building on results of 2 earlier trials, this enormous effort showed a significant reduction in the rate of cerebral palsy in the magnesium sulfate group (1.9% vs 3.5%; relative risk, 0.55; 95% confidence interval [CI], 0.32–0.95). Some viewed these results as definitive, but others remained skeptical. The ensuing ACOG Committee Opinion[2] straddled the fence, commenting that although none of the randomized trials of magnesium neuroprophylaxis demonstrated a significant effect on the primary outcome, they collectively suggested a reduction in cerebral palsy in surviving infants. This article attempts to resolve this through decision and cost-effectiveness analysis. These authors found that magnesium treatment resulted in lower costs and better outcomes, but the differences were modest and sensitive to estimates of the effect size. Treatment of all women with threatened preterm delivery before 32 weeks appeared to be more cost effective than limiting treatment to those at less than 28 weeks, but the model appears to assume equal efficacy across this range of gestational ages. The BEAM trial, however, found that magnesium significantly reduced the risk of moderate or severe CP in infants whose mothers were enrolled before 28 weeks of gestation (relative risk [RR], 0.45; 95% CI, 0.23–0.87) but not in those enrolled after 28 weeks (RR, 1.00; 95% CI, 0.38–2.65), suggesting that most or all of the benefit could be realized if magnesium is offered only to the 12 000 women a year in the United States who deliver before 28 weeks. Under those assumptions, it is difficult to imagine that treatment for threatened preterm delivery after 28 weeks could be cost effective. This analysis therefore leaves the matter of the optimal strategy for use of this treatment unresolved.

**W. E. Benitz, MD**

*References*

1. Rouse DJ, Hirtz DG, Thom E, et al. A randomized, controlled trial of magnesium sulfate for the prevention of cerebral palsy. *N Engl J Med.* 2008;359:895-905.
2. American College of Obstetricians and Gynecologists Committee on Obstetric Practice, Society for Maternal-Fetal Medicine. Committee Opinion No. 455: magnesium sulfate before anticipated preterm birth for neuroprotection. *Obstet Gynecol.* 2010; 115:669-671.

# 2 Epidemiology and Pregnancy Complications

---

**Improving Quality of Care for Maternal and Newborn Health: Prospective Pilot Study of the WHO Safe Childbirth Checklist Program**
Spector JM, Agrawal P, Kodkany B, et al (Harvard School of Public Health, Boston, MA; London School of Hygiene and Tropical Medicine, UK; Jawaharlal Nehru Med College, Karnataka, India; et al)
*PLoS One* 7:e35151, 2012

---

*Background.*—Most maternal deaths, intrapartum-related stillbirths, and newborn deaths in low income countries are preventable but simple, effective methods for improving safety in institutional births have not been devised. Checklist-based interventions aid management of complex or neglected tasks and have been shown to reduce harm in healthcare. We hypothesized that implementation of the WHO Safe Childbirth Checklist program, a novel childbirth safety program for institutional births incorporating a 29-item checklist, would increase delivery of essential childbirth practices linked with improved maternal and perinatal health outcomes.

*Methods and Findings.*—A pilot, pre-post-intervention study was conducted in a sub-district level birth center in Karnataka, India between July and December 2010. We prospectively observed health workers that attended to women and newborns during 499 consecutively enrolled birth events and compared these with observed practices during 795 consecutively enrolled birth events after the introduction of the WHO Safe Childbirth Checklist program. Twenty-nine essential practices that target the major causes of childbirth-related mortality, such as hand hygiene and uterotonic administration, were evaluated. The primary end point was the average rate of successful delivery of essential childbirth practices by health workers. Delivery of essential childbirth-related care practices at each birth event increased from an average of 10 of 29 practices at baseline (95% CI 9.4, 10.1) to an average of 25 of 29 practices afterwards (95% CI 24.6, 25.3; $p < 0.001$). There was significant improvement in the delivery of 28 out of 29 individual practices. No adverse outcomes relating to the intervention occurred. Study limitations are the pre-post design, potential Hawthorne effect, and focus on processes of care versus health outcomes.

23

*Conclusions.*—Introduction of the WHO Safe Childbirth Checklist program markedly improved delivery of essential safety practices by health workers. Future study will determine if this program can be implemented at scale and improve health outcomes.

▶ The use of checklists in health care has been linked to improved patient outcomes and safety, particularly in intensive care and surgical settings. As the number of institutional births increases in low-income settings, the opportunity arises to implement these initiatives in the perinatal setting worldwide. The World Health Organization (WHO) established a 29-item bedside checklist-based childbirth program in 2008 that was proven usable in 10 countries in Asia and Africa. In this pilot study, it is hypothesized that implementation of this checklist will significantly increase the rate of delivery of essential child birth practices that are linked to improved maternal, fetal, and neonatal outcomes in a low-income setting. Using a prospective preintervention and postintervention study design, the investigators determined that the use of the checklist was associated with enhanced adherence to accepted clinical practices (the number of essential practices delivered per birth event increased from 10 to 25). The study was not powered to detect differences in maternal deaths, stillbirth rate, and neonatal death; however, a trend for lower stillbirth rates was observed with the use of the checklist. A larger multicenter study is currently underway that will assess the impact of this program on maternal, fetal, and neonatal outcomes.

Despite the limitations of this pilot study, the potential impact of this relatively simple, low-cost intervention on health outcomes in low-income settings is enormous. Implementation of a checklist serves as the central component of a comprehensive educational and behavioral modification program. This needs to be sustainable and generalizable in order to transform evidence-based care and safety protocols into optimal health care delivery and adoption of best practices.

**H. Christou, MD**

---

**Use of alcohol-free antimicrobial mouth rinse is associated with decreased incidence of preterm birth in a high-risk population**
Jeffcoat M, Parry S, Gerlach RW, et al (Univ of Pennsylvania, Philadelphia; Procter and Gamble Co, Mason, OH)
*Am J Obstet Gynecol* 205:382.e1-382.e6, 2011

---

*Objective.*—We sought to determine if treatment of periodontal disease during pregnancy with an alcohol-free antimicrobial mouth rinse containing cetylpyridinium chloride impacts the incidence of preterm birth (PTB) in a high-risk population.

*Study Design.*—This single-blind clinical trial studied pregnant women (6-20 weeks' gestation) with periodontal disease who refused dental care. Subjects receiving mouth rinse were compared to designated controls who did not receive rinse (1 rinse:2 controls), balanced on prior PTB and smoking. Primary outcome was PTB < 35 weeks.

*Results.*—In all, 226 women were included in the analysis (71 mouth rinse subjects, 155 controls). Incidence of PTB < 35 weeks was lower in the rinse group compared to controls (5.6% and 21.9% respectively, $P < .01$); relative risk was 0.26 (95% confidence interval, 0.096–0.70). Gestational age and birthweight were significantly higher in the rinse group ($P < .01$).

*Conclusion.*—A nonalcohol antimicrobial mouth rinse containing cetylpyridinium chloride was associated with decreased incidence of PTB < 35 weeks.

▶ The association between maternal periodontal disease and infant prematurity is indisputable. What is open to question is whether treatment of periodontal disease before or during pregnancy reduces the risk of premature delivery. Further confusing the issue is the finding in some reviews that treatment is beneficial, whereas others fail to demonstrate benefit. Thus, the systematic review by Chambrone et al[1] of randomized trials revealed no decrease in preterm or low birth weight deliveries, whereas George et al[2] from Western Australia included 5645 pregnant women from 10 eligible trials, and the meta-analysis indicated that periodontal treatment significantly lowered preterm birth (odds ratio [OR] 0.65; 95% confidence interval [CI], 0.45–0.93; $P = .02$) and low birth weight (OR 0.53; 95% CI, 0.31–0.92; $P = .02$). Nonetheless, they were extremely cautious with their conclusion: "The cumulative evidence suggests that periodontal treatment during pregnancy may reduce preterm birth and low birth weight incidence. However, these findings need to be further validated through larger more targeted randomized control trials."

Polyzos et al[3] came to the conclusion that treatment of periodontal disease with scaling and root planing during pregnancy is inefficient, and that the treatment is unlikely to reduce preterm birth or low birth weight infants.

To add fuel to this fire, Matevosyan[4] has shown a relationship between periodontal disease and pre-eclampsia. It is therefore entirely logical to add care of periodontal disease prior to conception as an element in the prevention of premature delivery.

Jeffcoat et al[5] have been studying this problem for many years. They present a refreshing, cost-effective new approach (ie, nonalcohol antibacterial mouthwash on a daily basis) that in this small trial demonstrated efficacy. Both bleeding areas and depth of pockets between the teeth (evidence of inflammation) showed improvement with the oral mouthwash and further inflammation in the control group. The key is the type of the mouthwash, which contains neither alcohol nor antibiotics such as tetracyclines (common in mouthwashes), which can affect the teeth and bones of the fetus. It harms neither mother nor the fetus/neonate. Admittedly this is a relatively small trial, but the concept is certainly worth further study. We await the results of such trials.

**A. A. Fanaroff, MBBCh, FRCPE**

*References*

1. Chambrone L, Pannuti CM, Guglielmetti MR, Chambrone LA. Evidence grade associating periodontitis with preterm birth and/or low birth weight: II: a systematic review of randomized trials evaluating the effects of periodontal treatment. *J Clin Periodontol.* 2011;38:902-914.

2. George A, Shamim S, Johnson M, et al. Periodontal treatment during pregnancy and birth outcomes: a meta-analysis of randomised trials. *Int J Evid Based Healthc.* 2011;9:122-147.

3. Polyzos NP, Polyzos IP, Zavos A, et al. Obstetric outcomes after treatment of periodontaldisease during pregnancy: systematic review and meta-analysis. *BMJ.* 2010;341:c7017.

4. Matevosyan NR. Periodontal disease and perinatal outcomes. *Arch Gynecol Obstet.* 2011;283:675-686.

5. Jeffcoat MK, Geurs NC, Reddy MS, Cliver SP, Goldenberg RL, Hauth JC. Periodontal infection and preterm birth: results of a prospective study. *J Am Dent Assoc.* 2001;132:875-880.

## The Prediction and Cost of Futility in the NICU

Meadow W, Cohen-Cutler S, Spelke B, et al (The University of Chicago, IL; et al)

*Acta Paediatr* 101:397-402, 2012

*Aim.*—To quantify the cost and prediction of futile care in the Neonatal Intensive Care Unit (NICU).

*Methods.*—We observed 1813 infants on 100 000 NICU bed days between 1999 and 2008 at the University of Chicago. We determined costs and assessed predictions of futility for each day the infant required mechanical ventilation.

*Results.*—Only 6% of NICU expenses were spent on nonsurvivors, and in this sense, they were futile. If only money spent *after* predictions of death is considered, futile expenses fell to 4.5%. NICU care was preferentially directed to survivors for even the smallest infants, at the highest risk to die. Over 75% of ventilated NICU infants were correctly predicted to survive on every day of ventilation by every caretaker. However, predictions of 'die before discharge' were wrong more than one time in three. Attendings and neonatology fellows tended to be optimistic, while nurses and neonatal nurse practitioners tended to be pessimistic.

*Conclusions.*—Criticisms of the expense of NICU care find little support in these data. Rather, NICU care is remarkably well targeted to patients who will survive, particularly when contrasted with care in adult ICUs. We continue to search for better prognostic tools for individual infants.

▶ Amid important reports of successes and failures of neonatal therapies and exciting laboratory breakthroughs, this article is an important reminder that ethical questions sometimes have empirical answers. These authors at the University of Chicago continue to publish research and insights that should serve as a source of reassurance to all of us who grapple with the thorny ethical issues that accompany caring for extremely preterm infants in delivery rooms and newborn intensive care units (NICUs). For all those who worry that prolonged intensive care inflicts needless and invasive care for babies and saddles the health care system with a big bill for all of this care, this article should be a huge help. In a clear and concise manner, the authors walk us through their results and ensuing arguments to make a few key points. First, even the most accurate caretakers overestimate the likelihood that ventilated infants will die. Second, of all the money spent on mechanically ventilated infants in NICUs, very little is actually spent on nonsurvivors. Finally, if care is considered to be futile only after the point that caregivers predict nonsurvival, the relative cost of providing intensive care to these infants is even lower.

In their conclusions, the authors point out the two most important limitations of this work. The first is that death is not the only important outcome in the NICU, and data about long-term neurodevelopmental outcome are not available for this cohort of patients (although this group has studied and published long-term outcome data for a small subset of these patients with interesting results).[1] The other is that these data come from a single NICU with a rather homogenous patient population that may not resemble that served by many other institutions around the country. Validation in a large, multicenter study is clearly warranted, but communication with the authors suggests that efforts are under way to conduct such a study.

These limitations do not detract from the intellectual appeal of this kind of reasoning, and the research itself is striking in its intuitive and simple design. Simply put, these authors have been able to draw very important conclusions with an inexpensive and understandable study design that can easily be replicated at other institutions. By collecting predictions of death from NICU care providers each day infants are mechanically ventilated, along with very basic clinical outcome data (only survival and length of stay are used here), the authors are able to draw important conclusions, which may well be at odds with conventional thinking about extremely preterm infants.

**N. Laventhal, MD, MA**

*Reference*

1. Lagatta J, Andrews B, Caldarelli L, Schreiber M, Plesha-Troyke S, Meadow W. Early neonatal intensive care unit therapy improves predictive power for the outcomes of ventilated extremely low birth weight infants. *J Pediatr.* 2011;159:384-391.e1.

---

**Survival rates in extremely low birthweight infants depend on the denominator: avoiding potential for bias by specifying denominators**

Guillen Ú, DeMauro S, Ma L, et al (Children's Hosp of Philadelphia, PA; Hebei Provincial Children's Hosp, Shijiazhuang, China; et al)
*Am J Obstet Gynecol* 205:329.e1-329.e7, 2011

---

*Objective.*—The objective of the study was to assess whether recent data reporting survival of preterm infants introduce a bias from the use of varying denominators.

*Study Design.*—We performed a systematic review of hospital survival of infants less than 1000 g or less than 28 weeks. Included publications specified the denominator used to calculate survival rates.

*Results.*—Of 111 eligible publications only 51 (46%) specified the denominators used to calculate survival rates: 6 used all births, 25 used live births, and 20 used neonatal intensive care unit admissions. Overall rates of survival to hospital discharge ranged widely: from 26.5% to 87.8%. Mean survival varied significantly by denominator: 45.0% (±11.6) using a denominator of all births, 60.7% (±13.2) using live births, or 71.6% (±12.1) using used neonatal intensive care unit admissions ($P \leq .009$ or less for each of 3 comparisons).

*Conclusion.*—Variations in reported rates of survival to discharge for extremely low-birthweight (<1000 g) and extremely low-gestational-age (<28 weeks) infants reflect in part a denominator bias that dramatically affects reported data.

▶ This is a most important article, which draws attention to the importance of carefully examining the numbers. There is a huge bias introduced by varying the denominator. Guillen et al not only analyze the literature extensively but "demonstrate the magnitude of a continuing lack of clarity in current reports of neonatal survival outcomes and show that survival rate, a nonspecific single term, is really a range of rates that are derived from different denominators." It is concerning that their review showed that less than 50% of the studies reviewed reported the denominator that was used; hence, there is no way of knowing what type of survival was presented. The concepts emphasized by Guillen et al are neither new nor original but were highlighted by Evans and Levene over a decade ago.[1] They completed a systematic review of studies reporting survival in infants less than 28 weeks of gestation published from 1978 to 1998, and graded them according to cohort definition: A, stillbirths and live births; B, live births; C, neonatal unit admissions. Proportions of infants surviving to discharge were calculated for each week of gestation. Studies including only neonatal intensive care unit (NICU) admissions had significantly higher survival than those including stillbirths and live births or live births alone. They recommended the following: "To minimize the potential for overestimating survival around the limits of viability, future studies should endeavor to report the outcome of all pregnancies for each week of gestation (terminations, miscarriages, stillbirths, and all live births)." Similar bias in outcomes has been noted when comparing single centers, with regions or multicentered networks and national data. The lowest survival is observed with the national data.

Guillen et al refresh our memories and demonstrate that most reports do not heed Evans and Levene's recommendations. To intelligently and appropriately counsel parents about outcomes for impending deliveries at the borders of viability, it is imperative that each unit have accurate data, not just survival data for babies admitted alive into their NICU. Furthermore, long-term morbidity data should also be made available during this counseling process. I endorse Guillen's proposal that journals demand comprehensive data that include all births to not mislead clinicians by publishing apparently outstanding but misleading survival rates, when all the stillbirths and deaths in the delivery room have been excluded from the data set.

**A. A. Fanaroff, MBBCh, FRCPE**

*Reference*

1. Evans DJ, Levene MI. Evidence of selection bias in preterm survival studies: a systematic review. *Arch Dis Child Fetal Neonatal Ed.* 2001;84:79-84.

## Improving Survival of Extremely Preterm Infants Born Between 22 and 25 Weeks of Gestation

Kyser KL, Morriss FH Jr, Bell EF, et al (Univ of Iowa Hosp and Clinic, Iowa City; Univ of Iowa Carver College of Medicine, Iowa City)

*Obstet Gynecol* 119:795-800, 2012

---

*Objective.*—To estimate observed compared with predicted survival rates of extremely premature infants born during 2000−2009, to identify contemporary predictors of survival, and to determine if improved survival rates occurred during the decade.

*Methods.*—We conducted a retrospective cohort analysis of 237 inborn neonates without major congenital anomalies born from 2000 to 2009 after 22 to 25 completed weeks of gestation. Observed survival rates at each gestational age were compared with predicted survival rates based on gestational age, birth weight, sex, singleton or multiple gestation, and antenatal corticosteroid administration estimated by a Web-based calculator that was derived from 1998 to 2003 outcomes of a large national cohort. Multivariable logistic regression analysis was used to identify significant predictors of survival of the study cohort, including year of birth.

*Results.*—Survival rates for the decade by gestational age (compared with predicted rates) were: 22 weeks, 33% (compared with 19%); 23 weeks, 58% (compared with 38%); 24 weeks, 87% (compared with 58%); and 25 weeks, 85% (compared with 70%). Antenatal corticosteroids were administered in 96% of pregnancies. Variables that significantly predicted survival and their odds ratios (OR) with 95% confidence intervals (CI) are: antenatal corticosteroid administration (OR 5.27, CI 1.26−22.08); female sex (OR 3.21, CI 1.42−7.26); gestational age (OR 1.89, CI 1.27− 2.81); 1-minute Apgar score (OR 1.39, CI 1.15−1.69); and birth year (OR 1.17, CI 1.02−1.34). The number needed to treat with any antenatal corticosteroid therapy to prevent one death was 2.4.

*Conclusion.*—In this single-institution cohort treated aggressively (antenatal corticosteroid administration [even if less than 24 weeks], tocolysis until steroid course complete, cesarean for fetal distress) by perinatologists and neonatologists, survival rates at 22−25 weeks of gestation age for inborn infants during the 2000s exceeded predicted rates, with increasing odds of survival during the decade. Antenatal corticosteroid administration had a significant effect on survival.

*Level of Evidence.*—II.

▶ Is the National Institute of Child Health and Human Development's (NICHD) Neonatal Research Network (NRN) Outcomes Calculator[1] already out of date? This article from one of the centers that contributed to that analysis suggests that it may be. The data used to develop the calculator were gathered between 1998 and 2003. This article examines a single center experience from 2000 to 2009. Although there were no breakthrough advances in care during that decade, experience at that center suggests that more aggressive application of prenatal and postnatal measures might result in better survival rates at the very margins of viability. It is difficult to know how representative this may be of the broad swath of extremely premature infants across the country, but this observation has several important implications. First, as these authors suggest, it is important for individual centers to be aware of how their outcomes compare to those predicted by the calculator and to adjust parent counseling accordingly. Second, periodic updates of the NICHD NRN calculator would be highly desirable. Finally, reports of higher survival rates should not be the primary determinant of decisions about care. It is notable that both surviving infants born at 22 weeks gestation had neurodevelopmental impairment, as did half of those born at 23 weeks. These are not the outcomes hoped for by the parents of these babies. Thoughtful discussion of the quality of survival, as well as survival rates, is still required. Such discussions are exemplified by one detail mentioned in this article: grade IV intraventricular hemorrhage predicted a reduced likelihood of survival (odds ratio 0.14), but was removed from the regression model because the parents were (appropriately) offered discontinuation of intensive care for those infants. Tools such as the NICHD calculator remain important for framing estimates of probabilities of outcomes for extremely premature infants, although they may underestimate the probability of desirable outcomes. Individualized assessments and nuanced conversations with the parents of each infant remain essential.

**W. E. Benitz, MD**

*Reference*

1. Tyson JE, Parikh NA, Langer J, Green C, Higgins RD. Intensive care for extreme prematurity—moving beyond gestational age. N Engl J Med. 2008;358:1672-1681.

**Effect of Antenatal Corticosteroids on Fetal Growth and Gestational Age at Birth**
Murphy KE, for the Multiple Courses of Antenatal Corticosteroids for Preterm Birth Study Collaborative Group (Mount Sinai Hosp, Toronto, Ontario, Canada; et al)
*Obstet Gynecol* 119:917-923, 2012

*Objective.*—To estimate the effect of multiple courses of antenatal corticosteroids on neonatal size, controlling for gestational age at birth and other confounders, and to determine whether there was a dose—response relationship between number of courses of antenatal corticosteroids and neonatal size.
*Methods.*—This is a secondary analysis of the Multiple Courses of Antenatal Corticosteroids for Preterm Birth Study, a double-blind randomized controlled trial of single compared with multiple courses of antenatal corticosteroids in women at risk for preterm birth and in which fetuses administered multiple courses of antenatal corticosteroids weighed less, were shorter, and had smaller head circumferences at birth. All women (n = 1,858) and children (n = 2,304) enrolled in the Multiple Courses of

Antenatal Corticosteroids for Preterm Birth Study were included in the current analysis. Multiple linear regression analyses were undertaken.

*Results.*—Compared with placebo, neonates in the antenatal corticosteroids group were born earlier (estimated difference and confidence interval [CI]:−0.428 weeks, CI −0.10264 to −0.75336; $P =.01$). Controlling for gestational age at birth and confounding factors, multiple courses of antenatal corticosteroids were associated with a decrease in birth weight (−33.50 g, CI −66.27120 to −0.72880; $P =.045$), length (−0.339 cm, CI −0.6212 to −0.05676]; $P =.019$), and head circumference (−0.296 cm, −0.45672 to −0.13528; $P <.001$). For each additional course of antenatal corticosteroids, there was a trend toward an incremental decrease in birth weight, length, and head circumference.

*Conclusion.*—Fetuses exposed to multiple courses of antenatal corticosteroids were smaller at birth. The reduction in size was partially attributed to being born at an earlier gestational age but also was attributed to decreased fetal growth. Finally, a dose—response relationship exists between the number of corticosteroid courses and a decrease in fetal growth. The long-term effect of these findings is unknown.

*Clinical Trial Registration.*—ClinicalTrials.gov, www.clinicaltrials.gov, NCT00187382.

*Level of Evidence.*—II.

▶ The knowledge that antenatal glucocorticoids induce a maturational effect on the lung as well as other organs is now approximately 40 years old. Numerous studies in sheep, other mammals, and humans have supported this concept, and providing antenatal glucocorticoids to pregnant women at risk of preterm delivery is now considered standard care. In fact, these steroids are now administered to approximately 10% of pregnant women in the United States and Canada.[1] Although it is clear that some of the morbidities, such as respiratory distress syndrome (RDS) in preterm infants, can be ameliorated, more current evidence such as in this article suggests that there is a price paid in terms of stunting of growth, especially in those infants born to mothers who received multiple courses. In fact, this study showed a dose-response relationship between the degree of growth stunting and number of doses of the glucocorticoid. As pointed out by the authors, there have been previous studies suggesting increased neurodevelopmental problems in infants whose mothers received multiple doses of the corticosteroids. The authors warn about the risks of multiple doses of these corticosteroids. Here, I would like to present an additional caveat: these synthetic glucocorticoids have the capability to induce major epigenetic changes that may have an effect not only on the infant, but on generations to come. Recent research in pregnant guinea pigs[1] using luminometric methylation assays nicely demonstrates that treatment with synthetic glucocorticoids shows that there are organ-specific developmental trajectories of methylation in the fetus and newborn. These trajectories are substantially modified by intrauterine exposure to these glucocorticoids. These changes in DNA methylation remain into adulthood and are evident in the next generation. These data support the hypothesis that prenatal corticosteroid exposure leads to broad changes in important components of the epigenetic machinery that can be passed to subsequent generations.

Should we be more discriminate in treating so many mothers with these agents? Are these epigenetic effects seen in humans and, if so, do they induce a healthy or unhealthy phenotype? Is the dose we are using appropriate? To my knowledge, the minimum dose needed to elicit a response that decreases RDS is not known. Are there alternative preventative measures that we should consider that would not induce these epigenetic effects?

It appears that we need to go back to the drawing board.

**J. Neu, MD**

*Reference*

1. Crudo A, Petropoulos S, Moisiadis VG, et al. Prenatal synthetic glucocorticoid treatment changes DNA methylation states in male organ systems: multigenerational effects. *Endocrinology.* 2012 May 7. Epub ahead of print.

**Causes of Death Among Stillbirths**
The Stillbirth Collaborative Research Network Writing Group (Univ of Texas Med Branch at Galveston; Brown Univ School of Medicine, Providence, RI; Univ of Texas Health Science Ctr at San Antonio; et al)
*JAMA* 306:2459-2468, 2011

*Context.*—Stillbirth affects 1 in 160 pregnancies in the United States, equal to the number of infant deaths each year. Rates are higher than those of other developed countries and have stagnated over the past decade. There is significant racial disparity in the rate of stillbirth that is unexplained.

*Objective.*—To ascertain the causes of stillbirth in a population that is diverse by race/ethnicity and geography.

*Design, Setting, and Participants.*—A population-based study from March 2006 to September 2008 with surveillance for all stillbirths at 20 weeks or later in 59 tertiary care and community hospitals in 5 catchment areas defined by state and county boundaries to ensure access to at least 90% of all deliveries. Termination of a live fetus was excluded. Standardized evaluations were performed at delivery.

*Main Outcome Measures.*—Medical history, fetal postmortem and placental pathology, karyotype, other laboratory tests, systematic assignment of causes of death.

*Results.*—Of 663 women with stillbirth enrolled, 500 women consented to complete postmortem examinations of 512 neonates. A probable cause of death was found in 312 stillbirths (60.9%; 95% CI, 56.5%-65.2%) and possible or probable cause in 390 (76.2%; 95% CI, 72.2%-79.8%). The most common causes were obstetric conditions (150 [29.3%; 95% CI, 25.4%-33.5%]), placental abnormalities (121 [23.6%; 95% CI, 20.1%-27.6%]), fetal genetic/structural abnormalities (70 [13.7%; 95% CI, 10.9%-17.0%]), infection (66 [12.9%; 95% CI, 10.2%-16.2%]), umbilical cord abnormalities (53 [10.4%; 95% CI, 7.9%-13.4%]), hypertensive disorders (47 [9.2%; 95% CI, 6.9%-12.1%]), and other maternal medical conditions (40 [7.8%; 95% CI, 5.7%-10.6%]). A higher proportion of still-births in non-Hispanic black women compared with non-Hispanic white and Hispanic ones was associated with obstetric complications (43.5% [50] vs 23.7% [85]; difference, 19.8%; 95% CI, 9.7%-29.9%; P<.001) and infections (25.2% [29] vs 7.8% [28]; difference, 17.4%; 95% CI, 9.0%-25.8%; P<.001). Stillbirths occurring intrapartum and early in gestation were more common in non-Hispanic black women. Sources most likely to provide positive information regarding cause of death were placental histology (268 [52.3%; 95% CI, 47.9%-56.7%]), perinatal postmortem examination (161 [31.4%; 95% CI, 27.5%-35.7%]), and karyotype (32 of 357 with definitive results [9%; 95% CI, 6.3%-12.5%]).

*Conclusions.*—A systematic evaluation led to a probable or possible cause in the majority of stillbirths. Obstetric conditions and placental abnormalities were the most common causes of stillbirth, although the distribution differed by race/ethnicity.

▶ As neonatologists, we focus almost exclusively on events starting in the delivery room. Stillbirth, defined as fetal death at 20 weeks' gestation or later, is one of the most common adverse pregnancy outcomes in the United States and affects approximately 1 in 160 pregnancies.[1] These approximately 26 000 still-births per year are equivalent to the number of infant deaths.

Stillbirth rates in high-income countries declined dramatically from about 1940, but this decline has slowed or stalled over recent times.[2] Further reduction in stillbirth is definitely possible as evidenced by the continued variation in stillbirth rates across and within high-income countries.

In the United States, women who experienced stillbirth in their first pregnancy were more likely to be of advanced age, black, and obese and had higher rates of pregnancy-related complications. Previous stillbirth was associated with an elevated risk for subsequent infant mortality and neonatal mortality after adjustment for sociodemographic variables and pregnancy complications. Women with prior infant deaths, particularly white women, are about 3 times as likely to experience stillbirth in their subsequent pregnancy. "Overweight, obesity, and smoking are important modifiable risk factors for stillbirth, and advanced maternal age is also an increasingly prevalent risk factor. Intensified efforts are needed to ameliorate the effects of these factors on stillbirth rates."[3]

In classifying stillbirths, 6 broad categories are suggested,[4] including maternal medical conditions; obstetric complications; maternal or fetal hematologic conditions; fetal genetic, structural, and karyotypic abnormalities; placental infection, fetal infection or both; and placental pathologic findings. As noted in the article abstracted, these conditions account for the bulk of the stillbirths. There are still many stillbirths for which the underlying cause is not established either because of underinvestigation or inability to determine the cause. Education and more diligent investigations should resolve these mysteries.

The key is to prevent stillbirths, and a concerted effort is needed in this regard. Intrapartum-related neonatal deaths can be averted by prevention and management of preeclampsia, detection and management of intrapartum problems (eg, monitoring progress of labor with access to emergency obstetric care), and recognition and intervention for the neonate who is not breathing.[5] Avoidance of hyperthermia is also important for pregnant women, as there is a strong association between increased temperature and increased risk of stillbirth and shorter gestation.

Simple, affordable, and effective approaches are available for low-resource settings, including community-based strategies to increase skilled birth attendance and the widespread dissemination of the Help Babies Breathe Program.

**A. A. Fanaroff, MBBCh, FRCPE**

*References*

1. MacDorman MF, Kirmeyer S. Fetal and perinatal mortality, United States, 2005. *Natl Vital Stat Rep.* 2009;57:1-19.
2. MacDorman MF, Mathews TJ. Recent trends in infant mortality in the United States. *NCHS Data Brief.* 2008;9:1-8.
3. Flenady V, Middleton P, Smith GC, et al. Lancet's Stillbirths Series steering committee. Stillbirths: the way forward in high-income countries. *Lancet.* 2011; 377:1703-1717.
4. Dudley DJ, Goldenberg R, Conway D, et al. Stillbirth Research Collaborative Network. A new system for determining the causes of stillbirth. *Obstet Gynecol.* 2010;116:254-260.
5. Wall SN, Lee AC, Carlo W. Reducing intrapartum-related neonatal deaths in low- and middle-income countries-what works? *Semin Perinatol.* 2010;34:395-407.

---

**Assessing the Optimal Definition of Oligohydramnios Associated With Adverse Neonatal Outcomes**
Shanks A, Tuuli M, Schaecher C, et al (Washington Univ, St Louis, MO)
*J Ultrasound Med* 30:303-307, 2011

---

*Objectives.*—The purpose of this study was to compare the use of an amniotic fluid index (AFI) less than 5 cm to the use of an AFI less than the fifth percentile for gestational age in predicting adverse perinatal outcomes.

*Methods.*—This was a retrospective cohort study from 1998 to 2008. Patients with an AFI less than 5 cm and those with an AFI less than the fifth percentile were compared to patients with a normal AFI. The primary outcome measure was neonatal intensive care unit (NICU) admission.

*Results.*—A total of 17,887 patients had complete information for analysis. There were 145 NICU admissions in patients with an AFI less than 5 cm (relative risk, 2.2) compared to 235 in patients with an AFI less than the fifth percentile for gestational age (relative risk, 2.37). The sensitivity and specificity for NICU admission using an AFI less than 5 cm were 10.9% and 95.2% compared to 17.6% and 92.5% for an AFI less than the fifth percentile for gestational age.

*Conclusions.*—Oligohydramnios defined as an AFI less than the fifth percentile better predicts fetuses at risk for adverse perinatal outcomes compared to an AFI less than 5 cm.

▶ The amniotic fluid volume (AFV) is regulated by fetal production (fetal urine and lung fluid) and uptake (fetal swallowing) and the balance of fluid movement via osmotic gradients across the membranes. Amniotic fluid provides an ideal environment for normal fetal growth and development. It provides the fetus with a source of water, protects the fetus from trauma, allows for normal movements critical for anatomic development, and contributes to the development of the fetal lungs. During the 40-week period of human gestation, approximately 4 L of water accumulate with 2800 mL in the fetus, 400 mL in the placenta, and 800 mL in the amniotic fluid. Amniotic fluid is really a "magical liquor," as it both protects and nourishes the fetus while at the same time assisting in the development of the gastrointestinal tract, kidneys, and lungs, protecting the skin and protecting the fetus from infection. Indeed, the amniotic fluid also serves as an important source of nutrition and growth factors for the fetus. The rate of change in amniotic fluid volume (AVF) is a strong function of gestational age. There is a progressive AFV increase from 30 mL at 10 weeks' gestation to 190 mL at 16 weeks and to a mean of 780 mL at 32 to 35 weeks, after which a decrease occurs.[1] Decreased amniotic fluid is associated with increased risks of intrauterine growth restriction, pulmonary hypoplasia, congenital abnormalities, postdate pregnancy, meconium passage, abnormal fetal heart rate patterns, and lower Apgar scores, resulting in increased perinatal mortality. Pregnancies with decreased amniotic fluid index (AFI) between 24 and 34 weeks' gestation have significantly more major fetal malformations, and in the absence of malformations, the pregnancy is likely to be complicated by fetal growth restriction and preterm birth.[2]

Because oligohydramnios has such important clinical implications for the fetus, determination of the amniotic fluid volume is a critical measurement. For too long we have been wedded to the standard definition of less than 5 cm from the combined deepest pockets in the 4 quadrants of the uterus without taking into consideration gestational age.

Shanks et al make a strong case for changing the definition of oligohydramnios to a more dynamic one, taking into consideration gestational age. They have a large cohort to draw from, and they documented that an amniotic fluid index (AFI) less than the fifth percentile was a better predictor of adverse clinical events; it also better predicts fetuses at risk for adverse perinatal outcomes compared with an AFI less than 5 cm. Shanks concludes "The discovery of a decreased AFI in pregnancies should prompt the obstetrician to search for underlying causes and increase antenatal surveillance. Although heightened surveillance patterns in the form of weekly AFI checks and nonstress tests are frequently used in pregnancies with oligohydramnios defined as less than 5 cm, our results suggest that this strategy should be extended to patients with oligohydramnios defined as less than the fifth percentile for gestational age as well." My impression is that this is a small change with no additional costs or risks. However, habits that are ingrained change at glacial speeds, so it may be some time before this concept is broadly accepted.

Just when you think we are gaining a handle on the definitions of oligohydramnios, Magann et al,[3] in a state-of-the-art review of the subject, made the following observations: "The definition of normal AFV is hampered by inadequate data concerning AFV across gestation. There is no true gold standard and sonographic estimates of the AFV, correlate poorly with dye-determined or directly measured amniotic fluid which are invasive and time consuming."

Magann is of the opinion that neither color Doppler sonography nor the use of the AFI has improved the diagnostic accuracy of sonographic estimates of the AFV but instead has led to overdiagnosis of oligohydramnios, resulting in more labor inductions and operative deliveries without any improvement in perinatal outcomes. My final word is that there have been enough measurements made of AFI and amniotic fluid pockets that it is time for perinatologists to agree on the definitions of normal fluid volumes related to gestational age.

**A. A. Fanaroff, MBBCh, FRCPE**

*References*

1. Modena AB, Fieni S. Amniotic fluid dynamics. *Acta Biomed.* 2004;75:11-13.
2. Petrozella LN, Dashe JS, McIntire DD, Leveno KJ. Clinical significance of borderline amniotic fluid index and oligohydramnios in preterm pregnancy. *Obstet Gynecol.* 2011;117:338-342.
3. Magann EF, Sandlin AT, Ounpraseuth ST. Amniotic fluid and the clinical relevance of the sonographically estimated amniotic fluid volume: oligohydramnios. *J Ultrasound Med.* 2011;30:1573-1585.

---

**Antenatal Steroids for Treatment of Fetal Lung Immaturity After 34 Weeks of Gestation: An Evaluation of Neonatal Outcomes**

Kamath-Rayne BD, Defranco EA, Marcotte MP (Univ of Cincinnati School of Medicine, OH)

*Obstet Gynecol* 119:909-916, 2012

---

*Objective.*—To estimate whether antenatal corticosteroids given after fetal lung immaturity in pregnancies at 34 weeks of gestation or more would improve neonatal outcomes and, in particular, respiratory outcomes.

*Methods.*—We compared outcomes of 362 neonates born at 34 weeks of gestation or more after fetal lung maturity testing: 102 with immature fetal lung indices were treated with antenatal corticosteroids followed by planned delivery within 1 week; 76 with immature fetal lung indices were managed expectantly; and 184 were delivered after mature amniocentesis. Primary outcomes were composites of neonatal and respiratory morbidity.

*Results.*—Compared with corticosteroid-exposed neonates those born after mature amniocentesis had lower rates of adverse neonatal (26.5% compared with 14.1%, adjusted odds ratio [OR] 0.51, 95% confidence interval [CI] 0.27−0.96) and adverse respiratory outcomes (9.8% compared with 3.3%, adjusted OR 0.33, 95% CI 0.11−0.98); newborns born after expectant management had significantly less respiratory morbidity (1.3% compared with 9.8%, adjusted OR 0.11, 95% CI 0.01−0.92) compared with corticosteroid-exposed newborns.

*Conclusion.*—Administration of antenatal corticosteroids after immature fetal lung indices did not reduce respiratory morbidity in neonates born at 34 weeks of gestation or more. Our study supports prolonging gestation until delivery is otherwise indicated.

## Level of Evidence.—II.

▶ The administration of antenatal corticosteroids for the prevention of respiratory distress syndrome (RDS) and intracranial hemorrhage in fetuses at less than 34 weeks of gestation has been globally accepted since it was supported by the National Institutes of Health Consensus statement in 1994.[1] However, little information exists on the use of antenatal steroids to promote fetal lung maturation in women at risk of preterm birth beyond 34 weeks of gestation. In Sinclair's[2] analysis of the available data in 1995, he estimated that with the assumption of a baseline risk of RDS of 50% in neonates at 30 weeks of gestation or less, 5 neonates would need to be treated to prevent 1 case of RDS. However, at 34 weeks or beyond, the baseline risk of RDS is 15%, so the number needed to treat rises to 145. These authors in fact demonstrated that not only was there no respiratory advantage to administering corticosteroids beyond 34 weeks' gestation, but there was evidence of harm with a doubling of the incidence of hypoglycemia and a trebling of the need for a sepsis evaluation in the neonates. The true prevalence of benefit and harm will be determined in larger prospective randomized trials, which are ongoing.

Shanks et al,[3] in a small prospective trial, showed that administration of antennal corticosteroids to women after 34 weeks' gestation and evidence of lung immaturity on analysis of the amniotic fluid demonstrated some degree of maturation. The trial is far too small to draw any meaningful conclusions.

So the logical conclusion is that Mother Nature knows best, and until there is evidence to the contrary, awaiting maturation in utero without interference after 34 weeks is the appropriate course of action. Indeed the least morbidity was observed in the group not exposed to antenatal corticosteroids.

**A. A. Fanaroff, MBBCh, FRCPE**

### References

1. Effect of corticosteroids for fetal maturation on perinatal outcomes. *NIH Consensus Statement.* 1994;12:1-24.
2. Sinclair J. Meta-analysis of randomized controlled trials of antenatal corticosteroid for the prevention of respiratory distress syndrome: discussion. *Am J Obstet Gynecol.* 1995;173:335-344.
3. Shanks A, Gross G, Shim T, Allsworth J, Sadovsky Y, Bildirici I. Administration of steroids after 34 weeks of gestation enhances fetal lung maturity profiles. *Am J Obstet Gynecol.* 2010;203:47.e1-47.e5.

---

### Antenatal Steroids for Treatment of Fetal Lung Immaturity After 34 Weeks of Gestation: An Evaluation of Neonatal Outcomes

Kamath-Rayne BD, Defranco EA, Marcotte MP (Univ of Cincinnati School of Medicine, OH)
*Obstet Gynecol* 119:909-916, 2012

---

*Objective.*—To estimate whether antenatal corticosteroids given after fetal lung immaturity in pregnancies at 34 weeks of gestation or more would improve neonatal outcomes and, in particular, respiratory outcomes.

*Methods.*—We compared outcomes of 362 neonates born at 34 weeks of gestation or more after fetal lung maturity testing: 102 with immature fetal lung indices were treated with antenatal corticosteroids followed by planned delivery within 1 week; 76 with immature fetal lung indices were managed expectantly; and 184 were delivered after mature amniocentesis. Primary outcomes were composites of neonatal and respiratory morbidity.

*Results.*—Compared with corticosteroid-exposed neonates those born after mature amniocentesis had lower rates of adverse neonatal (26.5% compared with 14.1%, adjusted odds ratio [OR] 0.51, 95% confidence interval [CI] 0.27–0.96) and adverse respiratory outcomes (9.8% compared with 3.3%, adjusted OR 0.33, 95% CI 0.11–0.98); newborns born after expectant management had significantly less respiratory morbidity (1.3% compared with 9.8%, adjusted OR 0.11, 95% CI 0.01–0.92) compared with corticosteroid-exposed newborns.

*Conclusion.*—Administration of antenatal corticosteroids after immature fetal lung indices did not reduce respiratory morbidity in neonates born at 34 weeks of gestation or more. Our study supports prolonging gestation until delivery is otherwise indicated.

*Level of Evidence.*—II.

▶ This retrospective study attempted to examine the effects of later corticosteroid treatment of mothers whose fetuses had immature lung maturation indices in pregnancies beyond 34 weeks. The study population was assigned to 1 of 3 groups: mature amniocentesis (ages 34 weeks to 38 6/7 weeks), expectant management (34 4/7 weeks to 40 weeks), and steroid treatment following immature indices on amniocentesis (34 weeks to 38 6/7 weeks). Neonatal outcomes were significantly worse in the group treated with steroids. They were more immature; weighed less at birth; had worse composite and respiratory outcomes; had more neonatal intensive care unit admissions; and they required more supplemental oxygen, continuous positive airway pressure, time on respiratory support, treatment for hypoglycemia, sepsis evaluations, and treatment with antibiotics. Subgroup analyses revealed that most of these differences were attributed to late preterm infants. The authors concluded that expectant management to delay delivery was more beneficial than administration of corticosteroids and immediate delivery.

As a retrospective study, typical cautions need to be taken because of the non-randomized and nonmasked nature of the observation. Nevertheless, the authors did try to account for confounding variables and adjusted for factors known to influence neonatal outcomes. Their finding of a lack of benefit of corticosteroids raises a serious question to this continued practice, but this can only be answered by a prospective randomized clinical trial. Given the significant morbidities found in this observation, as well as the obvious increased cost of care, a trial of this nature does indeed seem justified.

**S. M. Donn, MD**

## Outcome of Extremely Low Birth Weight Infants Who Received Delivery Room Cardiopulmonary Resuscitation

Wyckoff MH, for the National Institute of Child Health and Human Development Neonatal Research Network (Univ of Texas Southwestern Med Ctr, Dallas; et al)

*J Pediatr* 160:239-244, 2012

*Objective.*—To determine whether delivery room cardiopulmonary resuscitation (DR-CPR) independently predicts morbidities and neurodevelopmental impairment (NDI) in extremely low birth weight infants.

*Study Design.*—We conducted a cohort study of infants born with birth weight of 401 to 1000 g and gestational age of 23 to 30 weeks. DR-CPR was defined as chest compressions, medications, or both. Logistic regression was used to determine associations among DR-CPR and morbidities, mortality, and NDI at 18 to 24 months of age (Bayley II mental or psychomotor index <70, cerebral palsy, blindness, or deafness). Data are adjusted ORs with 95% CIs.

*Results.*—Of 8685 infants, 1333 (15%) received DR-CPR. Infants who received DR-CPR had lower birth weight (708 ± 141 g versus 764 ± 146 g, $P < .0001$) and gestational age (25 ± 2 weeks versus 26 ± 2 weeks, $P < .0001$). Infants who received DR-CPR had more pneumothoraces (OR, 1.28; 95% CI, 1.48-2.99), grade 3 to 4 intraventricular hemorrhage (OR, 1.47; 95% CI, 1.23-1.74), bronchopulmonary dysplasia (OR, 1.34; 95% CI, 1.13-1.59), death by 12 hours (OR, 3.69; 95% CI, 2.98-4.57), and death by 120 days after birth (OR, 2.22; 95% CI, 1.93-2.57). Rates of NDI in survivors (OR, 1.23; 95% CI, 1.02-1.49) and death or NDI (OR, 1.70; 95% CI, 1.46-1.99) were higher for DR-CPR infants. Only 14% of DR-CPR recipients with 5-minute Apgar score <2 survived without NDI.

*Conclusions.*—DR-CPR is a prognostic marker for higher rates of mortality and NDI for extremely low birth weight infants. New DR-CPR strategies are needed for this population.

▶ Twenty years ago, cases of extremely low birth weight (ELBW) infants who required chest compressions or epinephrine in the delivery room always came to a bad end. In 1999, this belief was challenged by a review of experience across the Vermont Oxford Network (VON) from 1994 to 1996. That study demonstrated survival of 54% of infants who weighed less than 1000 g who had received cardiopulmonary resuscitation (CPR) in the delivery room, including 44% who survived without severe (grade 3 or 4) intraventricular hemorrhage. This report from the National Institute of Child Health and Human Development's Neonatal Research Network (NRN) confirms those observations but provides only a modest update, since it describes outcomes for infants enrolled in the NRN between 1996 and 2002. That limitation notwithstanding, there are remarkable similarities to the earlier results. A slightly higher proportion of infants (15.4 vs 9.7%) in this slightly later cohort were given CPR in the delivery room, suggesting that the earlier report may have encouraged less temerity in the approach to ELBW infants who seemed to qualify for CPR. CPR in the delivery room was associated with increased risks for several adverse outcomes, but the extent to which that might be attributable to CPR versus the reason that CPR was needed remains unclear. Rates of adverse outcomes mirrored the VON results: 58% of infants who received CPR survived to discharge, and only 25% of those who had head sonograms had grade 3 or 4 intraventricular hemorrhage. However, only 28% of infants who received delivery room CPR were alive without neurodevelopmental impairment at 18 to 22 months of age (compared with 46% of those who did not get CPR). Infants who got CPR and had Apgar scores less than 2 at 5 minutes of age fared particularly badly; only 14% were alive without neurodevelopmental impairment at 18 to 22 months of age. It is possible that circumstances may have changed since 2002, such that fewer ELBW infants need CPR or had better outcomes. Statistics for overall mortality rates in this population do not support this hypothesis, however. Investigations of resuscitation techniques specifically tailored for ELBW infants, possibly including different criteria for or timing of initiation of chest compressions or epinephrine administration and of strategies for postresuscitation hemodynamic, respiratory, and neuroprotective support are clearly needed. Our best hope is likely to lie in closer collaboration with our obstetrical colleagues to find ways to minimize the number of ELBW babies who might need such measures.

**W. E. Benitz, MD**

## Gestational Age at Birth and Mortality in Young Adulthood
Crump C, Sundquist K, Sundquist J, et al (Stanford Univ, CA; Lund Univ, Malmö, Sweden)
*JAMA* 306:1233-1240, 2011

*Context.*—Preterm birth is the leading cause of infant mortality in developed countries, but the association between gestational age at birth and mortality in adulthood remains unknown.

*Objective.*—To examine the association between gestational age at birth and mortality in young adulthood.

*Design, Setting, and Participants.*—National cohort study of 674 820 individuals born as singletons in Sweden in 1973 through 1979 who survived to age 1 year, including 27 979 born preterm (gestational age <37 weeks), followed up to 2008 (ages 29-36 years).

*Main Outcome Measures.*—All-cause and cause-specific mortality.

*Results.*—A total of 7095 deaths occurred in 20.8 million person-years of follow-up. Among individuals still alive at the beginning of each age range, a strong inverse association was found between gestational age at birth and mortality in early childhood (ages 1-5 years: adjusted hazard ratio [aHR] for each additional week of gestation, 0.92; 95% CI, 0.89-0.94; $P < .001$), which disappeared in late childhood (ages 6-12 years: aHR, 0.99; 95% CI, 0.95-1.03; $P = .61$) and adolescence (ages 13-17 years: aHR, 0.99; 95% CI, 0.95-1.03; $P = .64$) and then reappeared in young adulthood (ages 18-36 years: aHR, 0.96; 95% CI, 0.94-0.97; $P < 001$). In young adulthood, mortality rates (per 1000 person-years) by gestational age at birth were 0.94 for 22 to 27 weeks, 0.86 for 28 to 33 weeks, 0.65 for 34 to 36 weeks, 0.46 for 37 to 42 weeks (full-term), and 0.54 for 43 or more weeks. Preterm birth was associated with increased mortality in young adulthood even among individuals born late preterm (34-36 weeks, aHR, 1.31; 95% CI, 1.13-1.50; $P < 001$), relative to those born full-term. In young adulthood, gestational age at birth had the strongest inverse association with mortality from congenital anomalies and respiratory, endocrine, and cardiovascular disorders and was not associated with mortality from neurological disorders, cancer, or injury.

*Conclusion.*—After excluding earlier deaths, low gestational age at birth was independently associated with increased mortality in early childhood and young adulthood.

▶ Because large numbers of individuals who were born preterm are now surviving to adulthood, there is a heightened awareness that they continue to be at risk for a spectrum of diseases and early death. Earlier studies have explored the relationship between preterm birth and mortality in childhood, adolescence, and adulthood. Because fetal growth was not considered in these previous studies, the relative contribution of prematurity per se to increased mortality in later life is unknown.

The data in this report were abstracted from the Swedish Birth Registry and Death Registry and included individuals who were singleton births and who survived to age 1 year. Only 0.5% of the 678 528 individuals identified were excluded because of missing birth data. The model was adjusted for fetal growth measured as the number of standard deviations from mean birth weight for gestational age and sex from a Swedish reference growth curve.

The investigators found that low gestational age at birth was associated with an increased mortality in early childhood and early adulthood that was independent of fetal growth as well as other perinatal and socioeconomic factors. Congenital anomalies and respiratory and endocrine disorders were significant causes of death in both early childhood and young adulthood, whereas cardiovascular disorders were significant only in early adulthood. Interestingly, the association between gestational age at birth and mortality was no different for males and females. This study adds to the growing body of information indicating that prematurity is a chronic condition that requires the same degree of vigilant monitoring as other chronic medical problems.

**L. A. Papile, MD**

# 3 Genetics and Teratology

**Prenatal environmental risk factors for genital malformations in a population of 1442 French male newborns: a nested case–control study**
Gaspari L, Paris F, Jandel C, et al (CHU Montpellier et Université Montpellier 1, France; et al)
*Hum Reprod* 26:3155-3162, 2011

*Background.*—Over the past decades, an increasing trend in male external genital malformations such as cryptorchidism and hypospadias has led to the suspicion that environmental chemicals are detrimental to male fetal sexual development. Several environmental pollutants, including organochlorine pesticides, polychlorinated biphenyls, bisphenol A, phthalates, dioxins and furans have estrogenic and anti-androgenic activity and are thus considered as endocrine-disrupting chemicals (EDCs). Since male sex differentiation is critically dependent on the normal production and action of androgens during fetal life, EDCs may be able to alter normal male sex differentiation.

*Objective.*—The objective of this study was to determine the incidence of external genital malformations in a population of full-term newborn males in southern France. We also performed a case–control study to identify the risk factors for male external genital malformations, with a focus on parental occupational exposure to EDCs.

*Methods.*—Over a 16-month period, 1615 full-term newborn males with a birth weight above 2500 g were registered on a level-1 maternity ward, and the same pediatrician systematically examined 1442 of them (89%) for cryptorchidism, hypospadias and micropenis. For every male newborn with genital malformation, we enrolled nearly two males matched for age, parity and term. All parents of the case and control newborns were interviewed about pregnancy aspects, personal characteristics, lifestyle and their occupational exposure to EDCs using a detailed questionnaire.

*Results.*—We report 39 cases of genital malformation (2.70%), with 18 cases of cryptorchidism (1.25%), 14 of hypospadias (0.97%), 5 of micropenis (0.35%) and 2 of 46,XY disorders of sexual differentiation (DSD; 0.14%). We observed a significant relationship between newborn cryptorchidism, hypospadias or micropenis and parental occupational exposure to pesticides [odds ratio (OR) = 4.41; 95% confidence interval (95% CI), 1.21–16.00]. Familial clustering for male external genital malformations (OR = 7.25; 95% CI, 0.70–74.30) and medications taken by mothers during pregnancy (OR $= 5.87$; 95% CI, 0.93–37.00) were associated with the risk of cryptorchidism, hypospadias and micropenis, although the association was not statistically significant.

*Conclusions.*—Although the causes of male genital malformation are multifactorial, our data support the hypothesis that prenatal contamination by pesticides may be a potential risk factor for newborn male external genital malformation and it should thus be routinely investigated in all undervirilized newborn males.

▶ A prime example of the consequences of the exposure of the human fetus to hormonally active agents is the case of diethylstilbestrol (DES), a nonsteroidal estrogen and not an environmental pollutant. Many millions of women were prescribed this agent to prevent abortion and premature labor. It did neither but caused cervical anomalies and vaginal cancer as well as male anomalies. Furthermore, it affected the third generation. Compared with endocrine disruptors, which may produce anomalies in fish in parts per billion, the dose of DES was relatively high.

Endocrine disruptors are chemicals that interfere with the endocrine system in animals, including humans. These disruptions can cause birth defects, developmental disorders, and cancer. Specifically, they are known to cause learning disabilities, severe attention deficit disorder, cognitive and even developmental brain problems, deformations of the body (including limbs), sexual development problems, cryptorchidism, hypospadias, and feminization of males or masculine effects on females. Several environmental pollutants, including organochlorine pesticides (DDT), polychlorinated biphenyls, bisphenol A, phthalates, dioxins, and furans have estrogenic and antiandrogenic activity and are thus considered as endocrine-disrupting chemicals (EDCs). Because male sex differentiation is critically dependent on the normal production and action of androgens during fetal life, EDCs may be able to alter normal male sex differentiation. Toppari et al[1] report that cryptorchidism and hypospadias affect 2% to 9% and 0.2% to 1% of male newborns, respectively. The incidence of both defects shows large geographic variation, but in several countries there are increased numbers of these conditions reported. They are also interlinked to the risk of testis cancer and poor semen quality. Testicular dysgenesis syndrome (TDS) may underlie many cases of all these male reproductive health problems. Genetic defects in androgen production or action can cause both cryptorchidism and hypospadias, but these are not common. Toppari et al observe "Environmental effects appear to play a major role in TDS. Exposure to several persistent chemicals has been found to be associated with the risk of cryptorchidism, and exposure to anti-androgenic phthalates has been shown to be associated with hormonal changes predisposing to male reproductive problems." Torres-Sanchez et al[2] measured maternal serum levels of DDT metabolites (p,p'-DDE and p,p'-DDT) before and during each trimester of pregnancy by electron capture gas-liquid chromatography. They found that in boys, a doubling increase of maternal p,p'-DDE serum levels during the first trimester of pregnancy was associated with a significant reduction of the distance between the anus and perineum, a reflection of decreased androgen exposure in utero.

Gaspari et al make a compelling case to seek evidence of environmental exposure, including potential endocrine disruptors in all males with genital anomalies and lack of virilization.

**A. A. Fanaroff, MBBCh, FRCPE**

*References*

1. Toppari J, Virtanen HE, Main KM, Skakkebaek NE. Cryptorchidism and hypospadias as a sign of testicular dysgenesis syndrome (TDS): environmental connection. *Birth Defects Res A Clin Mol Teratol.* 2010;88:910-919.
2. Torres-Sanchez L, Zepeda M, Cebrián ME, et al. Dichlorodiphenyldichloroethylene exposure during the first trimester of pregnancy alters the anal position in male infants. *Ann N Y Acad Sci.* 2008;1140:155-162.

---

**Brain anomalies in children exposed prenatally to a common organophosphate pesticide**
Rauh VA, Perera FP, Horton MK, et al (Columbia Univ, NY; et al)
*Proc Natl Acad Sci U S A* 109:7871-7876, 2012

---

Prenatal exposure to chlorpyrifos (CPF), an organophosphate insecticide, is associated with neurobehavioral deficits in humans and animal models. We investigated associations between CPF exposure and brain morphology using magnetic resonance imaging in 40 children, 5.9–11.2 y, selected from a nonclinical, representative community-based cohort. Twenty high-exposure children (upper tertile of CPF concentrations in umbilical cord blood) were compared with 20 low-exposure children on cortical surface features; all participants had minimal prenatal exposure to environmental tobacco smoke and polycyclic aromatic hydrocarbons. High CPF exposure was associated with enlargement of superior temporal, posterior middle temporal, and inferior postcentral gyri bilaterally, and enlarged superior frontal gyrus, gyrus rectus, cuneus, and precuneus along the mesial wall of the right hemisphere. Group differences were derived from exposure effects on underlying white matter. A significant exposure × IQ interaction was derived from CPF disruption of normal IQ associations with surface measures in low-exposure children. In preliminary analyses, high-exposure children did not show expected sex differences in the right inferior parietal lobule and superior marginal gyrus, and displayed reversal of sex differences in the right mesial superior frontal gyrus, consistent with disruption by CPF of normal behavioral sexual dimorphisms reported in animal models. High-exposure children also showed frontal and parietal cortical thinning, and an inverse dose-response relationship between CPF and cortical thickness. This study reports significant associations of prenatal exposure to a widely used environmental neurotoxicant, at standard use levels, with structural changes in the developing human brain.

▶ According to the US Environmental Protection Agency,[1] a pesticide is any substance or mixture of substances intended for preventing, destroying, repelling, or mitigating any pest. Although often misunderstood to refer only to insecticides, the term pesticide also applies to herbicides, fungicides, and various other substances used to control pests. Because they are designed to kill or otherwise adversely affect living organisms, it comes as no surprise that pesticides can cause harm to humans, animals, or the environment. Pesticides can be potent neurotoxins; thus, the findings in humans, which link both prenatal and postnatal exposure to organophosphate pesticides to adverse effects on brain and neurologic development, come as no surprise.[2-4] A spectrum of developmental disabilities has been associated with these toxins, ranging from attention deficit hyperactivity disorder to learning disabilities, autism, and mental retardation. There have also been a variety of birth defects, including limb reduction defects, cleft palate, hypospadias, and cryptorchidism associated with pesticide exposure during pregnancy.

This report from Rauh et al addresses a previous gap in knowledge, that is, a detailed examination of the specific effects of organophosphate insecticides on brain structure. The exquisitely detailed cerebral anatomy permits many regional comparisons and explains some of the sex issues associated with these toxic exposures. It is of concern that these cerebral findings were observed at levels well below the threshold for any signs of acute exposure. Also, these differences were detected in such a small sample (40 children age 5.9 to 11.2 years of age). In an era in which many authorities are clamoring for organic products for children and adults alike, reports like this support such a cause.

**A. A. Fanaroff, MBBCh, FRCPE**

*References*

1. US Environmental Protection Agency. About pesticides. 2006. http://www.epa.gov/pesticides/about/index.htm. Accessed June 5, 2012.
2. Rosas LG, Eskenazi B. Pesticides and child neurodevelopment. *Curr Opin Pediatr.* 2008;20:191-197.
3. Eskenazi B, Rosas LG, Marks AR, et al. Pesticide Toxicity and the developing brain. *Basic Clin Pharmacol Toxicol.* 2008;102:228-336.
4. Stillerman KP, Mattison DR, Giudice LC, Woodruff TJ. Environmental exposures and adverse pregnancy outcomes: a review of the science. *Reprod Sci.* 2008;15:631-650.

**Complete Screening of 50 Patients with CHARGE Syndrome for Anomalies in the *CHD7* Gene Using a Denaturing High-Performance Liquid Chromatography–Based Protocol: New Guidelines and a Proposal for Routine Diagnosis**
Bilan F, Legendre M, Charraud V, et al (Poitiers Univ Hosp, France)
*J Mol Diagn* 14:46-55, 2012

Ocular coloboma, heart malformation, choanal atresia, retardation of growth and/or development, genital hypoplasia, and ear anomalies associated with deafness (CHARGE) syndrome is a rare, usually sporadic, autosomal dominant disorder, caused by mutations within the *CHD7* (chromodomain helicase DNA-binding protein 7) gene, in nearly 70% of cases. Because human *CHD7* is relatively large (38 exons encoding a 300-kDa protein), genetic analysis requires cost-effective and time-consuming techniques. Herein, we propose an alternative screening method to quickly detect *CHD7* mutations using mainly denaturing high-performance liquid chromatography. The entire coding region with exon-intron boundaries was amplified under the same experimental conditions. Each amplicon of the same *CHD7* region was subjected to denaturing high-performance liquid chromatography analysis, and resulting chromatograms were compared within small series of patients. Because a *CHD7* mutation differs generally from one patient to another, corresponding chromatograms exhibited a unique pattern that is significantly different from common polymorphisms. Only amplicons exhibiting a unique profile were subjected to DNA sequencing analysis. Intragenic rearrangements were investigated with only nine multiplex PCRs. In conclusion, using our protocol, we can quickly detect the right containing mutation amplicon and we provide a robust, rapid, and cheaper method to screen *CHD7* microrearrangements or an entire deletion (Figs 3 and 4).

▶ CHARGE syndrome (CS), first described in 1981, occurs in about 1 per 10 000 births and includes children with coloboma of the eye, heart defects, atresia of the choanae, retardation of growth or development, genital or urinary abnormalities, and ear abnormalities and deafness. Additional characteristic clinical features include cranial nerve defects (I, VII, IX, and X), many types of cardiovascular malformations, and tracheoesophageal fistula. Moreover, it is well established that arhinencephaly and semicircular canal hypoplasia or agenesis, resulting in vestibular areflexia, are 2 critical landmarks of CS.

These are the cold hard features of CS. The story comes to life, and one gains a better perception of what it means for the family when you visit the CHARGE Syndrome Foundation Web page.[1] They note "Babies with CS are often born with life-threatening birth defects, including complex heart defects and breathing problems. They spend many months in the hospital and undergo many surgeries and other treatments. Swallowing and breathing problems make life difficult even when they come home. Most have hearing loss, vision loss, and balance problems, which delay their development and communication. All are likely to require medical and educational intervention for many years. Despite these seemingly insurmountable obstacles, children with CHARGE syndrome often far surpass their medical, physical, educational, and social expectations."

Since 2004, it has been recognized that CS is caused by a mutation in a single regulatory gene, most often CHD7, located on the long arm of chromosome #8.[2] To date, most reports indicate that the genetic abnormality is detected in 70% of patients with CS. The landscape for genetic diagnosis is changing swiftly. This report from Bilan et al discusses a more rapid, less-expensive, but reliable approach to the genetic diagnosis of CHARGE and allied syndromes. The algorithm (Fig 4) presents a logical approach and the fluorescence *in situ* hybridization analysis of the CHD7 locus using the RP11-414L17 BAC probe (Fig 3) graphically demonstrates a missing locus in the child with CS when compared with both parents.

The genetics are complex, and I do not pretend to understand all the manipulations or graphs from the Denaturing High-Performance Liquid Chromatography

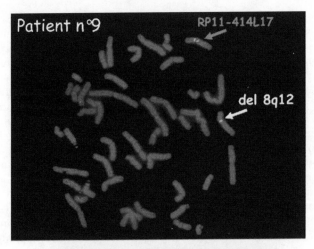

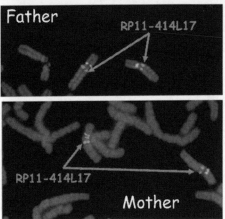

FIGURE 3.—FISH analysis of the *CHD7* locus using the RP11-414L17 BAC probe. Patient 9 (**top panel**) exhibits only one copy of the *CHD7* locus (one purple spot) compared with his mother and father, who exhibit two copies (two red spots on each **bottom panels**). For interpretation of the references to color in this figure legend, the reader is referred to web version of this article. (Reprinted from the Journal of Molecular Diagnostics, Bilan F, Legendre M, Charraud V, et al. Complete screening of 50 patients with CHARGE syndrome for anomalies in the *CHD7* gene using a denaturing high-performance liquid chromatography–based protocol: new guidelines and a proposal for routine diagnosis. *J Mol Diagn.* 2012;14:46-55. Copyright 2012 with permission from Elsevier.)

(DHPLC). In essence, they have developed a main DHPLC-based molecular analysis of the CHD7 gene, allowing easy screening for point mutations, small deletions/insertions, and more complex gene rearrangements. We identified causative disease mutations (or gene alterations) in two-thirds (33 of 50 [66%]) of the patients who were clinically diagnosed with CS. This ratio can be extended to more than four-fifths (84%) if we include the 9 orphan mutations characterized in this study. All mutations were private, except for c.2504_2508delATCTT, which was found in 2 unrelated patients, and all were scattered throughout

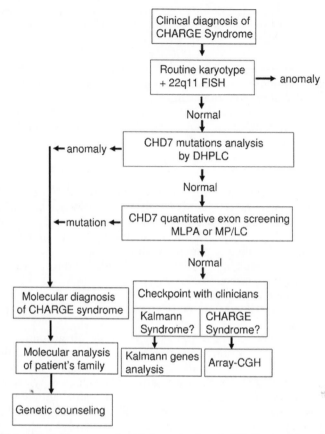

FIGURE 4.—Proposal for a new molecular diagnostic scheme for CS. (Reprinted from the Journal of Molecular Diagnostics, Bilan F, Legendre M, Charraud V, et al. Complete screening of 50 patients with CHARGE syndrome for anomalies in the *CHD7* gene using a denaturing high-performance liquid chromatography—based protocol: new guidelines and a proposal for routine diagnosis. *J Mol Diagn.* 2012;14:46-55. Copyright 2012 with permission from Elsevier.)

CHD7; however, some exons seemed more affected than others (eg, exons 2, 8, 31, and 34, with 6, 4, 4, and 4 mutations, respectively.)

Their concluding statement provides insight into the future of many genetic disorders. "This DHPLC-based protocol, dedicated for CS, could be easily transposed to any other inherited diseases, especially autosomal dominant disorders due to large genes. We also performed such analysis in recessive disorders, such as cystic fibrosis (private mutation screening on the whole CFTR gene) and familial pulmonary fibrosis (ABCA3 gene)."

**A. A. Fanaroff, MBBCh, FRCPE**

*References*

1. The CHARGE Syndrome Foundation. About CHARGE. http://chargesyndrome.org/about-charge.asp. Accessed June 7, 2012.

2. Vissers LE, van Ravenswaaij CM, Admiraal R, et al. Mutations in a new member of the chromodomain gene family cause CHARGE syndrome. *Nat Genet.* 2004; 36:955-957.

---

## Ichthyosis prematurity syndrome: Clinical evaluation of 17 families with a rare disorder of lipid metabolism

Khnykin D, Rønnevig J, Johnsson M, et al (Oslo Univ Hospitale—Rikshospitalet and Univ of Oslo, Norway; Norwegian Univ of Science and Technology, Trondheim, Norway; et al)
*J Am Acad Dermatol* 66:606-616, 2012

---

*Background.*—Ichthyosis prematurity syndrome (IPS) is classified as a syndromic congenital ichthyosis based on the presence of skin changes at birth, ultrastructural abnormalities in the epidermis, and extracutaneous manifestations. Recently, mutations in the fatty acid transporter protein 4 gene have been identified in patients with IPS.

*Objective.*—We sought to perform a detailed clinical evaluation of patients with IPS identified in Norway.

*Methods.*—Clinical examination and follow-up of all patients (n = 23) and light and electron microscopic examination of skin biopsy specimens were performed.

*Results.*—IPS was characterized prenatally by ultrasound findings of polyhydramnios, separation of membranes, echogenic amniotic fluid, and clear chorionic fluid. All patients were born prematurely with sometimes life-threatening neonatal asphyxia; this was likely caused by aspiration of corneocyte-containing amniotic fluid as postmortem examination of lung tissue in two patients revealed keratin debris filling the bronchial tree and alveoli. The skin appeared erythrodermic, swollen, and covered by a greasy, thick vernix caseosa-like "scale" at birth, and evolved rapidly to a mild chronic ichthyosis. Many patients subsequently had chronic, severe pruritus. Histopathologic and ultrastructural examination of skin biopsy specimens showed hyperkeratosis, acanthosis, dermal inflammation, and characteristic aggregates of curved lamellar structures in the upper epidermis. Peripheral blood eosinophilia was invariably present and most patients had increased serum immunoglobulin E levels. Over 70% of the patients had a history of respiratory allergy and/or food allergy.

*Limitations.*—The study included only 23 patients because of the rarity of the disease.

*Conclusion.*—IPS is characterized by defined genetic mutations, typical ultrastructural skin abnormalities, and distinct prenatal and postnatal clinical features.

▶ Despite the fact that the disorder ichthyosis prematurity syndrome (IPS) was described in 1982, this article represented my first encounter with this distinct disease, which has characteristic prenatal and postnatal clinical features. I will therefore attempt to summarize the key features of this disorder under the assumption that increased awareness of IPS is necessary to recognize the disorder; to provide the best perinatal and postnatal care for affected infants; and to make families aware of the genetic features of IPS.

IPS, a rare form of ichthyosis, is an autosomal recessive disorder, characterized by premature birth, nonscaly ichthyosis, and atopic manifestations. It is caused by mutations in the gene encoding the fatty acid transport protein 4 (FATP4) and a specific reduction in the incorporation of very long-chain fatty acids into cellular lipids.[1] FATP4 encodes a protein that functions both as a fatty acid transporter and an acyl coenzyme A synthetase. FATP4 is expressed in the suprabasal layer of the epidermis. Reduced function of this protein most likely leads to disturbance of the intercellular lipid layer of the stratum corneum as observed for other subtypes of ichthyosis.

IPS may be recognized in the fetus by the following combination of features: polyhydramnios (present in all cases where ultrasound is available), separation of the chorionic and amniotic membranes, echogenic sediment in the amniotic fluid, clear chorionic fluid (Fig 1), and debris filling the stomach. The separation of the amnion and the chorion appears to be very distinctive and the debris in the amniotic cavity unmistakable. Khnykin reported that all patients were born prematurely, and 15 of 17 patients had neonatal asphyxia primarily as a result of reduced lung function. Prenatal ultrasound findings suggested that reduced lung function was caused by aspiration of corneocyte-containing amniotic fluid. Autopsy examination of both patients who died within hours of birth revealed large keratin masses filling the bronchial tree and alveoli.

The skin appearance goes through a few phases. All patients were born with grossly abnormal-appearing skin. The entire skin surface, but most strikingly the head, was covered by a greasy, thick vernix caseosalike scale (Fig 3). The

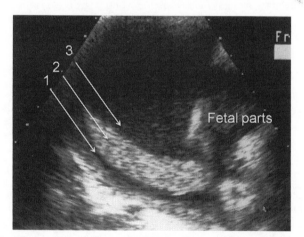

FIGURE 1.—Ultrasound image of fetus with ichthyosis prematurity syndrome at 29 weeks. Chorionic cavity with clear fluid (1), sediment (skin debris) in amniotic cavity (2), and amniotic fluid (3) are indicated by *arrows*. Note that amniotic and chorionic membranes are adherent in normal pregnancies. (Reprinted from the Journal of the American Academy of Dermatology, Khnykin D, Rønnevig J, Johnsson M, et al. Ichthyosis prematurity syndrome: Clinical evaluation of 17 families with a rare disorder of lipid metabolism. *J Am Acad Dermatol.* 2012;66:606-616. Copyright 2012, with permission from the American Academy of Dermatology.)

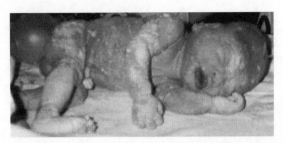

FIGURE 3.—Prematurely born infant with caseous vernixlike desquamation and erythrodermic skin. (Reprinted from the Journal of the American Academy of Dermatology, Khnykin D, Rønnevig J, Johnsson M, et al. Ichthyosis prematurity syndrome: Clinical evaluation of 17 families with a rare disorder of lipid metabolism. *J Am Acad Dermatol*. 2012;66:606-616. Copyright 2012, with permission from the American Academy of Dermatology.)

underlying skin was variably erythrodermic and swollen. A rapid improvement occurred in the first few days of life. The skin surface lost its vernixlike cover and passed through an erythrodermic phase. After a few weeks, the skin was no longer erythematous but was drier than normal. During infancy, the skin became red with handling, and red dermographism was always present. In many patients, this evolved into white dermographism later in life.

Sobol[2] screened probands from 5 families segregating IPS for mutations in the FATP4 gene. Four probands were compound heterozygous for 4 different mutations, of which 3 are novel. Four patients were heterozygous and 1 patient homozygous for the previously reported nonsense mutation p.C168X (c.504c > a). All patients had clinical characteristics of IPS and a similar clinical course. They concluded that missense mutations and nonsense mutations in FATP4 are associated with similar clinical features, suggesting that missense mutations have a severe impact on FATP4 function. The results broaden the mutational spectrum in FATP4 associated with IPS for molecular diagnosis of and further functional analysis of FATP4.

The disorder to date has mainly been described from Scandinavia, but it is an interesting clinical entity with many pearls for the clinicians. Advances in genetics quickly simplify the classification of such disorders.

**A. A. Fanaroff, MBBCh, FRCPE**

*References*

1. Klar J, Schweiger M, Zimmerman R, et al. Mutations in the fatty acid transport protein 4 gene cause the ichthyosis prematurity syndrome. *Am J Hum Genet*. 2009;85:248-253.
2. Sobol M, Dahl N, Klar J. FATP4 missense and nonsense mutations cause similar features in Ichthyosis Prematurity Syndrome. *BMC Res Notes*. 2011;4:90.

# 4 Labor and Delivery

**Effectiveness of pulse oximetry versus fetal electrocardiography for the intrapartum evaluation of nonreassuring fetal heart rate**
Valverde M, Puertas AM, Lopez-Gallego MF, et al (Virgen de las Nieves Univ Hosp, Granada, Spain; Santa Ana Hosp, Granada, Spain)
*Eur J Obstet Gynecol Reprod Biol* 159:333-337, 2011

*Objectives.*—To compare the effectiveness of pulse oximetry and fetal electrocardiography in the management of labor with nonreassuring fetal heart rate (NRFHR).

*Study Design.*—This randomized experimental study consisted of two arms. In group 1 we used pulse oximetry and in group 2 we used STAN® technology. The participants in each group were 90 pregnant women with a full-term singleton fetus in cephalic presentation and cardiotocographic tracings compatible with NRFHR. We compared the following variables: rate of cesarean delivery, indications for operative delivery due to NRFHR, and repercussions on the newborn's acid–base status.

*Results.*—The two groups differed significantly in the mode of delivery, with a cesarean delivery rate of 47.6% in group 1 vs. 30% in group 2 ($p = 0.032$). The groups did not differ in the indications for ending labor due to NRFHR (62% vs. 61%, NS). In terms of neonatal outcomes, the 1-min Apgar score was 6 or lower in 17.8% of the group 1 neonates vs. 4.44% of the group 2 neonates ($p < 0.001$). The groups also differed significantly in umbilical cord vein pH (7.23 vs. 7.27) and $pCO_2$ (57.27 vs. 46.86) at birth.

*Conclusions.*—Fetal electrocardiography with the STAN® 21 system was more effective in detecting good fetal status and thus in identifying cases in which labor could proceed safely. Intrapartum surveillance with the STAN® 21 system reduced the rate of emergency cesarean delivery.

▶ For decades, obstetricians have made their decisions to intervene for fetal distress mainly on the basis of fetal cardiotocography (CTG) tracings. This has resulted in many emergency interventions and operative deliveries for fetal distress only to deliver a vigorous infant with no biochemical evidence of fetal hypoxia. None of the randomized trials have proven this technology to be reliable or predictive of important fetal and neonatal outcomes, and there are many false-positive findings with CTG driving these deliveries. It is thus encouraging to learn that the fetal electrocardiogram (ECG) monitoring with the STAN® system reduces cesarean sections and improves pH at delivery. Furthermore, in this study, the ST analysis (STAN®) proved to be superior to pulse oximetry.

For those who need updated information on this technology, the following paragraph comes from the article, "Fetal ECG with the STAN® system combines standard internal (CTG) technology with measurements of the ST segment and T wave (ST) interval in the fetal ECG. The STAN® system for analysis of the ST segment records FHR, the changes in ST interval and the changes in the T/QRS ratio. Changes in the fetal ST interval, as in adults, provide reliable information about the capacity of the myocardium to respond to hypoxia. The fetal heart and brain are equally sensitive to oxygen deficiency, and therefore the data for myocardial functioning provide an indirect measure of the condition of the fetal brain during labor and delivery."

Westerhaus[1] reported that intrapartum monitoring by cardiotocography combined with ST analysis does not significantly reduce the incidence of metabolic acidosis calculated in the extracellular fluid compartment. It does reduce the incidence of metabolic acidosis calculated in blood and the need for fetal blood sampling without affecting the Apgar score, neonatal admissions, hypoxic-ischemic encephalopathy, or operative deliveries. However Doret,[2] from an analysis of 3112 women, noted that the cesarean section rate for suspected fetal distress was 9.5%. Acid-base status was available for 3067 (98.5%) neonates. There were 14 cases of fetal metabolic acidosis, including 11 who were not treated according to the STAN® guidelines. Sixty-two neonates (2%) had an umbilical pH ≤ 7.05 and normal extracellular base deficit, and 27 neonates had 5-minute Apgar scores ≤ 7. No cases of neonatal encephalopathy or fetal or neonatal death occurred.

STAN® monitoring without fetal blood sampling (FBS) support was associated with a low rate of fetal metabolic acidosis. Most cases of fetal metabolic acidosis were not managed in accordance with the STAN® guidelines. This study supports STAN® usage without FBS support. On the other hand, Becker[3] reported that baseline T/QRS has no added value in the prediction of adverse neonatal outcome or interventions for suspected fetal distress.

The state of the art with respect to fetal evaluation for distress is still evolving. A computer-assisted study[4] has been registered, and hopefully the data will shed further light on this complex and often confusing topic.

**A. A. Fanaroff, MBBCh, FRCPE**

*References*

1. Westerhuis ME, Visser GH, Moons KG, Zuithoff N, Mol BW, Kwee A. Cardiotocography plus ST analysis of fetal electrocardiogram compared with cardiotocography only for intrapartum monitoring: a randomized controlled trial. *Obstet Gynecol.* 2010;115:1173-1180.
2. Doret M, Massoud M, Constans A, Gaucherand P. Use of peripartum ST analysis of fetal electrocardiogram without blood sampling: a large prospective cohort study. *Eur J Obstet Gynecol Reprod Biol.* 2011;156:35-40.
3. Becker JH, Kuipers LJ, Schuit E, et al. Predictive value of the baseline T-QRS ratio of the fetal electrocardiogram in intrapartum fetal monitoring: a prospective cohort study. *Acta Obstet Gynecol Scand.* 2012;91:189-197.
4. Ayres-de-Campos D, Ugwumadu A, Banfield P, et al. A randomised clinical trial of intrapartum fetal monitoring with computer analysis and alerts versus previously monitoring. *BMC Pregnancy Childbirth.* 2010;28:10-71.

## Diversity of microbes in amniotic fluid

DiGiulio DB (Stanford Univ School of Medicine, CA)
*Semin Fetal Neonatal Med* 17:2-11, 2012

Recent polymerase chain reaction (PCR)-based studies estimate the prevalence of microbial invasion of the amniotic cavity (MIAC) to be ≥30–50% higher than that detected by cultivation-based methods. Some species that have been long implicated in causing MIAC remain among the common invaders (e.g. *Ureaplasma* spp., *Mycoplasma* spp., *Fusobacterium* spp. *Streptococcus* spp., *Bacteroides* spp. and *Prevotella* spp.). Yet we now know from studies based on PCR of the 16S ribosomal DNA that cultivation-resistant anaerobes belonging to the family Fusobacteriaceae (particularly *Sneathia sanguinegens*, and *Leptotrichia* spp.) are also commonly found in amniotic fluid. Other diverse microbes detected by PCR of amniotic fluid include as-yet uncultivated and uncharacterized species. The presence of some microbial taxa is associated with specific host factors (e.g. *Candida* spp. and an indwelling intrauterine device). It appears that MIAC is polymicrobial in 24–67% of cases, but the potential role of pathogen synergy is poorly understood. A causal relationship between diverse microbes, as detected by PCR, and preterm birth is supported by types of association (e.g. space, time and dose) proposed as alternatives to Koch's postulates for inferring causality from molecular findings. The microbial census of the amniotic cavity remains unfinished. A more complete understanding may inform future research directions leading to improved strategies for preventing, diagnosing and treating MIAC.

▶ This review is of interest in that it suggests a causal relationship between diverse microbes as detected by polymerase chain reaction (PCR) as microbial invasion of the intra-amniotic cavity (MIAC) to preterm delivery. One of the first studies done more than 30 years ago relating amniotic infections without rupture of membranes to prematurity used quantitative amniotic fluid cultures in 12 patients who delivered premature infants. Seven of the 10 women with preterm labor who had intact membranes had cultured bacterial colony counts greater than 1000/mL.[1] Over the next 3 decades, considerable additional data have emerged supporting the concept that microbial colonization of the amniotic fluid is a very significant risk factor for premature delivery.[2] However, the fact that these data were based on culture-based technology has caused some confusion, as intra-amniotic inflammation is often detected in the absence of infection diagnosed by culture. More recent studies using non–culture-based techniques are beginning to clarify this issue by revealing significant prevalence of microbes that cannot be readily cultured using standard laboratory techniques.[3,4] Studies by Dr Roberto Romero and his group used a PCR-based technique to detect and characterize the presence of bacteria in amniotic fluid without reliance on culture as the sole means of bacterial detection. The results have provided at least a partial explanation: in the amniotic fluid of many women who deliver prematurely, there are bacteria present that have not previously been cultured by standard techniques. Furthermore, the greater degree of prematurity is directly related to the 16SrRNA bacterial load in the amniotic fluid, even in the absence of ruptured membranes.[3] Other investigators have used closely related non–culture-based techniques and have also found noncultivatable and difficult-to-cultivate microbes in amniotic fluid of those who delivered prematurely,[4] thus, validating the previous studies. Both studies related the presence of these microbes to premature delivery via an inflammatory response but did not specifically address the origin of the inflammation. From these studies, it is beginning to appear that many cases of preterm labor are associated with microbial colonization. The evidence supports that these microbes are inducing an inflammatory response, but is the origin of this response the fetus or the mother or both? Studies are needed to better define this overall relationship and specific mechanisms involved.

**J. Neu, MD**

*References*

1. Bobitt JR, Ledger WJ. Unrecognized amnionitis and prematurity: a preliminary report. *J Reprod Med.* 1977;19:8-12.
2. Goldenberg RL, Culhane JF, Iams JD, Romero R. Epidemiology and causes of preterm birth. *Lancet.* 2008;371:75-84.
3. DiGiulio DB, Romero R, Amogan HP, et al. Microbial prevalence, diversity and abundance in amniotic fluid during preterm labor: a molecular and culture-based investigation. *PLoS One.* 2008;3:e3056.
4. Han YW, Shen T, Chung P, Buhimschi IA, Buhimschi CS. Uncultivated bacteria as etiologic agents of intra-amniotic inflammation leading to preterm birth. *J Clin Microbiol.* 2009;47:38-47.

---

**Neonatal Outcomes After Implementation of Guidelines Limiting Elective Delivery Before 39 Weeks of Gestation**
Ehrenthal DB, Hoffman MK, Jiang X, et al (Christiana Ctr for Outcomes Res, Newark, DE)
*Obstet Gynecol* 118:1047-1055, 2011

---

*Objective.*—To evaluate the association of a new institutional policy limiting elective delivery before 39 weeks of gestation with neonatal outcomes at a large community-based academic center.

*Methods.*—A retrospective cohort study was conducted to estimate the effect of the policy on neonatal outcomes using a before and after design. All term singleton deliveries 2 years before and 2 years after policy enforcement were included. Clinical data from the electronic hospital obstetric records were used to identify outcomes and relevant covariates. Multivariable logistic regression was used to account for independent effects of changes in characteristics and comorbidities of the women in the cohorts before and after implementation.

*Results.*—We identified 12,015 singleton live births before and 12,013 after policy implementation. The overall percentage of deliveries occurring before 39 weeks of gestation fell from 33.1% to 26.4% ($P < .001$); the greatest difference was for women undergoing repeat cesarean delivery or induction of labor. Admission to the neonatal intensive care unit (NICU) also decreased significantly; before the intervention, there were 1,116 admissions (9.29% of term live births), whereas after, there were 1,027 (8.55% of term live births) and this difference was significant ($P = .044$). However, an 11% increased odds of birth weight greater than 4,000 g (adjusted odds ratio 1.11; 95% confidence interval [CI] 1.01–1.22) and an increase in stillbirths at 37 and 38 weeks, from 2.5 to 9.1 per 10,000 term pregnancies (relative risk 3.67, 95% CI 1.02–13.15, $P = .032$), were detected.

*Conclusion.*—A policy limiting elective delivery before 39 weeks of gestation was followed by changes in the timing of term deliveries. This was associated with a small reduction in NICU admissions; however, macrosomia and stillbirth increased.

▶ The law of unintended consequences has not been repealed. Based on observational studies linking elective delivery between 37 and 39 weeks of gestation with increased neonatal morbidity, and noting that ACOG and the AAP have long recommended elective induction of labor or cesarean section only after 39 weeks of gestation, the Joint Commission adopted the rate of such births as a core outcome measure of hospital performance in 2010. This report provides the first data on the effects of implementation of strategies for compliance with these recommendations at a large regional medical center. Coincident with reduction in the proportion of these early-term births, these authors describe an unexpected increase in rates of stillbirth and macrosomia. Their data suggest occurrence of 1 additional stillbirth for every 9 avoided neonatal intensive care unit admissions—a high and probably unacceptable price. It is premature to rush to judgment with advocacy for reversal of this policy, however. These observations must be confirmed in other populations, and the reasons for stillbirth need further exploration to better delineate causes and potential approaches to prevention. Postmarketing surveillance for unanticipated adverse consequences is as essential for quality assurance measures as it is for novel therapies.

**W. E. Benitz, MD**

---

**Maternal and perinatal complications by day of gestation after spontaneous labor at 40–42 weeks of gestation**
Greve T, Lundbye-Christensen S, Nickelsen CN, et al (Univ of Copenhagen, Hvidovre, Denmark; Univ of Aarhus, Aalborg, Denmark)
*Acta Obstet Gynecol Scand* 90:852-856, 2011

---

*Objective.*—To evaluate pregnancy outcome after spontaneous labor by day of gestation between $40^{+0}$ and $41^{+6}$ weeks of gestation.

*Design.*—Evaluation of prospectively collected labor ward data.

*Setting.*—University Hospital, Denmark.

*Population.*—Unselected consecutive cohort of 14 678 spontaneously starting deliveries between 280 and 293 days of gestation during the years 2000–2006.

*Methods.*—Data were registered in a computer program after each delivery by a midwife and the entries further evaluated by a specialist in obstetrics. Complication rates were compared using Fisher's exact test.

*Main Outcome Measures.*—Maternal complication rates for each gestation day, including cesarean delivery, maternal blood transfusion, episiotomy, operative vaginal delivery, third and fourth degree perineal lacerations and perinatal morbidity.

*Results.*—The cesarean delivery rate increased from 6% on day 280 to 11% on day 293. Cesarean delivery increased from 40 to 41 weeks gestation (7.3 vs. 9.5%, $p < 0.005$), as did maternal transfusion (0.5 vs. 1.2%, $p < 0.001$) and cesarean section on the indication fetal distress (1.5 versus 2.4%, $p < 0.005$), but perineal lacerations did not. Likewise, there was an increase in episiotomy rates (3.0 vs. 3.5%, $p = 0.08$), operative vaginal delivery (5.8 vs. 6.5%, $p = 0.07$) and admission to neonatal intensive care (1.4 versus 2.0%, $p = 0.009$), but no increase in 5 minute Apgar scores < 7 or low umbilical artery acid—base values.

*Conclusions.*—Deliveries starting spontaneously in an unselected cohort showed an increase in maternal complications, meconium-stained amniotic fluid and admission to the neonatal intensive care unit.

▶ "It's not nice to fool Mother Nature." I was intrigued by this article from Denmark, which looked at maternal and perinatal complications by completed days of gestation in women who underwent spontaneous labor from 40 to 42 weeks. Data were collected prospectively from a population of nearly 15 000 women from 2000 to 2006.

The investigators found a progressive increase in the rate of cesarean section (6% on day 280, 11% on day 293), cesarean section for fetal distress (1.5% at 40 weeks, 2.4% at 41 weeks), incidence of meconium-stained amniotic fluid (22.4% at 41 weeks, 29% at 41 weeks), and admission of the infant to a neonatal intensive care unit (1.4% at 40 weeks, 2.0% at 41 weeks). However, there were no increases in the number of infants with a 5-minute Apgar score < 7 or abnormalities in umbilical artery pH, although a daily trend toward acidosis was seen.

These differences suggest the concept of progressive placental senescence as pregnancy advances, with an increasing incidence of utero-placental insufficiency as the pregnancy becomes more postdated, even in a population of women with no prior demonstrated complications. As the authors discuss, the study is not able to address the issue of whether risks to the mother or fetus/baby can be reduced by induction of labor at 41 completed weeks, but it does provide a signal for future prospective clinical trials.

**S. M. Donn, MD**

**Effect of delayed versus early umbilical cord clamping on neonatal outcomes and iron status at 4 months: a randomised controlled trial**
Andersson O, Hellström-Westas L, Andersson D, et al (Hosp of Halland, Halmstad, Sweden; Uppsala Univ, Sweden; et al)
*BMJ* 343:d7157, 2011

*Objective.*—To investigate the effects of delayed umbilical cord clamping, compared with early clamping, on infant iron status at 4 months of age in a European setting.
*Design.*—Randomised controlled trial.
*Setting.*—Swedish county hospital.
*Participants.*—400 full term infants born after a low risk pregnancy.
*Intervention.*—Infants were randomised to delayed umbilical cord clamping ($\geq$180 seconds after delivery) or early clamping ($\leq$10 seconds after delivery).
*Main Outcome Measures.*—Haemoglobin and iron status at 4 months of age with the power estimate based on serum ferritin levels. Secondary outcomes included neonatal anaemia, early respiratory symptoms, polycythaemia, and need for phototherapy.
*Results.*—At 4 months of age, infants showed no significant differences in haemoglobin concentration between the groups, but infants subjected to delayed cord clamping had 45% (95% confidence interval 23% to 71%) higher mean ferritin concentration (117 µg/L $v$ 81 µg/L, $P < 0.001$) and a lower prevalence of iron deficiency (1 (0.6%) $v$ 10 (5.7%), $P = 0.01$, relative risk reduction 0.90; number needed to treat $= 20$ (17 to 67)). As for secondary outcomes, the delayed cord clamping group had lower prevalence of neonatal anaemia at 2 days of age (2 (1.2%) $v$ 10 (6.3%), $P = 0.02$, relative risk reduction 0.80, number needed to treat 20 (15 to 111)). There were no significant differences between groups in postnatal respiratory symptoms, polycythaemia, or hyperbilirubinaemia requiring phototherapy.
*Conclusions.*—Delayed cord clamping, compared with early clamping, resulted in improved iron status and reduced prevalence of iron deficiency at 4 months of age, and reduced prevalence of neonatal anaemia, without demonstrable adverse effects. As iron deficiency in infants even without anaemia has been associated with impaired development, delayed cord clamping seems to benefit full term infants even in regions with a relatively low prevalence of iron deficiency anaemia.
*Trial Registration.*—Clinical Trials NCT01245296.

▶ More and more prospective parents are inquiring about when the umbilical cord should be clamped. With each successive publication, evidence mounts in favor of delayed cord clamping, variably defined as between 30 seconds and 3 minutes after delivery or waiting until the cord stops pulsating. The benefits, including decreased need for blood transfusions, more stable blood pressure (in preterm infants), less intraventricular hemorrhage, and decreased infections in addition to higher iron stores (still evident at 4 to 6 months), clearly outweigh the convenience factor that drives immediate clamping and cutting and the marginal increase in jaundice. Whereas the benefits may be demonstrated in term and preterm infants, it is the preterm infants who derive the greatest benefit from delayed cord clamping. Most groups, including the World Health Organization, recommend that delayed cord clamping should be the standard practice with the exception of emergency situations, including placental separation or major hemorrhage. Change, however, takes place under normal circumstances at a glacial pace, causing David Hutchon[1] to note: "Clamping the functioning umbilical cord at birth is an unproved intervention. Lack of awareness of current evidence, pragmatism, and conflicting guidelines are all preventing change. To prevent further injury to babies we would be better to rush to change."

Iron deficiency and iron deficiency anemia are major public health problems in young children around the world and are associated with poor neurodevelopment. Young children are at particular risk due to their high iron requirements during rapid growth. Delayed cord clamping could prevent iron deficiency, but concern about jaundice has postponed the widespread introduction of delayed cord clamping. These authors lay these concerns to rest in their study by demonstrating that babies who experienced delayed clamping had fewer cases of neonatal anemia and better iron levels at 4 months of age. They estimated that for every 20 babies who had delayed clamping, 1 case of iron deficiency would be prevented, regardless of whether the baby also had anemia. Extrapolating these numbers on a global basis produces staggering numbers. Furthermore, delayed cord clamping was not associated with any adverse health effects.

The authors conclude that delayed cord clamping "should be considered as standard care for full term deliveries after uncomplicated pregnancies." Van Rheenen,[2] in an accompanying editorial, concludes that enough evidence now exists to encourage delayed cord clamping. He states that "The balance of maternal risks and infant benefits of delayed cord clamping now clearly favors the child. How much more evidence is needed to convince obstetricians and midwives that it is worthwhile to wait for three minutes to allow for placental transfusion, even in developed countries?"

**A. A. Fanaroff, MBBCh, FRCPE**

*References*

1. Hutchon D. Why do obstetricians and midwives still rush to clamp the cord? *BMJ.* 2010;341:c5447.
2. van Rheenen P. Delayed cord clamping and improved infant outcomes. *BMJ.* 2011;343:d7127.

---

**Uterine Rupture With Attempted Vaginal Birth After Cesarean Delivery: Decision-to-Delivery Time and Neonatal Outcome**
Holmgren C, Scott JR, Porter TF, et al (Univ of Utah Med Ctr, Salt Lake City)
*Obstet Gynecol* 119:725-731, 2012

---

*Objective.*—To estimate the time from the diagnosis of uterine rupture to delivery that would prevent adverse neonatal sequelae.

*Methods.*—Cases of uterine rupture from January 1, 2000, to December 31, 2009, were identified in nine hospitals in the Intermountain Health Care system and at the University of Utah. Maternal demographics, labor characteristics, and neonatal outcomes were obtained. Primary adverse outcome was abnormal umbilical artery pH level less than 7.0 or 5-minute Apgar score less than 7. Adverse secondary outcome included fetal or neonatal death and neonatal neurologic injury attributed to uterine rupture.

*Results.*—Thirty-six cases of uterine rupture occurred during 11,195 trials of labor after cesarean delivery. Signs of uterine rupture were fetal (n = 24), maternal (n = 8), or a combination of maternal and fetal (n = 3). In one case, uterine rupture was not suspected. Mean time to delivery from the onset of symptoms or signs for the primary adverse outcome group (n = 13) was 23.3 (±10.8) minutes compared with 16.0 (±7.7) minutes for those without an adverse outcome (*P* = .02). No neonate delivered in fewer than 18 minutes had an umbilical pH level below 7.0. Three neonates delivered at more than 30 minutes met criteria for an adverse secondary outcome.

*Conclusion.*—The frequency of uterine rupture was 0.32% in patients attempting a trial of labor after cesarean delivery. Neonates delivered within 18 minutes after a suspected uterine rupture had normal umbilical pH levels or 5-minute Apgar scores greater than 7. Poor long-term outcome occurred in three neonates with a decision-to-delivery time longer than 30 minutes.

*Level of Evidence.*—II.

▶ The question of how much asphyxia a fetus or newborn can withstand without permanent brain injury has fascinated physicians since Little proposed in 1862 that cerebral palsy is caused by intrapartum asphyxia. It has long been evident that most cases of cerebral palsy have other causes, but asphyxial insults can and do occasionally cause perinatal brain injury. Animal experiments have shed some light on the relation between the severity and duration of asphyxia required to produce permanent injury, but data from human infants have been difficult to acquire. Our limited ability to time the onset or characterize the nature of intrapartum asphyxia insults in most instances is a major barrier. However, intrapartum uterine rupture is an exception in that the onset of the event (abrupt and often precisely timed) and its nature (complete cessation of placental gas exchange, particularly when there is coincident complete placental abruption) can often be reliably established. Because uterine rupture is a low frequency event, very large population-based databases are needed to identify sufficient cases for these analyses.

Drawing data from 10 hospitals over a 10-year period, this article extends and updates earlier reports of such experiments of nature.[1,2] Despite differences in criteria for inclusion, timing of onset, and the particulars of outcome measures, these reports suggest that infants delivered within 18 minutes of recognition of uterine rupture are at low (but nonzero) risk of neurodevelopmental sequelae. Impairments following shorter periods from apparent onset to delivery imply fetal compromise before the onset of the sentinel event.

Conversely, onset-to-delivery intervals greater than 30 minutes are more likely (but not certain) to result in permanent injury. In the setting of this severe asphyxial insult, the probability of permanent injury appears to exceed 50% (ie, the medicolegal threshold of more likely than not) only when the duration is longer than a critical period in the range of 22 to 30 minutes. Fortunately, adverse outcomes after these potentially catastrophic events are now relatively unusual ( < 10% in the current study). Although trials of labor after cesarean section are rarely complicated by this unpredictable event (0.32% in this report), the importance of timely delivery when it occurs dictates that they take place where staff can immediately provide an emergency cesarean delivery.

**W. E. Benitz, MD**

*References*

1. Leung AS, Leung EK, Paul RH. Uterine rupture after previous cesarean delivery: maternal and fetal consequences. *Am J Obstet Gynecol.* 1993;169:945-950.
2. Bujold E, Gauthier RJ. Neonatal morbidity associated with uterine rupture: what are the risk factors? *Am J Obstet Gynecol.* 2002;186:311-314.

---

**Intrapartum Temperature Elevation, Epidural Use, and Adverse Outcome in Term Infants**
Greenwell EA, Wyshak G, Ringer SA, et al (Harvard School of Public Health, Boston, MA; Harvard School of Public Health and Harvard Med School, Boston, MA; Brigham and Women's Hosp and Harvard Med School, Boston, MA; et al)
*Pediatrics* 129:e447-e454, 2012

---

*Objectives.*—To examine the association of intrapartum temperature elevation with adverse neonatal outcome among low-risk women receiving epidural analgesia and evaluate the association of epidural with adverse neonatal outcome without temperature elevation.

*Methods.*—We studied all low-risk nulliparous women with singleton pregnancies ≥37 weeks delivering at our hospital during 2000, excluding pregnancies where infants had documented sepsis, meningitis, or a major congenital anomaly. Neonatal outcomes were compared between women receiving ($n = 1538$) and not receiving epidural analgesia ($n = 363$) in the absence of intrapartum temperature elevation (≤99.5°F) and according to the level of intrapartum temperature elevation within the group receiving epidural ($n = 2784$). Logistic regression was used to evaluate neonatal outcome while controlling for confounders.

*Results.*—Maternal temperature >100.4°F developed during labor in 19.2% (535/2784) of women receiving epidural compared with 2.4% (10/425) not receiving epidural. In the absence of intrapartum temperature elevation (≤99.5°F), no significant differences were observed in adverse neonatal outcomes between women receiving and not receiving epidural. Among women receiving epidural, a significant linear trend was observed between maximum maternal temperature and all neonatal outcomes examined including hypotonia, assisted ventilation, 1- and 5-min Apgar scores <7, and early-onset seizures. In regression analyses, infants born to women with fever >101°F had a two- to sixfold increased risk of all adverse outcomes examined.

*Conclusions.*—The proportion of infants experiencing adverse outcomes increased with the degree of epidural-related maternal temperature elevation. Epidural use without temperature elevation was not associated with any of the adverse outcomes we studied.

▶ Building on their earlier work, these investigators at Brigham and Women's Hospital examine potential fetal consequences of epidural analgesia during labor. Several years ago, they described frequent elevation of the maternal temperature following epidural analgesia, pointing out that this may not be an indication for evaluation for possible infection. Among nulliparous women who had uncomplicated deliveries at term during the year 2000, they identified 3209 low-risk mother-infant pairs. It is remarkable that 87% (2784) of these women had intrapartum epidural analgesia. (National surveillance data for 2008 suggest a typical rate of about 60%.) Of those, nearly half (45%) experienced an elevated intrapartum temperature, which exceeded 100.5°F in 19% and 101.0°F in 9%. Epidural analgesia without fever was not associated with adverse neonatal events, but increasing peak maternal temperature with epidural analgesia was linearly related to the frequency of those findings. The significance of short-term effects, including hypotonia, lower Apgar scores, and requirement for resuscitation measures, is not clear, as those findings may or may not be associated with long-term sequelae in this setting. The statistically significant risk-adjusted odds ratio (6.5, 95% confidence interval [CI], 1.0—40.8) for neonatal seizures among infants born to women whose temperatures exceeded 101.0°F is more worrisome, however, even though the rates of seizures were quite low (only 1.3% in the highest risk group). Notably, all 4 of the infants of mothers with fever ≥100.5°F who had seizures had cerebral infarction (3) or intracranial hemorrhage (1). While it is well known that neonatal fever may be a sign of intracranial injury, it is not clear whether, why, or how such events might lead to intrapartum maternal fever or vice versa. It is unfortunate that the number of women who did not have epidural analgesia was insufficient to determine whether fever in that setting is similarly associated with seizures and intracranial pathology; without that comparison, the significance of these infrequent events and the strength of association with epidural analgesia remain uncertain.

The implications for practice are not clear. While it may be tempting to suggest that measures to control maternal temperature elevation during epidural analgesia are now indicated, it is not clear how that might be achieved. Acetaminophen is ineffective. Corticosteroids may be effective, but adverse effects for mother and fetus may outweigh potential benefits. Controlling fever without ameliorating the underlying inflammatory system activation may not prevent neonatal sequelae, particularly if fetal nervous system injury causes, rather than results from, maternal fever. These observations raise concern that fetal effects of intrapartum epidural analgesia may not be entirely benign, but much work remains to be done before we can know how to respond to these worries.

**W. E. Benitz, MD**

## Trends and Characteristics of Home Vaginal Birth After Cesarean Delivery in the United States and Selected States

Macdorman MF, Declercq E, Mathews TJ, et al (Natl Ctr for Health Statistics, Hyattsville, MD; Boston Univ School of Public Health, MA; Univ of California, San Francisco)
*Obstet Gynecol* 119:737-744, 2012

*Objective.*—To examine trends and characteristics of home vaginal birth after cesarean delivery (VBAC) in the United States and selected states from 1990–2008.

*Methods.*—Birth certificate data were used to track trends in home and hospital VBACs from 1990–2008. Data on planned home VBAC were analyzed by sociodemographic and medical characteristics for the 25 states reporting this information in 2008 and compared with hospital VBAC data.

*Results.*—In 2008, there were approximately 42,000 hospital VBACs and approximately 1,000 home VBACs in the United States, up from 664 in 2003 and 656 in 1990. The percentage of home births that were VBACs increased from less than 1% in 1996 to 4% in 2008, whereas the percentage of hospital births that were VBACs decreased from 3% in 1996 to 1% in 2008. Planned home VBACs had a lower risk profile than hospital VBACs with fewer births to teenagers, unmarried women, or smokers; fewer preterm or low-birth-weight deliveries; and higher maternal education levels.

*Conclusion.*—Recent increases in the proportion of U.S. women with a prior cesarean delivery mean that an increasing number of women are faced with the choice and associated risks of either VBAC or repeat cesarean delivery. Recent restrictions in hospital VBAC availability have coincided with increases in home VBACs; however, home VBAC remains rare, with approximately 1,000 occurrences in 2008.

*Level of Evidence.*—II.

▶ In 2008, more than half a million US women gave birth after a previous cesarean section delivery, representing more than 1 in 8 US births. Most of these women would have been eligible for a trial of labor for vaginal birth after cesarean (VBAC) delivery with their next pregnancy; however, approximately half of US physicians and one-third of US hospitals no longer offer VBAC. Thus, a substantial proportion of women desiring a hospital VBAC are unable to access one and are faced with the choice of either a repeat cesarean delivery or a home VBAC. That some women are choosing home VBAC is evident from the data presented in this article.

Home births are rare, representing only 0.67% of total US births. However, among VBACs, the percentage of home births is more than 3 times higher; 2.3% of all VBACs in the United States occurred at home in 2008, up from 0.7% in 1999. Also the percentage of home births that were VBACs increased over time from less than 1% to almost 4% in 2008, while the number of hospital VBACs steadily declined. Women opting for home VBACs were predominately non-Hispanic white (91%), married (96%), and 30 years or older (68%). Of concern is the fact that only 27% of home VBACs were attended by a certified nurse midwife or certified midwife. There were not enough cases in the current study for analysis of neonatal morbidity and mortality for home VBACs. As the authors state, additional research on outcomes in relation to home and hospital-based VBACs and repeat cesarean deliveries would help further inform women and health care providers about childbirth options after cesarean delivery.

**L. A. Papile, MD**

---

**Changes in labor patterns over 50 years**

Laughon SK, Branch DW, Beaver J, et al (*Eunice Kennedy Shriver* Natl Inst of Child Health and Human Development, Bethesda, MD; Univ of Utah, Salt Lake City; et al)

*Am J Obstet Gynecol* 206:419.e1-419.e9, 2012

---

*Objective.*—The objective of the study was to examine differences in labor patterns in a modern cohort compared with the 1960s in the United States.

*Study Design.*—Data from pregnancies at term, in spontaneous labor, with cephalic, singleton fetuses were compared between the Collaborative Perinatal Project (CPP, n = 39,491 delivering 1959-1966) and the Consortium on Safe Labor (CSL; n = 98,359 delivering 2002-2008).

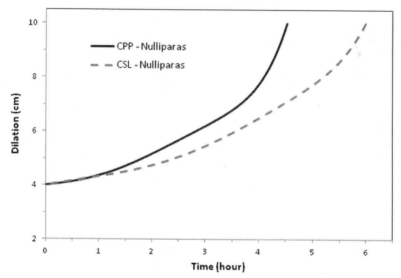

FIGURE 1.—Average labor curves for nulliparas (P0). Average labor curves for women by study with singleton term pregnancies presenting in spontaneous labor with vaginal delivery for nulliparas (P0). Curves were evaluated at the average values of the combined population for maternal age, maternal race, BMI at delivery, spontaneous rupture of membranes, gestational age, and birthweight. The CPP was conducted from 1959 to 1966; the CSL was conducted from 2002 to 2008. *BMI*, body mass index; *CSL*, Consortium on Safe Labor; *CPP*, Collaborative Perinatal Project. (Reprinted from American Journal of Obstetrics and Gynecology, Laughon SK, Branch DW, Beaver J, et al. Changes in labor patterns over 50 years. *Am J Obstet Gynecol.* 2012;206:419.e1-419.e9. Copyright 2012, with permission from Elsevier.)

*Results.*—Compared with the CPP, women in the CSL were older (26.8 ± 6.0 vs 24.1 ± 6.0 years), heavier (body mass index 29.9 ± 5.0 vs 26.3 ± 4.1 kg/m²), had higher epidural (55% vs 4%) and oxytocin use (31% vs 12%), and cesarean delivery (12% vs 3%). First stage of labor in the CSL was longer by a median of 2.6 hours in nulliparas and 2.0 hours in multiparas, even after adjusting for maternal and pregnancy characteristics, suggesting that the prolonged labor is mostly due to changes in practice patterns.

*Conclusion.*—Labor is longer in the modern obstetrical cohort. The benefit of extensive interventions needs further evaluation (Figs 1 and 2).

▶ It comes as no surprise, nor is it a revelation, that dramatic changes have occurred in labor patterns. However, it is still interesting to note these changes and to realize what accounts for such change. Understandable over the period of half a century, both maternal characteristics and obstetric practice have changed. We learn that among other things, women are older and heavier (higher body mass index [BMI]). Pharmacologic stimulation of uterine contractions is now commonplace (oxytocin) and alleviation of pain (epidural anesthesia) is used liberally. All of these factors alter the labor curves (Figs 1 and 2). The rate of vaginal operative deliveries has decreased, whereas cesarean sections have increased at an exponential rate from 10% of nulliparous women 50 years ago

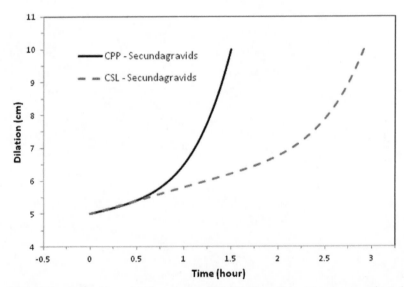

FIGURE 2.—Average labor curves for secundagravidas (P1). Average labor curves for women by study with singleton term pregnancies presenting in spontaneous labor with vaginal delivery for secundagravidas (P1). Curves were evaluated at the average values of the combined population for maternal age, maternal race, BMI at delivery, spontaneous rupture of membranes, gestational age, and birthweight. The CPP was conducted from 1959 to 1966; the CSL was conducted from 2002 to 2008. *BMI*, body mass index; *CSL*, Consortium on Safe Labor; *CPP*, Collaborative Perinatal Project. (Reprinted from American Journal of Obstetrics and Gynecology, Laughon SK, Branch DW, Beaver J, et al. Changes in labor patterns over 50 years. *Am J Obstet Gynecol.* 2012;206:419.e1-419.e9. Copyright 2012, with permission from Elsevier.)

to 66% in the modern era. The cesarean section rate was 4-fold higher, regardless of parity. The babies too are bigger but in better condition at birth as judged by fewer infants with Apgar scores less than 7 at 5 minutes.

Despite the obvious flaws inherent in 2 cohorts separated by such a long time period, apples were compared with apples, that is, the cohorts included women who presented in spontaneous labor, and neonatal outcomes may reflect improved neonatal care rather than changes in obstetric practice. There can be no doubt that labor takes longer, and with that costs are higher—again, no surprise.

Joesch et al[1] reported changes regarding cesarean sections. From 1979 to 2004, primary cesareans before labor contributed less to total cesareans than primary cesareans during labor and repeat cesareans without labor. Since 1998, primary prelabor cesareans have increased less than previously reported. This cannot be explained by changes in the frequency of pregnancy complications, women's age, insurance, or delivery hospital characteristics but may reflect changes in delivery practices regarding pregnancy complications. Another more recent change is the reluctance to offer a vaginal birth after a cesarean section (VBAC). Grobman et al[2] reported that from 1999 to 2002, the VBAC rate underwent a steady decline: 51.8% to 45.1% to 37.4% to 29.8% ($P < .001$). There is great fear concerning uterine rupture, and women are reluctant to undergo a trial of labor after cesarean section, electing for a repeat section.

So with a different pattern of labor, prolonged latent phase, and the increased use of epidural anesthesia, which slows labor, the neonatal team will have to be more patient until they get their call to action.

**A. A. Fanaroff, MBBCh, FRCPE**

*References*

1. Joesch JM, Gossman GL, Tanfer K. Primary cesarean deliveries prior to labor in the United States, 1979–2004. *Matern Child Health J*. 2008;12:323-331.
2. Grobman WA, Lai Y, Landon MB, et al. Eunice Kennedy Shriver National Institute of Child Health and Human Development Maternal-Fetal Medicine Units Network. The change in the rate of vaginal birth after caesarean section. *Paediatr Perinat Epidemiol*. 2011;25:37-43.

# 5 Infectious Disease and Immunology

**Estimating the Probability of Neonatal Early-Onset Infection on the Basis of Maternal Risk Factors**

Puopolo KM, Draper D, Wi S, et al (Brigham and Women's Hosp, Boston, MA; Univ of California, Santa Cruz; Kaiser Permanente Med Care Program, Oakland, CA; et al)

*Pediatrics* 128:e1155-e1163, 2011

*Objective.*—To develop a quantitative model to estimate the probability of neonatal early-onset bacterial infection on the basis of maternal intrapartum risk factors.

*Methods.*—This was a nested case-control study of infants born at ≥34 weeks' gestation at 14 California and Massachusetts hospitals from 1993 to 2007. Case-subjects had culture-confirmed bacterial infection at <72 hours; controls were randomly selected, frequency-matched 3:1 according to year and birth hospital. We performed multivariate analyses and split validation to define a predictive model based only on information available in the immediate perinatal period.

*Results.*—We identified 350 case-subjects from a cohort of 608 014 live births. Highest intrapartum maternal temperature revealed a linear relationship with risk of infection below 100.5°F, above which the risk rose rapidly. Duration of rupture of membranes revealed a steadily increasing relationship with infection risk. Increased risk was associated with both late-preterm and postterm delivery. Risk associated with maternal group B *Streptococcus* colonization is diminished in the era of group B *Streptococcus* prophylaxis. Any form of intrapartum antibiotic given > 4 hours before delivery was associated with decreased risk. Our model showed good discrimination and calibration ($c$ statistic = 0.800 and Hosmer-Lemeshow $P = .142$ in the entire data set).

*Conclusions.*—A predictive model based on information available in the immediate perinatal period performs better than algorithms based on risk-factor threshold values. This model establishes a prior probability for newborn sepsis, which could be combined with neonatal physical examination and laboratory values to establish a posterior probability to guide treatment decisions (Table 7).

▶ Because almost any sign of illness in a neonate can be an indication of neonatal sepsis, early-onset sepsis is the most common admitting diagnosis for our patients,

TABLE 7.—Comparison of Threshold Probability Approach to Individual Predictor Cutoffs When Applied to the Entire Newborn Population

| Risk Factor | Prevalence, % | Infected Infants Identified, % |
|---|---|---|
| Highest intrapartum temperature > 100.4°F | 4.73 | 30.0 |
| Highest intrapartum temperature > 101.4°F | 0.76 | 16.7 |
| ROM time ≥ 18 h | 8.66 | 23.1 |
| ROM time ≥ 24 h | 4.33 | 14.3 |
| Highest intrapartum temperature > 100.4°F and/or ROM ≥ 18 h and/or Broad-spectrum antibiotics and/or GBS prophylaxis-specific antibiotics < 4 h | 16.56 | 46.6 |
| Non-GBS intrapartum antibiotics or GBS prophylaxis-specific antibiotics < 4 h | 8.40 | 24.9 |
| Posterior rate per 1000 live births | | |
| Posterior rate ≥ 0.4 | 9.1 | 50.6 |
| Posterior rate ≥ 0.5 | 6.1 | 44.9 |
| Posterior rate ≥ 0.6 | 4.2 | 39.4 |
| Posterior rate ≥ 1.0 | 1.8 | 24.3 |
| Posterior rate ≥ 1.5 | 0.9 | 18.0 |

appearing in almost every initial differential diagnosis. Potential severe·consequences of untreated infection compel empiric initiation of antibiotic treatment in many babies, but sepsis is confirmed in only a small minority of treated infants. To reduce unnecessary exposure to antibiotics, a great deal of effort has gone into the search for better diagnostic tests for ascertainment of infection (or absence of infection), but a pathognomonic marker remains elusive. This report takes an alternative approach to the problem by attempting to use available clinical information to quantitatively estimate the probability of sepsis in individual babies. The resulting logistic regression model has a receiver operating characteristic $c$ statistic (area under the curve) of 0.80, which would generally be considered to fall at the border between fair and good as a measure of diagnostic performance. Despite performing better than individual predictors of risk (Table 7), the model appears to be somewhat insensitive, identifying only half of the infected infants at a cutoff value of a predicted (posterior) rate of 0.4 cases per 1000 births. The consequent low negative predictive value severely limits application of the model for exclusion of infants who do not need treatment. Treatment of all infants with a predicted risk in excess of 0.4 per 1000 would result in treatment of 310 infants for every one subsequently proven infected, reflecting a low positive predictive value. The current use of the model therefore appears to be confirmation of very low or very high predicted risks, with considerable uncertainty for cases at intermediate risk (ie, those for which clinical choices are not obvious). These limitations notwithstanding, the concept is sound, and this work provides an important proof of principle for this diagnostic methodology.

While this model is a significant step toward rationalizing the use of clinical data to guide therapeutic decisions, it is not sufficiently robust for immediate integration into routine practice. The authors' vision of integration of such models into the electronic medical record is nonetheless very attractive. As predictive models are refined, we should begin to insist on inclusion of complete descriptions of the regression equations and coefficients (with confidence intervals) in published reports to enable fulfillment of that vision.

W. E. Benitz, MD

## The Burden of Invasive Early-onset Neonatal Sepsis in the United States, 2005–2008

Weston EJ, Pondo T, Lewis MM, et al (Ctrs for Disease Control and Prevention, Atlanta, GA; et al)
*Pediatr Infect Dis J* 30:937-941, 2011

*Background.*—Sepsis in the first 3 days of life is a leading cause of morbidity and mortality among infants. Group B *Streptococcus* (GBS), historically the primary cause of early-onset sepsis (EOS), has declined through widespread use of intrapartum chemoprophylaxis. We estimated the national burden of invasive EOS cases and deaths in the era of GBS prevention.

*Methods.*—Population-based surveillance for invasive EOS was conducted in 4 of the Centers for Disease Control and Prevention's Active Bacterial Core surveillance sites from 2005 to 2008. We calculated incidence using state and national live birth files. Estimates of the national number of cases and deaths were calculated, standardizing by race and gestational age.

*Results.*—Active Bacterial Core surveillance identified 658 cases of EOS; 72 (10.9%) were fatal. Overall incidence remained stable during the 3 years (2005: 0.77 cases/1000 live births; 2008: 0.76 cases/1000 live births). GBS (~38%) was the most commonly reported pathogen followed by *Escherichia coli* (~24%). Black preterm infants had the highest incidence (5.14 cases/1000 live births) and case fatality (24.4%). Nonblack term infants had the lowest incidence (0.40 cases/1000 live births) and case fatality (1.6%). The estimated national annual burden of EOS was approximately 3320 cases (95% confidence interval [CI]: 3060–3580), including 390 deaths (95% CI: 300–490). Among preterm infants, 1570 cases (95% CI: 1400–1770; 47.3% of the overall) and 360 deaths (95% CI: 280–460; 92.3% of the overall) occurred annually.

*Conclusions.*—The burden of invasive EOS remains substantial in the era of GBS prevention and disproportionately affects preterm and black infants. Identification of strategies to prevent preterm births is needed to reduce the neonatal sepsis burden.

▶ The incidence and microbiology of neonatal early-onset sepsis (EOS) has changed with the evolution of obstetrical practices, including the widespread implementation of intrapartum antibiotic prophylaxis to prevent EOS caused by group B streptococcus (GBS). This article provides contemporary data on the epidemiology of EOS in the United States, using the Centers for Disease Control and Prevention active population-based surveillance from 2005 to 2008. The overall incidence of EOS during this period was 0.77 cases per

1000 live births. GBS remained the single most common microbial cause of EOS, accounting for 38% of all EOS. However, *Escherichia coli* had a higher case to fatality ratio than GBS, and two-thirds of *E coli* isolates tested were resistant to ampicillin. Significant race and gestational age disparities were noted: EOS incidence among black infants was approximately twice that of white infants, and among infants born at less than 37 weeks gestation, EOS incidence was approximately 4 times that reported for those born at 37 or more weeks. Disparities were also evident in EOS-attributable mortality; nearly 50% of EOS cases and 92% of sepsis-attributable deaths occurred among those born at less than 37 weeks' gestation, with mortality rates ranging from 1.6% among white term infants compared to 24% among black preterm infants. This information can assist the neonatal clinician in the development of EOS assessment and treatment strategies appropriate for their local care settings.

**K. Puopolo, MD**

---

**Cytokine screening identifies NICU patients with Gram-negative bacteremia**
Raynor LL, Saucerman JJ, Akinola MO, et al (Univ of Virginia School of Medicine, Charlottesville; Wake Forest Univ School of Medicine, Winston-Salem, NC)
*Pediatr Res* 71:261-266, 2012

---

*Introduction.*—Biomarkers and physiomarkers may be useful adjunct tests for sepsis detection in neonatal intensive care unit (NICU) patients. We studied whether measuring plasma cytokines at the time of suspected sepsis could identify patients with bacteremia in centers in which patients were undergoing continuous physiomarker screening using a heart rate characteristics (HRC) index monitor.

*Results.*—Six cytokines were higher in Gram-negative bacteremia (GNB) than in Gram-positive bacteremia or candidemia (GPBC). A cytokine score using thresholds for granulocyte colony—stimulating factor (G-CSF), interleukin (IL)-6, IL-8, and tumor necrosis factor (TNF)-$\alpha$ had 100% sensitivity and 69% positive predictive value (PPV) for GNB. A single cytokine marker, IL-6 <130 pg/ml, had 100% sensitivity and 52% PPV for sepsis ruled out (SRO). The average HRC index was abnormal in this cohort of patients with clinical suspicion of sepsis and did not discriminate between the final sepsis designations.

*Discussion.*—In summary, in NICU patients with suspected late-onset sepsis, plasma cytokines can identify those with SRO and those with GNB, potentially aiding in decisions regarding therapy.

*Methods.*—Seven cytokines were measured in 226 plasma samples from patients >3 d old with sepsis suspected based on clinical signs, abnormal HRC index, or both. Cases were classified as SRO, clinical sepsis (CS), GPBC, or GNB.

▶ Over the years, a number of sepsis screens have evolved. Their prevalence reflects the fact that none of them are effective enough to suit our needs. They are, as a whole, quite inadequate. Yet the morbidity and mortality of the very low-birth-weight (VLBW) infant in the neonatal intensive care unit remains a significant problem in terms of the cost of care of these infants and the burden eventually born by them and their families. The most appropriate antibiotics need to be used in the timeliest fashion, especially for those infants with the most virulent organisms—the Gram-negative bacteria—or the loss of life and future potential will be substantial. However, overtreatment of neonates who are merely "acting up" and not really septic leads to all the problems of antibiotic resistance and superinfection with yeast and other organisms.

Raynor and colleagues are attempting to address the needs of the neonatologist by developing a more effective screen for cytokines that will rise earlier in the onset of sepsis, possibly allowing nontreatment of some infants and more specific treatment of others. They have had some success. Gram-negative sepsis can be predicted with 100% sensitivity and 69% positive predictive value with just 4 of the 7 cytokines tested. In addition, culture-negative infants in this group were all seriously ill and also in need of effective antibiotics. Unfortunately, although the Sepsis Rule Out group was statistically different, it was not a clinically significant difference. Neither did the heart rate characteristics index monitor prove to be of usefulness, nor could the infants with clinical sepsis or Gram-positive bacteremia or candidemia be differentiated.

In short, the measurement of 4 cytokines may benefit clinicians, allowing more rapid identification of Gram-negative infection and more prompt initiation of treatment. However, these results need to be verified in repeat studies with larger numbers in other institutions, the tests need to be widely available in hospitals at a reasonable cost using a small amount of blood, and they need to have a quick turnaround time to be valuable. Let us hope there is some light on the horizon for caregivers of the VLBW infant.

**J. E. Baley, MD**

---

**Mortality Reduction by Heart Rate Characteristic Monitoring in Very Low Birth Weight Neonates: A Randomized Trial**

Moorman JR, Carlo WA, Kattwinkel J, et al (Univ of Virginia, Charlottesville; Univ of Alabama at Birmingham, et al)
*J Pediatr* 159:900-906, 2011

*Objective.*—To test the hypothesis that heart rate characteristics (HRC) monitoring improves neonatal outcomes.

*Study Design.*—We conducted a two-group, parallel, individually randomized controlled clinical trial of 3003 very low birth weight infants in 9 neonatal intensive care units. In one group, HRC monitoring was displayed; in the other, it was masked. The primary outcome was number of days alive and ventilator-free in the 120 days after randomization. Secondary outcomes were mortality, number of ventilator days, neonatal intensive care unit stay, and antibiotic use.

*Results.*—The mortality rate was reduced in infants whose HRC monitoring was displayed, from 10.2% to 8.1% (hazard ratio, 0.78; 95% CI,

0.61-0.99; $P = .04$; number needed to monitor $= 48$), and there was a trend toward increased days alive and ventilator-free (95.9 of 120 days compared with 93.6 in control subjects, $P = .08$). The mortality benefit was concentrated in infants with a birth weight <1000 g (hazard ratio, 0.74; 95% CI, 0.57-0.95; $P = .02$; number needed to monitor $= 23$). There were no significant differences in the other outcomes.

*Conclusion.*—HRC monitoring can reduce the mortality rate in very low birth weight infants.

▶ Early diagnostic tests for neonatal sepsis were based on the hematological response to bacterial infection. Because of their low sensitivity and specificity, particularly early in the course of the illness, more recent efforts have attempted to extract diagnostic information from measurements of the immune response, including circulating levels of cytokines (eg, interleukin [IL]-6, IL-8) and related factors (eg, C-reactive protein). Serum concentrations of these mediators do not lend themselves easily to continuous measurement, so they have been used as snapshots in time. The authors have developed another approach to using biological responses to infection: monitoring heart rate as an indicator of autonomic nervous system integration of internal responses to evolving infection. Their previous studies have demonstrated 2 important advantages: heart rate characteristic (HRC) changes can be identified before other diagnostic markers have changed, and they can be continuously monitored. In this randomized trial involving more than 3000 very low birth weight babies, they demonstrate a statistically significant and clinically substantial reduction in mortality rates associated with use of this monitoring. This benefit was limited to extremely low birth weight infants (birth weight < 1000 g), for whom the hazard ratio for mortality was 0.74 in the monitored group relative to the unmonitored group. The raw mortality rate was reduced from 17.6% to 13.2%. Such an impact for a therapy would likely result in a rush to universal adoption. So why shouldn't HRC be mandatory now? These observations should be confirmed before we all rush to adoption. We also need an understanding of why benefit is not evident in larger infants, who presumably have more mature autonomic nervous system function and might be expected to produce more informative signals. Perhaps a different analytical algorithm will be needed for signal detection in larger or more mature infants. Nonetheless, this is a very significant result, strongly suggesting that integration of internal biological signals by the baby's own nervous system—if skillfully interrogated—can provide diagnostic information that is timely and valuable. We should look forward to continued maturation of this technology and its incorporation into routine practice.

**W. E. Benitz, MD**

## Fluconazole Prophylaxis in Extremely Low Birth Weight Infants and Neurodevelopmental Outcomes and Quality of Life at 8 to 10 Years of Age

Kaufman DA, Cuff AL, Wamstad JB, et al (Univ of Virginia School of Medicine, Charlottesville; et al)
*J Pediatr* 158:759-765, 2011

*Objective.*—To examine the long-term effects of fluconazole prophylaxis in extremely low birth weight infants.

*Study Design.*—Neurodevelopmental status and quality of life of survivors from a randomized, placebo-controlled trial of fluconazole prophylaxis were evaluated at 8 to 10 years of life using the Vineland Adaptive Behavior Scales-II (VABS-II) and the Child Health Questionnaire Parent-Completed Form 28 (CHQ-PF28), respectively.

*Results.*—VABS-II Domain Scores for the fluconazole-treated (n = 21; 9.1 ± 0.7 years) compared with the placebo group (n = 17; 9.3 ± 0.8 years) were similar for communication [94.6 (± 14.8) versus 92.6 (± 12.6), $P = .65$], daily living skills [87.9 (± 10.6) versus 87.4 (± 9.3), $P = .89$], socialization [97.2 (± 9.2) versus 94.4 (± 7.9), $P = .31$], and motor skills [92.1 (± 17.8) versus 95.1 (± 14.6), $P = .57$]. Internalizing and externalizing behaviors and maladaptive behavior index were also similar. The CHQ-PF28 revealed no differences between the two groups regarding quality of life. Survivors were also happy or satisfied with school (90% versus 100%, $P = .49$), friendships (90% versus 88%, $P = 1.00$), and life (95% versus 100%, $P = 1.00$). Self esteem scores were 87.3 ± 15.7 versus 89.7 ± 10.4 ($P = .59$). There were also no differences between groups regarding emotional difficulties or behavior problems.

*Conclusions.*—Fluconazole prophylaxis for the prevention of invasive Candida infections is safe in extremely low birth weight infants and does not appear to be associated with any long-term adverse effects on neurodevelopment and quality of life at 8 to 10 years of life.

▶ Multiple trials have demonstrated that neonatal invasive fungal infection can be prevented by the prophylactic administration of fluconazole to extremely low birth weight infants. Widespread adoption of this practice has been limited by poor pharmacokinetic data and a lack of long-term safety data. In this article, the authors report on neurodevelopmental, behavioral, and health outcomes of infants enrolled in their previously published trial of fluconazole prophylaxis. The original trial enrolled 100 infants with birth weight less than 1000 g, which was conducted from 1998 to 2000.[1] Eighty-six infants survived to neonatal intensive care unit discharge, and this article reports on outcomes of 38 of the 86, at 8 to 10 years of age. No significant differences were found in neurodevelopmental and adaptive behaviors, quality of life, growth, or liver function between fluconazole-treated and placebo-treated patients. The study was limited by sample size, although the authors demonstrate that the neonatal characteristics of the evaluated and nonevaluated survivors were similar. This article presents the first evidence for long-term safety of neonatal fluconazole prophylaxis and may thus offer some reassurance to neonatal providers considering use of this preventative measure.

**K. Puopolo, MD, PhD**

*Reference*

1. Kaufman D, Boyle R, Hazen KC, Patrie JT, Robinson M, Donowitz LG. Fluconazole prophylaxis against fungal colonization and infection in preterm infants. *N Engl J Med.* 2001;345:1660-1666.

---

**Ohio Statewide Quality-Improvement Collaborative to Reduce Late-Onset Sepsis in Preterm Infants**
Kaplan HC, for the Ohio Perinatal Quality Collaborative (Cincinnati Children's Hosp Med Ctr, OH)
*Pediatrics* 127:427-435, 2011

---

*Objective.*—We aimed to reduce late-onset bacterial infections in infants born at 22 to 29 weeks' gestation by using collaborative quality-improvement methods to implement evidence-based catheter care. We hypothesized that these methods would result in a 50% reduction in nosocomial infection.

*Patients and Methods.*—We conducted an interrupted time-series study among 24 Ohio NICUs. The intervention began in September 2008 and continued through December 2009. Sites used the Institute for Healthcare Improvement Breakthrough Series quality-improvement model to facilitate implementation of evidence-based catheter care. Data were collected monthly for all catheter insertions and for at least 10 observations of indwelling catheter care. NICUs also submitted monthly data on catheter-days, patient-days, and episodes of infection. Data were analyzed by using statistical process control methods.

*Results.*—During the intervention, NICUs submitted information on 1916 infants. Of the 242 infections reported, 69% were catheter associated. Compliance with catheter-insertion components was > 90% by April 2009. Compliance with components of evidence-based indwelling catheter care reached 80.4% by December 2009. There was a significant reduction in the proportion of infants with at least 1 late-onset infection from a baseline of 18.2% to 14.3%.

*Conclusions.*—There was a 20% reduction in the incidence of late-onset infection after the intervention, but the magnitude was less than hypothesized, perhaps because compliance with components of evidence-based care of indwelling catheters remained < 90%. Because nearly one-third of infections were not catheter associated, improvement may require attention to other aspects of care such as skin integrity and nutrition.

▶ The adoption of interventions with demonstrated efficacy in low-bias study designs such as randomized trials has often been slow in medicine. In the past decade, the tools of quality improvement have increasingly been used to speed dissemination and address quality gaps at the local level. This article is an important milestone in that process for several reasons. First, it shows the successful application of these techniques to a problem—late-onset bacterial infections—which for many years was thought to be a refractory and necessary part of intensive care medicine. In 2012, there are now many examples at the local level of prolonged eradication of central line infections in neonatal intensive care units (NICUs). In contrast to local efforts, however, these authors apply the approach on a grand scale, in 24 NICUs in a statewide quality improvement collaborative. In addition to successfully lowering the late-onset bacterial infection rate by 20%, they thus show the feasibility of quality-improvement efforts at the population level, a trend that has now been adopted in more than 10 states in the United States. Even at this large scale, they adhere to a rigorous study design and apply some of the more sophisticated techniques of improvement science to confirm that the observed signal is valid.

**J. Zupancic, MD**

## Prolonged Initial Empirical Antibiotic Treatment is Associated with Adverse Outcomes in Premature Infants

Kuppala VS, Meinzen-Derr J, Morrow AL, et al (Cincinnati Children's Hosp Med Ctr, OH)
*J Pediatr* 159:720-725, 2011

*Objective.*—To investigate the outcomes after prolonged empirical antibiotic administration to premature infants in the first week of life, and concluding subsequent late onset sepsis (LOS), necrotizing enterocolitis (NEC), and death.

*Study Design.*—Study infants were ≤32 weeks gestational age and ≤1500 g birth weight who survived free of sepsis and NEC for 7 days. Multivariable logistic regression was conducted to determine independent relationships between prolonged initial empirical antibiotic therapy (≥5 days) and study outcomes that control for birth weight, gestational age, race, prolonged premature rupture of membranes, days on high-frequency ventilation in 7 days, and the amount of breast milk received in the first 14 days of life.

*Results.*—Of the 365 premature infants who survived 7 days free of sepsis or NEC, 36% received prolonged initial empirical antibiotics, which was independently associated with subsequent outcomes: LOS (OR, 2.45 [95% CI, 1.28-4.67]) and the combination of LOS, NEC, or death (OR, 2.66 [95% CI, 1.12-6.3]).

*Conclusions.*—Prolonged administration of empirical antibiotics to premature infants with sterile cultures in the first week of life is associated with subsequent severe outcomes. Judicious restriction of antibiotic use should be investigated as a strategy to reduce severe outcomes for premature infants.

▶ This important article provides another reminder that even treatments that seem innocuous may come at a price. These authors establish that postnatal exposure to antibiotics, especially if prolonged for 5 days or more, is associated with increased rates of late-onset sepsis, necrotizing enterocolitis (NEC), and death. Although this retrospective analysis cannot prove that these relationships are causal, they are robust to adjustment for several variables known to be predictive of these outcomes and which may be surrogates for severity of illness (birth weight, gestational age, 5-minute Apgar < 5, race, prolonged premature rupture of membranes, number of days on mechanical or high-frequency ventilation in first week of life, amount of breast milk received in first 14 days of life). A similar association between duration of antibiotics, including an apparent dose-response relationship showing increasing risk of NEC with increasing duration of initial antibiotic exposure, has been reported by others.[1] These observations should be sufficiently worrisome to compel assiduous consideration to the necessity for both initiation and continuation of antibiotics in very low-birth-weight infants. We need better tools for assessment of the likelihood of early-onset sepsis, and we need to become more comfortable relying on the negative predictive value of negative cultures and normal levels of acute-phase reactants, so that empiric antibiotics can at least be stopped as early as possible. Until prospective trials, as suggested by these authors, demonstrate that judicious restriction of early antibiotic treatment does not reduce the risk of late-onset sepsis, NEC, and death for premature infants, it is no longer acceptable to believe that extended antibiotic treatment courses are acceptable, because uncertainty about the possibility of infection outweighs the negligible risk of a few extra days of treatment.

**W. E. Benitz, MD**

*Reference*

1. Alexander VN, Northrup V, Bizzarro MJ. Antibiotic exposure in the newborn intensive care unit and the risk of necrotizing enterocolitis. *J Pediatr.* 2011;159: 392-397.

---

**Relationship Between Maternal and Neonatal *Staphylococcus aureus* Colonization**

Jimenez-Truque N, Tedeschi S, Saye EJ, et al (Vanderbilt Univ Med Ctr, Nashville, TN; Brigham and Women's Hosp, Boston, MA; et al)
*Pediatrics* 129:e1252-e1259, 2012

---

*Objective.*—The study aimed to assess whether maternal colonization with *Staphylococcus aureus* during pregnancy or at delivery was associated with infant staphylococcal colonization.

*Methods.*—For this prospective cohort study, women were enrolled at 34 to 37 weeks of gestation between 2007 and 2009. Nasal and vaginal swabs for culture were obtained at enrollment; nasal swabs were obtained from women and their infants at delivery and 2- and 4-month postbirth visits. Logistic regression was used to determine whether maternal colonization affected infant colonization.

*Results.*—Overall, 476 and 471 mother-infant dyads had complete data for analysis at enrollment and delivery, respectively. Maternal methicillin-resistant *S aureus* (MRSA) colonization occurred in 10% to 17% of mothers, with the highest prevalence at enrollment. Infant MRSA colonization peaked at 2 months of age, with 20.9% of infants colonized. Maternal staphylococcal colonization at enrollment increased the odds of infant staphylococcal colonization at birth (odds ratio; 95% confidence interval: 4.8; 2.4—9.5), hospital discharge (2.6; 1.3—5.0), at 2 months of life (2.7; 1.6—4.3), and at 4 months of life (2.0; 1.1—3.5). Similar results were observed for maternal staphylococcal colonization at delivery. Fifty maternal-infant dyads had concurrent MRSA colonization: 76% shared isolates of the same pulsed-field type, and 30% shared USA300 isolates. Only 2 infants developed staphylococcal disease.

*Conclusions.*—*S aureus* colonization (including MRSA) was extremely common in this cohort of maternal-infant pairs. Infants born to mothers with staphylococcal colonization were more likely to be colonized, and early postnatal acquisition appeared to be the primary mechanism.

▶ Methicillin-sensitive and methicillin-resistant *Staphylococcus aureus* (MSSA and MRSA) infections emerged in the past decade as significant causes of soft-tissue and invasive infections among neonates and infants in the United States. Little is known about the relative contribution of mother—infant vertical, mother—infant horizontal, and community—infant horizontal transmission of *Staphylococcal* colonization. This article reports the results of a prospective study of maternal, neonatal, and infant MSSA and MRSA colonization in 2 obstetrical care settings in Tennessee. Using careful microbiologic enrichment techniques to isolate MSSA and MRSA, 471 mother—infant dyads were assessed for colonization at 34 to 36 weeks' gestation; at delivery; and at 2 and 4 months of infant age. The study revealed that 38.6% of women were colonized with MSSA and 16.6% with MRSA at third trimester enrollment; 9.3% of neonates were colonized with MSSA and 2.5% with MRSA at birth. Infant colonization peaked at 2 months of age, with 38.9% colonized with MSSA and 20.9% with MRSA but only 2 noninvasive infections were diagnosed during the study period. Clinical correlation of colonization status and molecular analyses of concordant mother—infant pairs revealed that horizontal mother—infant transmission was the dominant source of infant colonization, although vertical transmission and non-maternal horizontal transmission were evident as well. The study is limited to one geographic area and may not represent the national community burden of *Staphylococcal* colonization. This article does, however, provide insight into the potentially high frequency of maternal *Staphylococcal* colonization, as well as to the complexity of infant transmission. This study provides important information that must be considered in the design of hospital nursery, neonatal intensive care unit—based and pediatric office—based *Staphylococcal* infection control programs.

**K. Puopolo, MD, PhD**

## Topical application of chlorhexidine to neonatal umbilical cords for prevention of omphalitis and neonatal mortality in a rural district of Pakistan: a community-based, cluster-randomised trial

Soofi S, Cousens S, Imdad A, et al (Aga Khan Univ, Karachi, Pakistan; et al)
*Lancet* 379:1029-1036, 2012

*Background.*—Umbilical cord infection (omphalitis) is a risk factor for neonatal sepsis and mortality in low-resource settings where home deliveries are common. We aimed to assess the effect of umbilical-cord cleansing with 4% chlorhexidine (CHX) solution, with or without handwashing with antiseptic soap, on the incidence of omphalitis and neonatal mortality.

*Methods.*—We did a two-by-two factorial, cluster-randomised trial in Dadu, a rural area of Sindh province, Pakistan. Clusters were defined as the population covered by a functional traditional birth attendant (TBA), and were randomly allocated to one of four groups (groups A to D) with a computer-generated random number sequence. Implementation and data collection teams were masked to allocation. Liveborn infants delivered by participating TBAs who received birth kits were eligible for enrolment in the study. One intervention comprised birth kits containing 4% CHX solution for application to the cord at birth by TBAs and once daily by family members for up to 14 days along with soap and educational messages promoting handwashing. One intervention was CHX solution only and another was handwashing only. Standard dry cord care was promoted in the control group. The primary outcomes were incidence of neonatal omphalitis and neonatal mortality. The trial is registered with ClinicalTrials.gov, number NCT00682006.

*Findings.*—187 clusters were randomly allocated to one of the four study groups. Of 9741 newborn babies delivered by participating TBAs, factorial analysis indicated a reduction in risk of omphalitis with CHX application (risk ratio [RR] = 0·58, 95% CI 0·41-0·82; $p = 0·002$) but no evidence of an effect of handwashing (RR = 0·83, 0·61−1·13; $p = 0·24$). We recorded strong evidence of a reduction in neonatal mortality in neonates who received CHX cleansing (RR = 0·62, 95% CI 0·45−0·85; $p = 0·003$) but no evidence of an effect of handwashing promotion on neonatal mortality (RR = 1·08, 0·79-1·48; $p = 0·62$). We recorded no serious adverse events.

*Interpretation.*—Application of 4% CHX to the umbilical cord was effective in reducing the risk of omphalitis and neonatal mortality in rural Pakistan. Provision of CHX in birth kits might be a useful strategy for the prevention of neonatal mortality in high-mortality settings (Fig 2).

▶ Current recommendations for cord care are chiefly based on research in hospital nurseries in developed countries. In developing countries, preventable infections, including omphalitis and neonatal tetanus, contribute significantly to high neonatal mortality rates. Prevention necessitates global education, clean cord care, and avoidance of harmful practices, such as cutting the cord with dirty blades/scissors or placing foreign substances such as dung on the cord, and by increasing tetanus toxoid immunization. Rooming with their mothers,

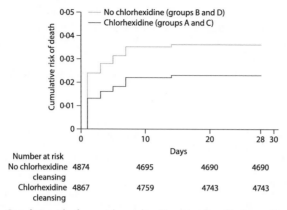

Number at risk

| | | | | |
|---|---|---|---|---|
| No chlorhexidine cleansing | 4874 | 4695 | 4690 | 4690 |
| Chlorhexidine cleansing | 4867 | 4759 | 4743 | 4743 |

FIGURE 2.—Cumulative risk of neonatal mortality. (Reprinted from The Lancet, Soofi S, Cousens S, Imdad A, et al. Topical application of chlorhexidine to neonatal umbilical cords for prevention of omphalitis and neonatal mortality in a rural district of Pakistan: a community-based, cluster-randomised trial. *Lancet.* 2012;379:1029-1036. Copyright © 2012, with permission from Elsevier.)

skin-to-skin contact, and early and frequent breast feeding may also reduce the risk of cord infection.

While there is general consensus that clean cord care decreases the risk of cord infection, the application of topical antimicrobials to the cord stump is more controversial. The World Health Organization recommends dry cord care for newborns,[1] but this recommendation may not be optimal in low-resource settings where most births take place in an unclean environment, and infections account for a high proportion of neonatal deaths. Each year, about one-third of the 3.3 million annual neonatal deaths occurring worldwide is attributed to infections. Approximately 500 000 infants die of neonatal tetanus and a further 460 000 die as a consequence of severe bacterial infection.[2] A substantial proportion of deaths from infection are due to cord infections.

Soofi et al demonstrate beyond reasonable doubt in a large cluster randomized trial that topical application of chlorhexidine reduces omphalitis and mortality in rural Pakistan (Fig 2). The treatment is simple and inexpensive and does not appear to interfere with local cultural practices. In fact, local practices of applying foreign substances to the cord continued. The study was effectively and efficiently carried out with the assistance of traditional birth attendants. As would be anticipated the next steps are to continue this practice on a broader scale. There is no reason to believe that it will not be effective because in a parallel community-based, cluster-randomized trial in Sylhet, Bangladesh, investigators[3] reported similar outcomes, eg, decreased mortality and infection from a very large cohort of 29 760 newborn babies (10 329, 9423, and 10 008 in the multiple-cleansing [with Chlorhexidine], single-cleansing, and dry cord care groups, respectively). Whereas they had no doubts that Chlorhexidine cleansing of a neonate's umbilical cord could be life saving, they remained uncertain of the optimum frequency with which to apply the chlorhexidine.

The inability to demonstrate the benefits of hand washing in the Soofi trial is both surprising and disappointing. The failure is attributed to the continued local practice of applying other traditional materials, such as surma, an eye cosmetic containing lead, to the cord at birth. This may lead to a local reaction, which serves as a substrate for bacterial growth and invasion.

Overall, it is encouraging to learn that keeping the cord clean not only reduces infection but mortality too.

**A. A. Fanaroff, MBBCh, FRCPE**

*References*

1. WHO Care of the Umbilical Cord-A review of the evidence. World Health Organization, 1999. https://www.apps.who.int/rht/documents/MSM98-4/MSM-98-4.htm#REFERENCES.
2. Lawn JE, Cousens S, Zupan J. 4 million neonatal deaths: when? Where? Why? *Lancet.* 2005;365:891-900.
3. Arifeen SE, Mullany LC, Shah R, et al. The effect of cord cleansing with chlorhexidine on neonatal mortality in rural Bangladesh: a community-based, cluster-randomised trial. *Lancet.* 2012;379:1022-1028.

---

## Treatment of Neonatal Sepsis with Intravenous Immune Globulin

The INIS Collaborative Group (Univ of Oxford, UK; et al)
*N Engl J Med* 365:1201-1211, 2011

---

*Background.*—Neonatal sepsis is a major cause of death and complications despite antibiotic treatment. Effective adjunctive treatments are needed. Newborn infants are relatively deficient in endogenous immunoglobulin. Meta-analyses of trials of intravenous immune globulin for suspected or proven neonatal sepsis suggest a reduced rate of death from any cause, but the trials have been small and have varied in quality.

*Methods.*—At 113 hospitals in nine countries, we enrolled 3493 infants receiving antibiotics for suspected or proven serious infection and randomly assigned them to receive two infusions of either polyvalent IgG immune globulin (at a dose of 500 mg per kilogram of body weight) or matching placebo 48 hours apart. The primary outcome was death or major disability at the age of 2 years.

*Results.*—There was no significant between-group difference in the rates of the primary outcome, which occurred in 686 of 1759 infants (39.0%) who received intravenous immune globulin and in 677 of 1734 infants (39.0%) who received placebo (relative risk, 1.00; 95% confidence interval, 0.92 to 1.08). Similarly, there were no significant differences in the rates of secondary outcomes, including the incidence of subsequent sepsis episodes. In follow-up of 2-year-old infants, there were no significant differences in the rates of major or nonmajor disability or of adverse events.

*Conclusions.*—Therapy with intravenous immune globulin had no effect on the outcomes of suspected or proven neonatal sepsis. (Funded by the United Kingdom Medical Research Council and others; INIS Current Controlled Trials number, ISRCTN94984750.)

▶ Quantitative deficiency of immunoglobulin and complement, combined with immaturity of neutrophil defenses, is thought to contribute to the susceptibility of neonates to invasive bacterial infection. Systematic reviews of prior studies of intravenous immunoglobulin (IVIG) to treat neonatal sepsis have provided conflicting results. This report describes the outcomes of the International Neonatal Immunotherapy Study (INIS), an international, multicenter, randomized, placebo-controlled trial of the adjuvant use of IVIG to treat suspected or proven bacterial infection among primarily very low birth weight infants. The study was designed for simplicity of entry and administration; infants were eligible for enrollment if receiving antibiotics for proven or suspected serious infection with at least 1 of the following characteristics: a birth weight less than 1500 g; culture-proven infection in blood, cerebrospinal fluid, or other usually sterile body fluid; or need for mechanical ventilation. Infants with prior IVIG treatment or severe congenital anomaly were excluded. Two doses of IVIG or placebo were administered at a dose of 500 mg/kg every 48 hours. A total of 3493 infants were enrolled, of whom approximately 40% had blood culture—proven infection. There were no differences found in the primary outcome of death or the presence of major disability at 2 years of age (observed in 39% of IVIG and placebo-treated infants) nor any difference observed in multiple other prespecified secondary outcomes. The straightforward design of the trial, which was conducted in a variety of different resource settings, as well as the survey-based determination of major disability, can be seen as both strengths and limitations of the study. The results clearly show that there is no evidence of benefit for the adjuvant administration of IVIG to treat suspected or proven bacterial infection among very low birth weight infants.

**K. Puopolo, MD, PhD**

## Treatment of Neonatal Sepsis with Intravenous Immune Globulin
The INIS Collaborative Group (Univ of Oxford, UK; et al)
*N Engl J Med* 365:1201-1211, 2011

*Background.*—Neonatal sepsis is a major cause of death and complications despite antibiotic treatment. Effective adjunctive treatments are needed. Newborn infants are relatively deficient in endogenous immunoglobulin. Meta-analyses of trials of intravenous immune globulin for suspected or proven neonatal sepsis suggest a reduced rate of death from any cause, but the trials have been small and have varied in quality.

*Methods.*—At 113 hospitals in nine countries, we enrolled 3493 infants receiving antibiotics for suspected or proven serious infection and randomly assigned them to receive two infusions of either polyvalent IgG immune globulin (at a dose of 500 mg per kilogram of body weight) or matching placebo 48 hours apart. The primary outcome was death or major disability at the age of 2 years.

*Results.*—There was no significant between-group difference in the rates of the primary outcome, which occurred in 686 of 1759 infants (39.0%) who received intravenous immune globulin and in 677 of 1734 infants (39.0%) who received placebo (relative risk, 1.00; 95% confidence interval, 0.92 to 1.08). Similarly, there were no significant differences in the rates of secondary outcomes, including the incidence of subsequent sepsis episodes. In follow-up of 2-year-old infants, there were no significant differences in the rates of major or nonmajor disability or of adverse events.

*Conclusions.*—Therapy with intravenous immune globulin had no effect on the outcomes of suspected or proven neonatal sepsis. (Funded by the United Kingdom Medical Research Council and others; INIS Current Controlled Trials number, ISRCTN94984750.)

▶ This international randomized controlled trial evaluated the effectiveness of intravenous immune globulin (IVIG) in reducing death or major disability at age 2 among infants on antibiotics for proven or suspected infection who met 1 of the following criteria: birth weight less than 1500 g; evidence of infection via blood culture, cerebrospinal fluid, or other bodily fluid; or need for respiratory support via an endotracheal tube. The infants were randomized to receive 2 doses of placebo or polyvalent immunoglobulin G IG at a dose of 500 mg/kg 48 hours apart. The study enrolled 3493 infants in 9 countries. Analyses detected no difference between study groups in the primary or any secondary outcome, including subsequent episodes of infection. Approximately one-quarter of the study population comprised infants who were born at or above 1500 g; however, there were no differences in results of analyses stratified by birth weight or other subgroups, such as gestational age, size for gestational age, sex, or presence or absence of chorioamnionitis. Although meta-analysis of prior studies[1] suggests preterm or low birth weight (LBW) infants treated with IVIG might see a modest (3% to 4%) reduction in infection rates, there has been no published evidence that LBW or a broader population of infants[2] derives additional short-term or long-term clinical benefits from IVIG prophylaxis. The addition of data from this current large and rigorously conducted study to the IVIG evidence base should soundly discourage routine neonatal IVIG prophylaxis.

**L. J. Van Marter, MD, MPH**

*References*

1. Ohlsson A, Lacey J. Intravenous immunoglobulin for preventing infection in preterm and/or low-birth-weight infants. *Cochrane Database Syst Rev.* 2004;(1): CD000361.
2. Ohlsson A, Lacey J. Intravenous immunoglobulin for suspected or subsequently proven infection in neonates. *Cochrane Database Syst Rev.* 2010;(3):CD001239.

---

**Treatment of Neonatal Sepsis with Intravenous Immune Globulin**
The INIS Collaborative Group (Univ of Oxford, UK; et al)
*N Engl J Med* 365:1201-1211, 2011

---

*Background.*—Neonatal sepsis is a major cause of death and complications despite antibiotic treatment. Effective adjunctive treatments are needed. Newborn infants are relatively deficient in endogenous immunoglobulin. Meta-analyses of trials of intravenous immune globulin for suspected or proven neonatal sepsis suggest a reduced rate of death from any cause, but the trials have been small and have varied in quality.

*Methods.*—At 113 hospitals in nine countries, we enrolled 3493 infants receiving antibiotics for suspected or proven serious infection and randomly assigned them to receive two infusions of either polyvalent IgG immune globulin (at a dose of 500 mg per kilogram of body weight) or matching placebo 48 hours apart. The primary outcome was death or major disability at the age of 2 years.

*Results.*—There was no significant between-group difference in the rates of the primary outcome, which occurred in 686 of 1759 infants (39.0%) who received intravenous immune globulin and in 677 of 1734 infants (39.0%) who received placebo (relative risk, 1.00; 95% confidence interval, 0.92 to 1.08). Similarly, there were no significant differences in the rates of secondary outcomes, including the incidence of subsequent sepsis episodes. In follow-up of 2-year-old infants, there were no significant differences in the rates of major or nonmajor disability or of adverse events.

*Conclusions.*—Therapy with intravenous immune globulin had no effect on the outcomes of suspected or proven neonatal sepsis. (Funded by the United Kingdom Medical Research Council and others; INIS Current Controlled Trials number, ISRCTN94984750.)

▶ The potential role of intravenous immunoglobulin for treatment or prevention of neonatal sepsis has been an enduring source of fascination since the 1980s. The rationale is compelling because low immunoglobulin levels in preterm infants correlate with increased rates of neonatal sepsis in general and lack of specific opsonizing antibody is a major risk factor for both early-onset and late-onset group B streptococcal sepsis. It stands to reason that correction of immunoglobulin deficiency should reduce rates of bacterial infection in this at-risk population. This large well-designed controlled trial marks the twentieth attempt to prove that. Previous trials have produced disappointing and some-times conflicting results, and this one continues in that vein. Lack of benefit or demonstration of only small benefits in prior trials has been attributed to failures of trial design or conduct, but such concerns do not seem to account for the complete lack of benefit from immunoglobulin demonstrated in this study. In addition to having no effect on the primary outcome of death or major disability at 2 years of age (relative risk [RR], 1.00; 95% confidence interval [CI], 0.92-1.08), immunoglobulin had no effect on death in hospital (RR, 1.00; 95% CI, 0.86-1.16), death by 2 years (RR, 1.04; 95% CI, 0.90-1.20), disability at 2 years (RR, 0.98; 95% CI, 0.86-1.10), or confirmed sepsis after trial entry (RR, 0.99; 95% CI, 0.89-1.11). There were no differences in rates of infection caused by coagulase-negative *Staphylococci*, other gram-positive organisms, gram-negative organisms, or fungi. Exogenous immunoglobulin does not seem to be an adequate replacement for maternal immunoglobulin acquired transpla-centally. Whether this results from specificity of a mother's antibody for bacteria that colonize her own infant or from concurrent functional maturation of the immune system will have to await further studies. In any case, it seems to be safe to abandon intravenous immunoglobulin as treatment or prophylaxis for neonatal sepsis.

**W. E. Benitz, MD**

---

**Oral Acyclovir Suppression and Neurodevelopment after Neonatal Herpes**
Kimberlin DW, for the National Institute of Allergy and Infectious Diseases Collaborative Antiviral Study Group (Univ of Alabama at Birmingham; et al)
*N Engl J Med* 365:1284-1292, 2011

---

*Background.*—Poor neurodevelopmental outcomes and recurrences of cutaneous lesions remain unacceptably frequent among survivors of neonatal herpes simplex virus (HSV) disease.

*Methods.*—We enrolled neonates with HSV disease in two parallel, identical, double-blind, placebo-controlled studies. Neonates with central nervous system (CNS) involvement were enrolled in one study, and neonates with skin, eye, and mouth involvement only were enrolled in the other. After completing a regimen of 14 to 21 days of parenteral acyclovir, the infants were randomly assigned to immediate acyclovir suppression (300 mg per square meter of body-surface area per dose orally, three times daily for 6 months) or placebo. Cutaneous recurrences were treated with open-label episodic therapy.

*Results.*—A total of 74 neonates were enrolled—45 with CNS involvement and 29 with skin, eye, and mouth disease. The Mental Development Index of the Bayley Scales of Infant Development (in which scores range from 50 to 150, with a mean of 100 and with higher scores indicating better neurodevelopmental outcomes) was assessed in 28 of the 45 infants with CNS involvement (62%) at 12 months of age. After adjustment for covariates, infants with CNS involvement who had been randomly assigned to acyclovir suppression had significantly higher mean Bayley mental-development scores at 12 months than did infants randomly assigned to placebo (88.24 vs. 68.12, $P = 0.046$). Overall, there was a trend toward more neutropenia in the acyclovir group than in the placebo group ($P = 0.09$).

*Conclusions.*—Infants surviving neonatal HSV disease with CNS involvement had improved neurodevelopmental outcomes when they received suppressive therapy with oral acyclovir for 6 months. (Funded by the National Institute of Allergy and Infectious Diseases; CASG 103 and CASG 104 ClinicalTrials.gov numbers, NCT00031460 and NCT00031447, respectively.)

▶ Neonatal herpes simplex virus (HSV) infection can present as skin, eye, and mouth, central nervous system, or disseminated disease. Nearly one-third of infants with disseminated disease die, and although the mortality rate is lower in central nervous system (CNS) disease, there is a high rate (approximately 70%) of neurological impairment following neonatal CNS HSV infection.[1] This article reports the results of parallel randomized clinical trials of acyclovir suppression therapy among 2 populations: the first comprising infants with skin, eye, and mouth disease (N = 29) and the other with CNS disease, plus or minus disseminated disease (N = 45). The infants were first treated with 2 to 3 weeks of acyclovir, then randomized to 6 months of acyclovir suppressive treatment. Among the 62% of infants with CNS disease who returned for follow-up, 6 months of acyclovir suppressive therapy resulted in improved neurodevelopmental outcomes. Assessments by Bayley Scales of Infant Development-II at age 12 months showed overall outcomes among the acyclovir suppression group: 69% were normal, 6% had mild impairment, 6% had moderate impairment, and 19% had severe impairment; among the control subjects the respective percentages were 33%, 8%, 25%, and 33%. The challenges of studies of such low prevalence disorders make this an especially valuable contribution to the evidence base guiding treatment of infants with HSV. I find the evidence encouraging in that at least early neurodevelopmental outcomes of neonatal CNS HSV infection can be improved by administration of 6 months of suppressive acyclovir therapy. These data make it imperative that we remain vigilant for HSV and, whenever it is among our differential diagnoses, that we perform a lumbar puncture to submit cerebrospinal fluid for HSV polymerase chain reaction and culture, in addition to bacterial culture and other routine studies.

**L. J. Van Marter, MD, MPH**

*Reference*

1. Kimberlin DW, Lin CY, Jacobs RF, et al. Safety and efficacy of high-dose intravenous acyclovir in the management of neonatal herpes simplex virus infections. *Pediatrics.* 2001;108:230-238.

## Oral Acyclovir Suppression and Neurodevelopment after Neonatal Herpes

Kimberlin DW, for the National Institute of Allergy and Infectious Diseases Collaborative Antiviral Study Group (Univ of Alabama at Birmingham; et al)
*N Engl J Med* 365:1284-1292, 2011

*Background.*—Poor neurodevelopmental outcomes and recurrences of cutaneous lesions remain unacceptably frequent among survivors of neonatal herpes simplex virus (HSV) disease.

*Methods.*—We enrolled neonates with HSV disease in two parallel, identical, double-blind, placebo-controlled studies. Neonates with central nervous system (CNS) involvement were enrolled in one study, and neonates with skin, eye, and mouth involvement only were enrolled in the other. After completing a regimen of 14 to 21 days of parenteral acyclovir, the infants were randomly assigned to immediate acyclovir suppression (300 mg per square meter of body-surface area per dose orally, three times daily for 6 months) or placebo. Cutaneous recurrences were treated with open-label episodic therapy.

*Results.*—A total of 74 neonates were enrolled — 45 with CNS involvement and 29 with skin, eye, and mouth disease. The Mental Development Index of the Bayley Scales of Infant Development (in which scores range from 50 to 150, with a mean of 100 and with higher scores indicating better neurodevelopmental outcomes) was assessed in 28 of the 45 infants with CNS involvement (62%) at 12 months of age. After adjustment for covariates, infants with CNS involvement who had been randomly assigned to acyclovir suppression had significantly higher mean Bayley mental-development scores at 12 months than did infants randomly assigned to placebo (88.24 vs. 68.12, $P = 0.046$). Overall, there was a trend toward more neutropenia in the acyclovir group than in the placebo group ($P = 0.09$).

*Conclusions.*—Infants surviving neonatal HSV disease with CNS involvement had improved neurodevelopmental outcomes when they received suppressive therapy with oral acyclovir for 6 months. (Funded by the National Institute of Allergy and Infectious Diseases; CASG 103 and CASG 104 ClinicalTrials.gov numbers, NCT00031460 and NCT00031447, respectively.)

▶ Therapeutic studies of a rare disease such as neonatal herpes simplex virus (HSV) present unique challenges. As in this study, it may take a decade or longer to enroll a sufficient number of subjects. In addition, clinicians may have been reluctant to refer eligible infants for this trial after the publication in 2005 of a small, uncontrolled study that suggested long-term oral acyclovir therapy is associated with improved neurodevelopmental outcome.[1]

It is disappointing that data for the primary endpoint are available for only 58% of enrolled infants and 62% of the subset of infants with central nervous system HSV disease. This substantial attrition tempers the interpretation of neurodevelopmental outcome among infants with central nervous system HSV who started oral acyclovir suppression at the end of intravenous therapy. Additionally, the data can only suggest that ongoing neurologic injury occurs in infants who survive neonatal central nervous system HSV disease and that it can be mitigated by long-term antiviral suppression.

Long-term oral acyclovir decreased the number of recurrences of cutaneous lesions among all infants with neonatal HSV disease by 36%. Because the recurrence of skin lesions necessitates an evaluation for central nervous system involvement, there may be a positive socioeconomic effect in the prevention of skin recurrences, such as the need for fewer medical evaluations.

**L. A. Papile, MD**

*Reference*

1. Tiffany KF, Benjamin DK Jr, Palasanthiran P, O'Donnell K, Gutman LT. Improved neurodevelopmental outcomes following long-term high-dose oral acyclovir therapy in infants with central nervous system and disseminated herpes simplex disease. *J Perinatol.* 2005;25:156-161.

## Long-term outcome in preterm children with human cytomegalovirus infection transmitted via breast milk

Bevot A, Hamprecht K, Krägeloh-Mann I, et al (Univ Children's Hosp Tübingen, Germany; Univ Hosp, Tübingen, Germany; et al)
*Acta Paediatr* 101:e167-e172, 2012

*Aim.*—To investigate neurodevelopmental outcome and hearing in preterm children with breast milk transmitted human cytomegalovirus (HCMV) infection.

*Methods.*—Forty-one preterm children (born before 32 weeks of gestation or birth weight <1500 g; 20 HCMV positive, 21 HCMV negative) from an original cohort of 44 children were examined at school age. Assessments included neurological examination, assessment of motor [Movement Assessment Battery for Children (M-ABC)] and cognitive function [Kaufman Assessment Battery for Children (K-ABC)], audiological tests and anthropometric measures.

*Results.*—In both groups, irrespective of the presence or absence of a history of HCMV infection, performance in assessments of cognitive and motor function was within the normal range. However, significant differences between the HCMV-positive and the HCMV-negative group were found in both motor and cognitive function, with poorer performance in the HCMV-positive group. There were no significant differences in anthropometric parameters, and all 20 HCMV-positive children had normal hearing function.

*Conclusions.*—In this study, cognitive and motor function in preterm children with early postnatally acquired HCMV infection transmitted via breast milk was within the normal range. However, the findings suggest that their outcome is poorer than outcome in preterm children without HCMV infection. These findings need to be replicated in larger scale studies.

▶ One percent of newborns delivered in the United States (ie, 40 000 babies annually) are infected with cytomegalovirus (CMV) in utero. Only 10% of these infants are symptomatic at birth, but 80% of these will suffer neurodevelopmental sequelae. The majority (90%) of those with congenital CMV infection appear well at birth and are indistinguishable from the other healthy newborns in the well-baby nursery. Unfortunately, 10% to 15% of these asymptomatic infants will go on to suffer serious sequelae. Congenital CMV infection is the most frequently known viral cause of mental retardation and the leading nongenetic cause of sensorineural hearing loss in the United States and other developed countries.[1] Perinatal CMV infection, in contrast to congenital CMV, refers to newborns who acquire the virus after vaginal delivery through an infected birth canal, through consumption of infected breast milk, or transfusion of blood from a CMV-positive donor.

Hamprecht showed that more than 96% of seropositive mothers have viral reactivation during lactation.[2] CMV transmission via breast milk can be as high as 38%, and up to 18% of exposed infants are likely to be infected. Only a small percent (9.3%) of preterm infants receiving breast milk from seropositive mothers develop symptomatic CMV infection. Less than 1% will develop severe clinical disease. Freezing and thawing of breast milk reduces the viral load in infected breast milk, but does not reliably prevent disease in the newborn. Pasteurization does kill the virus, but it also alters the immunologic properties of human milk and restricts any plans to transition a baby to breastfeeding.[3]

Available studies indicate that in full-term infants who acquire CMV from maternal breast milk, the risk for impaired development is no higher than in children without CMV infection. The risk for neurodevelopmental sequelae in premature infants < 32 weeks with perinatal CMV infection is less clear, however. In the first article by Bevot et al, 41 preterm infants (21 CMV positive, 20 CMV negative) from an original cohort of 44 VLBW ( < 32 weeks' gestation; < 1500 gm at birth) were evaluated at 8 years of age. The infected and control infants were well matched for prematurity issues such as birthweight, gender, intraventricular hemorrhage, sepsis, bronchopulmonary dysplasia, and socioeconomical/educational status of the parents. Assessment of cognitive and motor functions was within normal limits in both groups, but in several subtests of motor and cognition the children with breast milk acquired CMV showed poorer performance. Furthermore, 9/14 of the CMV-positive children who had started school required special help in the classroom, whereas only 4/16 CMV-negative children required such intervention, suggesting that the postnatally infected preterms may not have recovered unscathed. Neurodevelopmental testing of this same cohort at 2 to 4.5 years of age had not found any difference between the 2 groups.[4] Hearing loss was not worse in the CMV-positive premie cohort, either at 2 or 8 years of age. Most of the CMV-positive premies in this study were infected before 35 weeks' corrected age while brain development is far from complete. The authors note that although neuronal migration and proliferation are complete by this stage, processes of neuronal organization, glial proliferation and differentiation as well as myelination remain in flux.

The second manuscript by Scott et al catalogs an impressive list of proinflammatory cytokines, chemokines, and growth factors found in the amniotic fluid of fetuses infected with CMV, but not in most uninfected controls. One particular cytokine—CXCL10—was elevated in the amniotic fluid and serum of pregnant women with CMV infection. These findings heighten the concern for neurodevelopmental disadvantage in growing very low birthweight preterms infected with CMV before completed gestation, whether inside or out of the uterus.

The diligence of these investigators in following this unique cohort through 8 years is commendable. Though their numbers are small, I was encouraged that these very low birthweight infants with breast milk—acquired CMV were doing as well as they were at 8 years of age. Even in this vulnerable cohort, breast milk—acquired CMV appears to have fewer long-term sequelae than congenital CMV.

**E. K. Stork, MD**

*References*

1. Oliver SE, Cloud GA, Sánchez PJ; National Institute of Allergy and Infectious Diseases Collaborative Antiviral Study Group. Neurodevelopmental outcomes following ganciclovir therapy in symptomatic congenital cytomegalovirus infections involving the central nervous system. *J Clin Virol.* 2009;46:S22-S26.

2. Hamprecht K, Maschmann J, Vochem M, Dietz K, Speer CP, Jahn G. Epidemiology of transmission of cytomegalovirus from mother to preterm infant by breastfeeding. *Lancet.* 2001;17:513-518.
3. Rhodes J. Cytomegalovirus transmission to preterm infants via breast milk: issues in research and practice. *Neonatal Intensive Care.* 2012;25:17-19.
4. Vollmer B, Seibold-Weiger K, Schmitz-Salue C, et al. Postnatally acquired cytomegalovirus infection via breast milk: effects on hearing and development in preterm infants. *Pediatr Infect Dis J.* 2004;23:322-327.

## Association of Prenatal and Postnatal Exposure to Lopinavir-Ritonavir and Adrenal Dysfunction Among Uninfected Infants of HIV-Infected Mothers

Simon A, for the ANRS French Perinatal Cohort Study Group (Unité d'Endocrinologie Pédiatrique, Paris, France; et al)

*JAMA* 306:70-78, 2011

*Context.*—Lopinavir-ritonavir is a human immunodeficiency virus 1 (HIV-1) protease inhibitor boosted by ritonavir, a cytochrome p450 inhibitor. A warning about its tolerance in premature newborns was recently released, and transient elevation of 17-hydroxyprogesterone (17OHP) was noted in 2 newborns treated with lopinavir-ritonavir in France.

*Objective.*—To evaluate adrenal function in newborns postnatally treated with lopinavirritonavir.

*Design, Setting, and Participants.*—Retrospective cross-sectional analysis of the database from the national screening for congenital adrenal hyperplasia (CAH) and the French Perinatal Cohort. Comparison of HIV-1—uninfected newborns postnatally treated with lopinavir-ritonavir and controls treated with standard zidovudine.

*Main Outcome Measures.*—Plasma 17OHP and dehydroepiandrosterone-sulfate (DHEA-S) concentrations during the first week of treatment. Clinical and biological symptoms compatible with adrenal deficiency.

*Results.*—Of 50 HIV-1—uninfected newborns who received lopinavir-ritonavir at birth for a median of 30 days (interquartile range [IQR], 25-33), 7 (14%) had elevated 17OHP levels greater than 16.5 ng/mL for term infants (> 23.1 ng/mL for preterm) on days 1 to 6 vs 0 of 108 controls having elevated levels. The median 17OHP concentration for 42 term newborns treated with lopinavir-ritonavir was 9.9 ng/mL (IQR, 3.9-14.1 ng/mL) vs 3.7 ng/mL (IQR, 2.6-5.3 ng/mL) for 93 term controls (*P* < .001). The difference observed in median 17OHP values between treated newborns and controls was higher in children also exposed in utero (11.5 ng/mL vs 3.7 ng/mL; *P* < .001) than not exposed in utero (6.9 ng/mL vs 3.3 ng/mL; *P* = .03). The median DHEA-S concentration among 18 term newborns treated with lopinavir-ritonavir was 9242 ng/mL (IQR, 1347-25 986 ng/mL) compared with 484 ng/mL (IQR, 218-1308 ng/mL) among 17 term controls (*P* < .001). The 17OHP and DHEA-S concentrations were positively correlated (*r*=0.53; *P* = .001). All term newborns treated with lopinavir-ritonavir were asymptomatic, although 3 premature new borns experienced life-threatening symptoms compatible with adrenal insufficiency, including hyponatremia and hyperkalemia with, in 1 case, cardiogenic shock. All symptoms resolved following completion of the lopinavir-ritonavir treatment.

*Conclusion.*—Among newborn children of HIV-1–infected mothers exposed in utero to lopinavir-ritonavir, postnatal treatment with a lopinavir-ritonavir–based regimen, compared with a zidovudine-based regimen, was associated with transient adrenal dysfunction.

▶ Antepartum and perinatal management of maternal human immunodeficiency virus (HIV) infection has markedly reduced vertical transmission of the infection. In our focus on the fetal and neonatal benefits of perinatal HIV management, it is tempting to dismiss the potential toxicities of the pharmaceuticals that are used in the effort to reduce vertical transmission of HIV. This study contributes to what currently are sparse data on anti-HIV therapies beyond zidovudine, reporting the association of prenatal or postnatal exposure to the combination lopinavir-ritonavir (trade name Kaletra) and adrenal insufficiency. Among the study population of 50 HIV-uninfected newborns who received the drug at a higher than recommended dose for an average of 30 days, 14% had higher than normal 17-hydroxyprogesterone (17-OHP) levels that were greatest among infants who also were exposed in utero. Elevated 17-OHP levels correlated with elevated dehydroepiandrosterone sulfate (DHEA-S) levels as much as 64-times greater than normal. All term infants were asymptomatic; however, 3 preterm infants experienced life-threatening complications, including 1 infant who developed cardiogenic shock. Laboratory values and clinical signs improved following discontinuation of the therapy. The mechanism of these effects is unknown; however, the authors speculate that a relative adrenal insufficiency present during the neonatal period is worsened by cytochrome inhibition, leading to acute electrolyte abnormalities and cardiovascular collapse. Alternatively, the propylene glycol and ethanol present in the oral solution could be responsible. A 2011 US Food and Drug Administration warning reports additional cases of life-threatening events in preterm infants treated with lopinavir-ritonavir.[1] Lopinavir-ritonavir currently is approved for treatment of HIV-infected infants who are older than 14 days of age. This study raises the question of whether, in addition to standard monitoring of 17-OHP levels from routine newborn metabolic screening tests, these and other lopinavir-ritonavir–treated infants should undergo especially close monitoring of adrenal function.

**L. J. Van Marter, MD, MPH**

*Reference*

1. Kaletra (lopinavir-ritonavir): label change: serious health problems in premature babies. US Food and Drug Administration. http://www.fda.gov/safety/medwatch/safetyinformation/safetyalertsforhumanmedicalproducts/ucm246167.htm. Accessed June 28, 2012.

## Antibiotic Exposure in the Newborn Intensive Care Unit and the Risk of Necrotizing Enterocolitis

Alexander VN, Northrup V, Bizzarro MJ (Yale Univ School of Medicine, New Haven, CT; Yale Ctr for Analytical Sciences, New Haven, CT)
*J Pediatr* 159:392-397, 2011

*Objective.*—To determine whether duration of antibiotic exposure is an independent risk factor for necrotizing enterocolitis (NEC).

*Study Design.*—A retrospective, 2:1 control-case analysis was conducted comparing neonates with NEC to those without from 2000 through 2008. Control subjects were matched on gestational age, birth weight, and birth year. In each matched triad, demographic and risk factor data were collected from birth until the diagnosis of NEC in the case subject. Bivariate and multivariate analyses were used to assess associations between risk factors and NEC.

*Results.*—One hundred twenty-four cases of NEC were matched with 248 control subjects. Cases were less likely to have respiratory distress syndrome ($P = .018$) and more likely to reach full enteral feeding ($P = .028$) than control subjects. Cases were more likely to have culture-proven sepsis ($P < .0001$). Given the association between sepsis and antibiotic use, we tested for and found a significant interaction between the two variables ($P = .001$). When neonates with sepsis were removed from the cohort, the risk of NEC increased significantly with duration of antibiotic exposure. Exposure for >10 days resulted in a nearly threefold increase in the risk of developing NEC.

*Conclusions.*—Duration of antibiotic exposure is associated with an increased risk of NEC among neonates without prior sepsis.

▶ A prospective cohort study published in 2009 by the National Institute of Child Health and Human Development's Neonatal Research Network demonstrated an increased risk of death and necrotizing enterocolitis (NEC) among infants with birth weight less than 1000 g who received 5 or more days of empiric antibiotic therapy in the first week of life.[1] In this case-control study, the authors address the role of duration of any prior antibiotic exposure on the risk of developing NEC among infants with birth weight less than 1500 g. At a ratio of 1 case infant to 2 control infants, the authors matched infants on gestational age, birth weight, and postnatal age at diagnosis of NEC. No differences were found for sex, the proportion of small for gestational age infants, prenatal corticosteroid exposure, 5-minute Apgar score, umbilical catheter use, the timing of first enteral feeding, or the diagnosis of bronchopulmonary dysplasia among the cases and controls. A higher proportion of control infants had a history of surfactant deficiency or patent ductus arteriosus, and a higher proportion of case infants achieved full volume enteral feeding compared to controls. The study eliminated infants with culture-proven sepsis from the final comparison. Multivariate analysis demonstrated a small but significant ($P = .015$) increased risk of NEC with any prior antibiotic exposure compared to no exposure (odds ratio [OR] 1.10; 95% confidence interval, 1.02, 1.19) and also demonstrated an increasing risk with increasing duration of prior exposure, with an OR of 2.94 with more than

10 days of exposure. This study was limited by the relatively small sample size and cannot distinguish between the effects of antibiotic exposure and the concern that prolonged empiric antibiotic exposure may simply be a marker of severity of illness. This article adds to a growing concern about the relative risks and benefits of prolonged antibiotic exposure for culture-negative sepsis among very low birth weight infants.

**K. Puopolo, MD**

*Reference*

1. Cotten CM, Taylor S, Stoll B, et al. Prolonged duration of initial empirical antibiotic treatment is associated with increased rates of necrotizing enterocolitis and death for extremely low birth weight infants. *Pediatrics.* 2009;123:58-66.

**Saliva Polymerase-Chain-Reaction Assay for Cytomegalovirus Screening in Newborns**
Boppana SB, for the National Institute on Deafness and Other Communication Disorders CHIMES Study (Univ of Alabama at Birmingham; et al)
*N Engl J Med* 364:2111-2118, 2011

*Background.*—Congenital cytomegalovirus (CMV) infection is an important cause of hearing loss, and most infants at risk for CMV-associated hearing loss are not identified early in life because of failure to test for the infection. The standard assay for newborn CMV screening is rapid culture performed on saliva specimens obtained at birth, but this assay cannot be automated. Two alternatives—real-time polymerase-chain-reaction (PCR)—based testing of a liquid-saliva or dried-saliva specimen obtained at birth—have been developed.

*Methods.*—In our prospective, multicenter screening study of newborns, we compared real-time PCR assays of liquid-saliva and dried-saliva specimens with rapid culture of saliva specimens obtained at birth.

*Results.*—A total of 177 of 34,989 infants (0.5%; 95% confidence interval [CI], 0.4 to 0.6) were positive for CMV, according to at least one of the three methods. Of 17,662 newborns screened with the use of the liquid-saliva PCR assay, 17,569 were negative for CMV, and the remaining 85 infants (0.5%; 95% CI, 0.4 to 0.6) had positive results on both culture and PCR assay. The sensitivity and specificity of the liquid-saliva PCR assay were 100% (95% CI, 95.8 to 100) and 99.9% (95% CI, 99.9 to 100), respectively, and the positive and negative predictive values were 91.4% (95% CI, 83.8 to 96.2) and 100% (95% CI, 99.9 to 100), respectively. Of 17,327 newborns screened by means of the dried-saliva PCR assay, 74 were positive for CMV, whereas 76 (0.4%; 95% CI, 0.3 to 0.5) were found to be CMV-positive on rapid culture. Sensitivity and specificity of the dried-saliva PCR assay were 97.4% (95% CI, 90.8 to 99.7) and 99.9% (95% CI, 99.9 to 100), respectively. The positive and negative predictive values were 90.2% (95% CI, 81.7 to 95.7) and 99.9% (95% CI, 99.9 to 100), respectively.

*Conclusions.*—Real-time PCR assays of both liquid- and dried-saliva specimens showed high sensitivity and specificity for detecting CMV infection and should be considered potential screening tools for CMV in newborns. (Funded by the National Institute on Deafness and Other Communication Disorders.)

▶ Cytomegalovirus (CMV) is a major cause of hearing loss in infancy. Early treatment of neonatal CMV infection may prevent or ameliorate hearing loss; however, many congenital or neonatal CMV infections go undetected until hearing loss is permanent. In this article, the authors report a new method for quick detection of CMV: a polymerase chain reaction (PCR) assay conducted on a sample of the infant's saliva. The study enrolled and prospectively studied 34 989 infants, detecting 177 infants with CMV documented by standard culture methods. The PCR test detected 74 of 76 CMV saliva culture-documented infected infants, with high sensitivity, specificity, and positive and negative predictive values. Further more, the assay identified additional infants later shown to be CMV infected and was shown to work on saliva specimens whether fresh or dry. I find this report exciting because this new method of testing for CMV offers a more sensitive, rapid, and noninvasive method for detecting CMV infection. If made cost-effective, PCR assays could be used to screen for asymptomatic congenital as well as neonatal CMV. Although 60% of infants symptomatic with congenital CMV develop hearing impairment, those acquiring the infection in the first 6 months of postnatal life are at a 7% risk of hearing loss. It would be wonderful to incorporate CMV testing as a component of routine newborn screening and to monitor it periodically during the first 6 postnatal months.

**L. J. Van Marter, MD, MPH**

---

**Unrecognized Ingestion of *Toxoplasma gondii* Oocysts Leads to Congenital Toxoplasmosis and Causes Epidemics in North America**
Boyer K, other members of the Toxoplasmosis Study Group (Rush Univ Med Ctr, Chicago, IL; et al)
*Clin Infect Dis* 53:1081-1089, 2011

---

*Background.*—Congenital toxoplasmosis presents as severe, life-altering disease in North America. If mothers of infants with congenital toxoplasmosis could be identified by risks, it would provide strong support for educating pregnant women about risks, to eliminate this disease. Conversely, if not all risks are identifiable, undetectable risks are suggested. A new test detecting antibodies to sporozoites demonstrated that oocysts were the predominant source of *Toxoplasma gondii* infection in 4 North American epidemics and in mothers of children in the National Collaborative Chicago-based Congenital Toxoplasmosis Study (NCCCTS). This novel test offered the opportunity to determine whether risk factors or demographic characteristics could identify mothers infected with oocysts.

*Methods.*—Acutely infected mothers and their congenitally infected infants were evaluated, including in-person interviews concerning risks and evaluation of perinatal maternal serum samples.

*Results.*—Fifty-nine (78%) of 76 mothers of congenitally infected infants in NCCCTS had primary infection with oocysts. Only 49% of these mothers identified significant risk factors for sporozoite acquisition. Socioeconomic status, hometown size, maternal clinical presentations, and ethnicity were not reliable predictors.

*Conclusions.*—Undetected contamination of food and water by oocysts frequently causes human infections in North America. Risks are often unrecognized by those infected. Demographic characteristics did not identify oocyst infections. Thus, although education programs describing hygienic measures may be beneficial, they will not suffice to prevent the suffering and economic consequences associated with congenital toxoplasmosis. Only a vaccine or implementation of systematic serologic testing of pregnant women and newborns, followed by treatment, will prevent most congenital toxoplasmosis in North America.

▶ To avoid acquisition of *Toxoplasma gondii* infection, pregnant women are routinely counseled to avoid ingestion of undercooked meat and exposure to cat feces. However, neither the relative contributions of those sources of infection nor the efficacy of those measures has been well characterized. This report takes advantage of a novel immunoassay to begin to address those questions. Antibodies to sporozoites are present only after infection with *T gondii* oocysts (which are formed in cats, passed in feces, and acquired by ingestion of contaminated food or soil) but do not develop when infection results from ingestion of bradyzoites (tissue cysts) in undercooked meat. Presence of sporozoite antibody is therefore a reliable indicator of oocyst ingestion. In this case series, 59 of 76 mothers of congenitally infected infants (78%) enrolled in the Chicago-based Congenital Toxoplasmosis Study had primary infection with oocysts. Only half of these mothers reported cleaning a cat's litter box, gardening, contact with a sandbox, or close sustained contact with a kitten. These authors are therefore appropriately skeptical that education about and avoidance of cat exposures during pregnancy will be effective in prevention of *Toxoplasma* infections. Substantial reduction in the rate of *Toxoplasma* infection, estimated at 500 to 5000 cases per year in the United States, will therefore require adoption of a systematic serological screening program (as is the standard in France), followed by treatment of women who seroconvert during pregnancy. Although data from large randomized trials demonstrating efficacy are lacking, experts recommend treatment with spiramycin prior to 18 weeks' gestation and conversion to a combination of pyrimethamine, sulfadiazine, and folinic acid after 18 weeks of gestation.[1] Consultation with an expert in management of *Toxoplasma* infections is strongly recommended in these situations.

**W. E. Benitz, MD**

*Reference*

1. Montoya JG, Remington JS. Management of Toxoplasma gondii infection during pregnancy. *Clin Infect Dis.* 2008;47:554-566.

**The long quest for neonatal screening for severe combined immunodeficiency**

Buckley RH (Duke Univ Med Ctr, Durham, NC)
*J Allergy Clin Immunol* 129:597-604, 2012

Early recognition of severe combined immunodeficiency (SCID) is a pediatric emergency because a diagnosis before live vaccines or nonirradiated blood products are given and before development of infections permits life-saving unfractionated HLA-identical or T cell–depleted haploidentical hematopoietic stem cell transplantation, enzyme replacement therapy, or gene therapy. The need for newborn screening for this condition has been recognized for the past 15 years. However, implementation of screening required development of an assay for T-cell lymphopenia that could be performed on dried bloodspots routinely collected from newborn infants for the past 48 years. This was accomplished 6 years ago, and there have already been 7 successful pilot studies. A recommendation to add SCID to the routine newborn-screening panel was approved by the Secretary's Advisory Committee on Heritable Disorders of Newborns and Children in 2010 and was soon after approved by the Secretary of Health and Human Services. It is important for allergists, immunologists, and other health care providers to take an active role in promoting newborn screening for SCID and other T-lymphocyte abnormalities in their states. Even more important will be their roles in establishing accurate diagnoses for infants with positive screen results and in ensuring that they are given the best possible treatment (Fig 3).

▶ In 2010, the national Advisory Committee on Heritable Disorders recommended addition of severe combined immunodeficiency (SCID) to the growing list of conditions for which newborn infants should be routinely screened, so knowledge about this has become a necessity for neonatologists and pediatricians. This article provides a concise and lucid summary of the science behind this

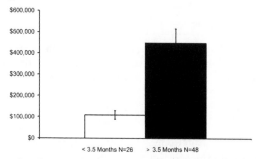

FIGURE 3.—Cost of treatment for 74 infants with SCID undergoing transplantation at Duke University Medical Center from 1998-2006, comparing costs for those who underwent transplantation before 3.5 months of life with the costs for those undergoing transplantation after age 3.5 months. (Reprinted from The Journal of Allergy and Clinical Immunology, Buckley RH. The long quest for neonatal screening for severe combined immunodeficiency. *J Allergy Clin Immunol.* 2012;129:597-604. Copyright 2012, with permission from Elsevier.)

advance, which will rapidly become a standard component of neonatal care. Recent technical innovations have made it feasible to do rapid screening using dried bloodspots, which are not suitable for lymphocyte counts, the previous best initial test. Pilot studies in several states have demonstrated that infants with SCID can be identified before they become symptomatic. Using real-time polymerase chain reaction analysis of dried bloodspots, the current technology detects SCID by testing for the absence of T-cell receptor recombination excision circles (TRECs), chunks of genomic DNA excised in the process by which T-cell receptor gene rearrangement leads to clonal antigen specificity. Because SCID is characterized by paucity or absence of T cells, all variants—independent of the underlying defect—are identified by the absence of TRECs. Neonates with a positive screening test (low or absent TRECs) should be urgently referred to a pediatric immunologist for complete immunological evaluation, including testing to quantify naive (CD45RA1) and memory (CD45RO1) T cells and to assess T-cell function. Patients with SCID, variant SCID, or complete DiGeorge syndrome have little or no T-cell function and may need hematopoietic stem cell or thymus transplantation or gene therapy. If transplantation is needed, prompt referral to a center with experience with transplantation for SCID or complete DiGeorge syndrome is essential. Patients with depressed T-cell numbers associated with partial DiGeorge syndrome have a significant number of naive T cells and normal or near-normal T-cell function, so treatment is not required. Pilot studies have already identified several other causes of relative T-cell deficiency, and we will likely learn of more as experience accrues, so not all infants with positive screens will require heroic therapies.

At first glance, it might seem that screening for a rare disease for which treatment costs are enormous would not be cost-effective. Economic analyses show otherwise. Although transplantation is undeniably costly, the alternative—treatment of infants not diagnosed until after acquisition of a serious infection—is even greater, sometimes exceeding $2 million per case. Earlier diagnosis and treatment before age 3.5 months is associated with substantially lower costs (see Fig 3), presumably because it avoids bone marrow chemoablation and severe infections requiring prolonged intensive care unit and hospital stays.

**W. E. Benitz, MD**

---

## Effect of a partially hydrolyzed whey infant formula at weaning on risk of allergic disease in high-risk children: A randomized controlled trial

Lowe AJ, Hosking CS, Bennett CM, et al (Univ of Melbourne, Australia; John Hunter Children's Hosp, Newcastle, Australia; et al)
*J Allergy Clin Immunol* 128:360-365, 2011

---

*Background.*—Partially hydrolyzed whey formula (pHWF) has been recommended for infants with a family history of allergic disease at the cessation of exclusive breast-feeding to promote oral tolerance and prevent allergic diseases.

*Objective.*—To determine whether feeding infants pHWF reduces their risk of allergic disease.

*Methods.*—A single-blind (participant) randomized controlled trial was conducted to compare allergic outcomes between infants fed a conventional cow's milk formula, a pHWF, or a soy formula. Before birth, 620 infants with a family history of allergic disease were recruited and randomized to receive the allocated formula at cessation of breast-feeding. Skin prick tests to 6 common allergens (milk, egg, peanut, dust mite, rye grass, and cat dander) were performed at 6, 12, and 24 months. The primary outcome was development of allergic manifestations (eczema and food reactions) measured 18 times in the first 2 years of life.

*Results.*—Follow-up was complete for 93% (575/620) at 2 years and 80% (495/620) at 6 or 7 years of age. There was no evidence that infants allocated to the pHWF (odds ratio, 1.21; 95% CI, 0.81-1.80) or the soy formula (odds ratio, 1.26; 95% CI, 0.84-1.88) were at a lower risk of allergic manifestations in infancy compared with conventional formula. There was also no evidence of reduced risk of skin prick test reactivity or childhood allergic disease.

*Conclusion.*—Despite current dietary guidelines, we found no evidence to support recommending the use of pHWF at weaning for the prevention of allergic disease in high-risk infants.

▶ What formula to place babies on after they conclude breast feeding, especially if they are at risk for allergic diseases, has been a source of considerable controversy. Based on a Cochrane meta-analysis,[1] and a large trial from Germany—the GINI trial,[2] suggesting that partially hydrolyzed formulas reduce allergies in at-risk babies—some highly respected agencies have supported the use of partially hydrolyzed whey formulas after breast-feeding has been discontinued. The meta-analysis upon which these recommendations are based is questioned in this study because of a suggestion that there may be bias because only published reports are analyzed. The GINI trial[2] is also scrutinized because an intention-to-treat analysis for the data in this trial failed to show benefit of partially hydrolyzed whey formula compared with conventional cow's milk formula. When intention-to-treat was incorporated, the statistical significance in the GINI trial was no longer detected at 3 years of life. This study, a large trial done over nearly 2 decades, compares soy formula with partially hydrolyzed protein formula and cow's milk formula. This study showed no effect on atopy, allergy, or other allergy-associated disorders among the 3 groups in either the first 2 years or at 6 to 7 years of age. In a subsequent editorial, concerns about the methodology used in this study were raised,[3] most of which were addressed by the authors.[4]

Why are the results of this study important? One issue is that a couple of highly respected agencies have suggested that the use of these formulas is appropriate for follow-up after breast-feeding in allergy-prone individuals. This study is a large trial raising serious questions. Second, partially hydrolyzed formulas tend to be considerably more expensive than regular formulas and the question of their palatability (taste) has been raised. Finally, if there is a recommendation for these formulas to be used in susceptible individuals, and since susceptibility is somewhat subjective, what is to say that pediatricians will not support the routine use of these formulas for a much wider, not highly susceptible group of infants who will not benefit from the use of these more costly products?

Overall, this was a reasonably well-done large study that deserves to be considered in any future agency's (eg, US Food and Drug Administration) decisions for health claims as well as additional systematic reviews.

**J. Neu, MD**

*References*

1. Osborn DA, Sinn J. Formulas containing hydrolysed protein for prevention of allergy and food intolerance in infants. *Cochrane Database Syst Rev.* 2006;(4): CD003664.
2. von Berg A, Koletzko S, Grübl A, et al. The effect of hydrolyzed cow's milk formula for allergy prevention in the first year of life: the German Infant Nutritional Intervention Study, a randomized double-blind trial. *J Allergy Clin Immunol.* 2003; 111:533-540.
3. Haschke FJ. Effect of partially hydrolyzed whey infant formula and prolonged breast-feeding on the risk of allergic disease in high-risk children. *J Allergy Clin Immunol.* 2011;128:688-689.
4. Hill D, Lowe AJ, Hoskins CS, et al. Reply. *J Allergy Clin Immunol.* 2011;3:689.

# 6 Cardiovascular System

**Birth Prevalence of Congenital Heart Disease Worldwide: A Systematic Review and Meta-Analysis**
van der Linde D, Konings EEM, Slager MA, et al (Erasmus Med Ctr, Rotterdam, the Netherlands)
*J Am Coll Cardiol* 58:2241-2247, 2011

Congenital heart disease (CHD) accounts for nearly one-third of all major congenital anomalies. CHD birth prevalence worldwide and over time is suggested to vary; however, a complete overview is missing. This systematic review included 114 papers, comprising a total study population of 24,091,867 live births with CHD identified in 164,396 individuals. Birth prevalence of total CHD and the 8 most common subtypes were pooled in 5-year time periods since 1930 and in continent and income groups since 1970 using the inverse variance method. Reported total CHD birth prevalence increased substantially over time, from 0.6 per 1,000 live births (95% confidence interval [CI]: 0.4 to 0.8) in 1930 to 1934 to 9.1 per 1,000 live births (95% CI: 9.0 to 9.2) after 1995. Over the last 15 years, stabilization occurred, corresponding to 1.35 million newborns with CHD every year. Significant geographical differences were found. Asia reported the highest CHD birth prevalence, with 9.3 per 1,000 live births (95% CI: 8.9 to 9.7), with relatively more pulmonary outflow obstructions and fewer left ventricular outflow tract obstructions. Reported total CHD birth prevalence in Europe was significantly higher than in North America (8.2 per 1,000 live births [95% CI: 8.1 to 8.3] vs. 6.9 per 1,000 live births [95% CI: 6.7 to 7.1]; $p < 0.001$). Access to health care is still limited in many parts of the world, as are diagnostic facilities, probably accounting for differences in reported birth prevalence between high- and low-income countries. Observed differences may also be of genetic, environmental, socioeconomical, or ethnic origin, and there needs to be further investigation to tailor the management of this global health problem (Fig 4).

▶ This is a timely and comprehensive literature review and analysis pertaining to congenital heart disease (CHD) and its impact on a worldwide basis. As noted by the authors, the increase in reported total CHD birth prevalence over time may be caused by changes in diagnostic methods and screening modalities rather than representing a true increase. Surely underreporting and underrecognition account

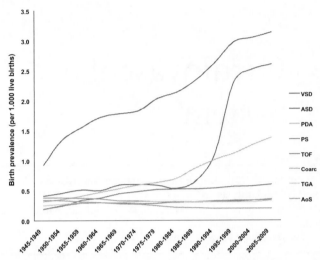

FIGURE 4.—Birth Prevalence of CHD Subtypes Over Time. Time course of birth prevalence of the 8 most common CHD subtypes from 1945 until 2010. AoS = aortic stenosis; ASD = atrial septal defect; Coarc = coarctation; PDA = patent ductus arteriosus; PS = pulmonary stenosis; TGA = transposition of the great arteries; TOF = tetralogy of Fallot; VSD = ventricular septal defect. (Reprinted from the Journal of the American College of Cardiology, van der Linde D, Konings EEM, Slager MA, et al. Birth prevalence of congenital heart disease worldwide: a systematic review and meta-analysis. *J Am Coll Cardiol.* 2011;58:2241-2247. Copyright 2011, with permission from the American College of Cardiology.)

for the very low rates in the 1930s. However, the burden globally from CHD is staggering, in excess of a million babies per year. It is also notable that there are significant differences in the prevalence among the various continents, which would point to a combination of genetic, social, and environmental effects.

From a recognition perspective, echocardiography, first introduced in the 1970s, and more recently, magnetic resonance imaging, both prenatally and after delivery, have simplified the identification of structural changes in both symptomatic and asymptomatic neonates. The widespread use of echocardiography probably explains the increased birth prevalence of total CHD in the 1970s as well as the increase in specific groups, such as patients with ventricular septal defect, atrial septal defect, and patent ductus arteriosus (PDA) (Fig 4). The survival of extremely preterm infants makes PDA a very commonplace condition with ongoing debate as to when and how to manage a PDA in these infants.

Few new risk factors have been identified for CHD, and the impact of global warming and industrialization on CHD have not been measured. Factors associated with an increased risk of CHD include maternal diabetes mellitus, phenylketonuria, febrile illness during pregnancy, infections (eg, rubella), various therapeutic drug exposures, vitamin A use, marijuana use, and exposure to organic solvents. Advances in genetics, including the recognition of babies with microdeletions of chromosome 22, Turner syndrome, and male Turner syndrome, permit better classification of these babies with CHD. Further genetic mutations may be anticipated.

Fetal cardiac anomalies are common, with half of them being lethal or requiring complex surgeries. A routine antenatal ultrasound scan performed between 18 and 22 weeks enables detection of most of these malformations. Early detection of these anomalies enables early referral to tertiary care centers with adequate expertise; however, termination of pregnancy for fetuses with severe cardiac anomalies is not uncommon. The impact of increased use of fetal echocardiography and pregnancy termination may reduce the prevalence of CHD in the next time periods. On the other hand, the introduction of routine evaluation for CHD using pulse oximetry screening may well increase the prevalence in North America,[1] and improved survival in developing countries may also increase the prevalence of CHD.

**A. A. Fanaroff, MBBCh, FRCPE**

*Reference*

1. Mahle WT, Martin GR, Beekman RH 3rd, Morrow WR; Section on Cardiology and Cardiac Surgery Executive Committee. Endorsement of Health and Human Services recommendation for pulse oximetry screening for critical congenital heart disease. *Pediatrics.* 2012;129:190-192.

---

**Strategies for Implementing Screening for Critical Congenital Heart Disease**

Kemper AR, Mahle WT, Martin GR, et al (Duke Univ, Durham, NC; Emory Univ School of Medicine, Atlanta, GA; Children's Natl Med Ctr, Washington, DC; et al)
*Pediatrics* 128:e1259-e1267, 2011

---

*Background.*—Although newborn screening for critical congenital heart disease (CCHD) was recommended by the US Health and Human Services Secretary's Advisory Committee on Heritable Disorders in Newborns and Children to promote early detection, it was deemed by the Secretary of the HHS as not ready for adoption pending an implementation plan from HHS agencies.

*Objective.*—To develop strategies for the implementation of safe, effective, and efficient screening.

*Methods.*—A work group was convened with members selected by the Secretary's Advisory Committee on Heritable Disorders in Newborns and Children, the American Academy of Pediatrics, the American College of Cardiology Foundation, and the American Heart Association.

*Results.*—On the basis of published and unpublished data, the work group made recommendations for a standardized approach to screening and diagnostic follow-up. Key issues for future research and evaluation were identified.

*Conclusions.*—The work-group members found sufficient evidence to begin screening for low blood oxygen saturation through the use of pulse-oximetry monitoring to detect CCHD in well-infant and intermediate care nurseries. Research is needed regarding screening in special populations (eg, at high altitude) and to evaluate service infrastructure and delivery strategies (eg, telemedicine) for nurseries without on-site echocardiography.

Public health agencies will have an important role in quality assurance and surveillance. Central to the effectiveness of screening will be the development of a national technical assistance center to coordinate implementation and evaluation of newborn screening for CCHD.

▶ There is a strong consensus regarding the need for screening for congenital cardiovascular malformations (CCVMs). They are relatively common, with a prevalence of 5 to 10 per 1000 live births and are the major cause of death due to birth defects, which cause most neonatal mortalities in the United States.[1] Delayed or missed diagnoses can result in significant morbidity and mortality.[2] A writing group appointed by the American Heart Association and the American Academy of Pediatrics reviewed the available literature addressing current detection methods for critical congenital heart disease (CCHD), burden of missed or delayed diagnosis of CCHD, rationale of oximetry screening, and clinical studies of oximetry in otherwise asymptomatic newborns.[3] They completed an exhaustive literature search and reviewed the evidence. In an analysis of pooled studies of oximetry assessment performed after 24 hours of life, the estimated sensitivity for detecting CCHD was 69.6%, and the positive predictive value was 47.0%; false-positive screens that required further evaluation occurred in only 0.035% of infants. They concluded "Currently, CCHD is not detected in some newborns until after their hospital discharge, which results in significant morbidity and occasional mortality. Furthermore, routine pulse oximetry performed on asymptomatic newborns after 24 hours of life, but before hospital discharge, may detect CCHD. Routine pulse oximetry performed after 24 hours in hospitals that have on-site pediatric cardiovascular services incurs very low cost and risk of harm. Future studies in larger populations and across a broad range of newborn delivery systems are needed to determine whether this practice should become standard of care in the routine assessment of the neonate."[3]

In September 2011, Health and Human Services Secretary Sebelius approved adding CCHD to the Recommended Uniform Screening Panel and outlined specific tasks assigned to National Institutes of Health, Centers for Disease Control and Prevention (CDC), and Health Resources and Services Administration. Pulse oximetry has been proposed by the CDC and endorsed by the American Academy of Pediatrics and American Heart Association as the method of choice to identify newborns with critical CCVMs. According to the CDC Website[4] "A screen is considered positive if (1) any oxygen saturation measure is < 90% (in the initial screen or in repeat screens); (2) oxygen saturation is < 95% in the right hand and foot on three measures, each separated by one hour; or (3) a > 3% absolute difference exists in oxygen saturation between the right hand and foot on three measures, each separated by one hour. Any screening that is ≥95% in the right hand or foot with a ≤3% absolute difference in oxygen saturation between the right hand or foot is considered a negative screen and screening would end Fig 1."

Any infant with a positive screen should have a diagnostic echocardiogram, which would involve an echocardiogram within the hospital or birthing center, transport to another institution for the procedure, or use of telemedicine for remote evaluation. The infant's pediatrician should be notified immediately

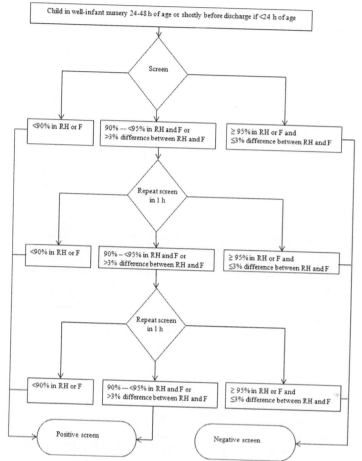

**FIGURE 1.**—The proposed pulse-oximetry monitoring protocol based on results from the right hand (RH) and either foot (F). (Reproduced with permission from Pediatrics, Kemper AR, Mahle WT, Martin GR, et al. Strategies for implementing screening for critical congenital heart disease. *Pediatrics.* 2011;128:e1259-e1267. Copyright © 2011 by the American Academy of Pediatrics.)

and the infant might need to be seen by a cardiologist for follow-up." The estimated cost of the screening is less than $10, but this does not take into account the positive screens that require echocardiography.

Not all congenital heart disease will be detected with pulse oximetry screening after 24 hours of life. The major defects identified with pulse oximetry screening include hypoplastic left heart syndrome, pulmonary atresia (with intact septum), tetralogy of Fallot, total anomalous pulmonary venous return, transposition of the great vessels, tricuspid atresia, and truncus arteriosus. These 7 CCHDs represent about 17% to 31% of all congenital heart disease. All of these defects require some type of intervention—often involving a surgical procedure—soon after birth.

The strategic approach and rationale for screening are discussed by Kemper. The difficulties and pitfalls are not underestimated. However, this is a step in the right direction. "To ensure that screening is implemented in a safe and effective manner, the work group strongly endorsed the development and funding of a national technical assistance center to disseminate best practices; to partner with public health agencies to monitor the impact of screening; to evaluate and make recommendations regarding workforce and related infrastructure needs; and to coordinate research to help answer the important unanswered questions regarding screening thresholds and optimal strategies for diagnosis and follow-up."

The application of pulse oximetry as a screening tool for CCHD is timely and appropriate. In contrast to the blood spots, the feedback is instant, and appropriate follow-up can be undertaken in a timely manner. This should substantially reduce morbidity and mortality in this group of infants.

**A. A. Fanaroff, MBBCh, FRCPE**

*References*

1. Centers for Disease Control and Prevention (CDC). Racial differences by gestational age in neonatal deaths attributable to congenital heart defects — United States, 2003-2006. *MMWR Morb Mortal Wkly Rep.* 2010;59:1208-1211.
2. Chang RK, Gurvitz M, Rodriguez S. Missed diagnosis of critical congenital heart disease. *Arch Pediatr Adolesc Med.* 2008;162:969-974.
3. Mahle WT, Newburger JW, Matherne GP, et al. Role of pulse oximetry in examining newborns for congenital heart disease: a scientific statement from the AHA and AAP. *Pediatrics.* 2009;124:823-836.
4. Centers for Disease Control and Prevention. Screening for critical congenital heart defects. http://www.cdc.gov/ncbddd/pediatricgenetics/pulse.html. Accessed June 7, 2012.

**Targeted Neonatal Echocardiography in the Neonatal Intensive Care Unit: Practice Guidelines and Recommendations for Training: Writing group of the American Society of Echocardiography (ASE) in collaboration with the European Association of Echocardiography (EAE) and the Association for European Pediatric Cardiologists (AEPC)**

Mertens L, Seri I, Marek J, et al (The Hosp for Sick Children, Toronto, Ontario, Canada; Children's Hosp Los Angeles, CA; Great Ormond Street Hosp, London, UK; et al)
*J Am Soc Echocardiogr* 24:1057-1078, 2011

*Background.*—Neonatologists can assess the hemodynamic stability of infants using echochardiography. Once significant congenital heart disease (CHD) is ruled out, the clinician can perform more focused studies (targeted neonatal echocardiography [TNE]) for specific indications. With the increased availability of echocardiography and miniaturization of technology, neonatal intensive care units (NICUs) around the world are able to not just diagnose or monitor CHD and screen for patent ductus arteriosus (PDA) but also to monitor the process of therapy. The current indications for TNE, the recommendations for its performance, and training requirements for those performing and interpreting TNE were documented.

*Indications.*—TNE with standard imaging is indicated for clinically suspected PDA, especially in very low birth weight (VLBW) neonates at least 24 hours of age; to assess perinatal asphyxia; for abnormal cardiovascular adaption manifest as hypotension, lactic acidosis, or oliguria during the first 24 postnatal hours or later in VLBW infants to diagnose low systemic blood flow; if persistent pulmonary hypertension is suspected in neonates; and for congenital diaphragmatic hernia (CDH). TNE with focused imaging is indicated if effusion (pericardial or pleural) is suspected; when a central line is placed; and for extracorporeal membrane oxygenation (ECMO) cannulation.

*Recommendations.*—If CHD or arrhythmia is strongly suspected clinically in a newborn, comprehensive echocardiography is done and interpreted by a pediatric cardiologist. Hemodynamically unstable newborns with no clinical suspicion of CHD undergo a comprehensive study done by a core TNE person and interpreted by an advanced TNE person, with interpretation by a pediatric cardiologist in a reasonable time. Children with no CHD are assessed by standard TNE as a targeted functional study.

Ultrasound systems used for TNE are optimized for imaging neonatal hearts, with special care when imaging a potentially unstable or VLBW infant to prevent infection, maintain body temperature, and monitor cardiorespiratory function. Quantitative assessment of left ventricular (LV) systolic function requires estimating LV dimensions from M-mode or two-dimensional (2D) measurements; measuring LV end-diastolic dimension and septal and posterior wall thickness; and determining shortening fraction (SF) if no regional wall motion or septal motion abnormalities occur. If either of these is abnormal, ejection fraction (EF) is calculated. Ideally the assessment of diastolic function and filling pressures are part of TNE, although no evidence supports the use of TNE data in the fluid management of neonates and infants. Assessing right ventricle (RV) size and function are also part of the TNE, with qualitative visual assessment the most commonly used technique. 2D measurements can aid quantitative serial follow-up. TNE should also include assessing the presence, size and direction of atrial-level shunting.

TNE can be used to determine the presence of a PDA, direction and characteristics of the shunt across the duct, and pressure gradient between the aorta and the pulmonary artery (PA).Hemodynamic significance is further evaluated using degree of volume overload by LV measurements.

TNE includes the estimation of RV systolic pressure (RVSp) and PA pressures and a measurement of cardiac index using the LV output method. Acquisition and analysis must be well standardized and optimized to guarantee maximal reproducibility. LV does not indicate systemic blood flow if a PDA is present. The superior vena cava (SVC) method can be used to follow changes in cardiac output with PDA, but interpretation must be done cautiously.

Pericardial effusion is measured from the epicardial surface of the heart to the maximal dimension on 2D imaging at end-diastole. Effusions should be measured by assessing maximal dimension at end-diastole and identifying the site.

All neonates clinically suspected to have PDA should undergo a comprehensive echocardiographic study before starting medical or surgical treatment to exclude ductal-dependent congenital heart defects and define arch sidedness. Standard TNE done subsequently defines the PDA's hemodynamic significance and documents spontaneous closure or treatment effects. TNE can also help identify the cause of hemodynamic instability in preterm infants after ductus ligation.

Comprehensive echocardiography is indicated for neonates with perinatal asphyxia and clinical or biochemical signs of cardiovascular compromise. Standard TNE helps optimize therapy, but its usefulness for monitoring cooling and rewarming phases of hypothermia care requires further study. TNE may also help define the underlying causes and medical management for hypotensive neonates who have no structural heart disease.

If pulmonary hypertension is suspected, comprehensive echocardiography can rule out structural heart disease. PA pressure, RV function, and shunt direction at the atrial and ductal levels can be determined using TNE in neonates with persistent pulmonary hypertension of the newborn (PPHN). In addition, all children with CDH should have comprehensive echocardiography to rule out CHD and assess PPHN severity. The effect of treatment on PA pressure, RV function, and shunt direction at atrial and ductal levels can be monitored, with focused TNE helping with line placement or ECMO use.

TNE with focused imaging can help diagnose pericardial and pleural effusions, assess their hemodynamic impact, and guide interventions. Comprehensive echocardiography is done after hemodynamic stabilization for infants with pericardial effusion. Focused TNE helps monitor treatment and can be used to identify catheter tip position after line placement or potential complications such as line thrombosis or infection. A pediatric cardiologist must perform or interpret echocardiographic procedures to rule out vegetations. Every child on ECMO must have comprehensive echocardiography. Focused TNE with focused imaging helps especially with assessing cannula position. The impact of venoarterial ECMO on ventricular filling must be considered when assessing PA pressure and ventricular performance.

*Training Requirements.*—The US and European training requirements for echocardiography are designed to cover individuals performing comprehensive pediatric and congenital echocardiography. The core or basic level includes the ability to perform comprehensive transthoracic echocardiography in neonates and children and the ability to distinguish normal from abnormal. Practitioners at the advanced or expert levels must be able to perform fetal echocardiography and transesophageal echocardiography (TEE) as well as diagnose complex disease and supervise and train core or basic practitioners. Specific cognitive and technical skills must be acquired during these training processes. Competence and quality assurance for TNE are maintained by having neonatal echocardiographers continue to perform a minimum of 100 echocardiographic studies per year and regularly participating in echocardiographic conferences or training courses.

▶ The background to this article is the political tension that surrounds the evolution of ultrasound from the consultative into the point of care (POC), with the former performed by imaging specialists and the latter by acute care doctors directly involved in the treatment of the patient. Some aspects of this tension are universal, such as concerns about training standards and diagnostic error; some are more parochial and relate to perceptions of ownership; and some relate to fear of loss of remuneration. These tensions are not unique to neonatology but have led to restrictive ultrasound practice, particularly in North America from where this document largely emanates. Against this background, there is much to applaud in this document; however, it falls short of delivering a realistic training model for neonatologists and rather than solve the problems, I fear it may just fossilize the current restrictive ultrasound practice.

There is a pressing need for training structures in POC ultrasound and there is also a need to define scope of practice; however, these must be relevant to the needs of the specialty. This can only happen if specialists collaborate on an equal footing with an agenda that is entirely focused on the patient. Although the group behind this statement consisted of cardiologists and neonatologists, the latter group was outnumbered and it shows in the result. The tensions show in the disconnect between the text, which gives a mainly balanced overview of the use of POC cardiac ultrasound within the neonatal intensive care unit (NICU), and the table of methods, which pointedly excludes hemodynamic measures widely used and researched within neonatology (superior vena cava flow, right ventricular output) yet includes traditional measures which provide little useful information in the sick newborn (eg, left ventricular wall thickness/contractility and pulmonary regurgitation).[1,2]

The involvement of cardiologists in training of neonatologists would be of great value, particularly in institutions where there are limited neonatal POC ultrasound skills. However, this statement pulls that training firmly into the consultative cardiology paradigm. I suspect 4 to 6 months in an echocardiology laboratory will be unattainable for most neonatal trainees notwithstanding the questionable relevance to their eventual skill needs within a critical care area. These proposals will only work with a greater recognition of the need for involvement of those neonatologists who have POC ultrasound skills and a shift in the balance of training back into the NICU.

Training requirements for any specialty should be self-determined and should not leave that specialty beholden to another. No one owns an organ or a technology. With or without diagnostic technologies, we all have a responsibility to work together in the best interests of our patients. Australia and New Zealand have addressed the issue of POC ultrasound training with the development of the neonatal Certificate in Clinician Performed Ultrasound (CCPU).[3] The process has been driven by neonatologists with input from other specialties, not the other way around; it reflects that neonatal POC ultrasound is not just about the heart; it allows flexibility in the provision of accredited supervision; it defines scope of practice; and is relevant and realistic to the needs of neonatal trainees. Developing this has not been without its challenges, but the CCPU provides a template on which others could build their neonatal POC ultrasound training.

If the proposals in this consensus statement are a first step from which neonatal POC ultrasound training evolves, it will be a significant achievement. If no such evolution occurs, neonatal POC ultrasound within North America will continue to lag behind much of the rest of the developed world.

**N. Evans, DM, MRCPCH**

*References*

1. Kluckow M, Seri I, Evans N. Functional echocardiography: an emerging clinical tool for the neonatologist. *J Pediatr.* 2007;150:125-130.
2. Tanke RB, Daniëls O, van Lier HJ, van Heyst AF, Festen C. Neonatal pulmonary hypertension during extracorporeal membrane oxygenation. *Cardiol Young.* 2000; 10:130-139.
3. ASUM: Promoting excellence in ultrasound. http://www.asum.com.au/newsite/Files %5CDocuments%5CEducation%5CCCCPU%5CNewCCPU%5C4.%20Freqently %20Asked%20Questions%5CCCCPU%20FAQ.pdf. Accessed August 13, 2012.

---

**Cardiac biomarkers in neonatal hypoxic ischaemia**
Sweetman D, Armstrong K, Murphy JFA, et al (Natl Maternity Hosp, Dublin, Ireland)
*Acta Paediatr* 101:338-343, 2012

---

Following a perinatal hypoxic—ischaemic insult, term infants commonly develop cardiovascular dysfunction. Troponin-T, troponin-I and brain natriuretic peptide are sensitive indicators of myocardial compromise. The longterm effects of cardiovascular dysfunction on neurodevelopmental outcome following perinatal hypoxic ischaemia remain controversial. Follow-up studies are warranted to ensure optimal cardiac function in adulthood.

*Conclusion.*—Cardiac biomarkers may improve the diagnosis of myocardial injury, help guide management, estimate mortality risk and may also aid in longterm neurodevelopmental outcome prediction following neonatal hypoxic-ischaemia.

▶ This article was a review of biomarkers useful in the assessment of myocardial injury, including troponin-T, troponin-I, creatine kinase-MB, and B-type natriuretic peptide. The authors seem to put great faith in the ability to use this information in clinical decision making in the setting of hypoxic-ischemic brain injury in the intrapartum period.

Unlike our counterparts in adult medicine, we have no baseline of past performance. However, information provided by measurement of biomarkers—when they are positive—is buttressed by the electrocardiogram, echocardiogram, and even cardiac catheterization. Our problem in the neonatal intensive care unit is that we have no gold standard and a rather nonuniform way in which we deal with affected infants. Moreover, the degree of myocardial injury may be very dependent upon the nature of the insult. Patterns of injury differ for prolonged, partial asphyxia and near-total asphyxia. Although this information might be a useful adjunct, a lot more work is needed before we can rely on it clinically.

Perhaps the best application will be in clinical research as a monitoring tool as we advance beyond hypothermia and start to add pharmacologic therapies. But let's not put the cart before the horse.

**S. M. Donn, MD**

---

### B-Type Natriuretic Peptide and Rebound during Treatment for Persistent Pulmonary Hypertension

Vijlbrief DC, Benders MJNL, Kemperman H, et al (Univ Med Ctr Utrecht/ Wilhelmina Children's Hosp, The Netherlands)
*J Pediatr* 160:111-115, 2012

---

*Objective.*—To investigate whether serum B-type natriuretic peptide (BNP) is a useful biomarker in evaluating the course of persistent pulmonary hypertension of the newborn (PPHN) and the effectiveness of treatment.

*Study Design.*—Prospective follow-up study of infants with clinical and echocardiographic signs of PPHN, who were treated with inhaled nitric oxide (iNO). Of 24 patients with PPHN who were treated, serum BNP levels were determined longitudinally in 21. BNP levels were compared between infants with (n = 6) and without rebound PPHN (n = 15).

*Results.*—BNP levels in all infants with PPHN were not significantly different at the initial start of iNO. BNP levels decreased in both groups during iNO treatment. In the infants in whom rebound PPHN developed after weaning from iNO, a significantly higher increase was found in BNP (283 pmol/L to 1232 pmol/L) compared with that in infants without rebound (98 pmol/L to 159 pmol/L). This occurred before the onset of clinical deterioration. BNP again decreased significantly after iNO treatment was restarted.

*Conclusions.*—BNP, a biomarker of cardiac ventricular strain, proved to be useful in evaluating the efficacy of PPHN treatment, and moreover, BNP helps to predict a rebound of PPHN (Fig 1).

▶ Measurement of serum levels of B-type natriuretic peptide (BNP) has been, to a large extent, a diagnostic test in search of a neonatal application. Because BNP is released by the cardiac ventricles in response to increased ventricular volume, pressure, or wall tension, it has been considered a potential indicator of hemodynamic decompensation in several settings. This study adds persistent pulmonary hypertension to congestive heart failure and patent ductus arteriosus as potential conditions in which measurement of this biomarker may prove useful. These preliminary observations in a small cohort of infants with diverse underlying diagnoses suggest that an increase in serum BNP levels following discontinuation of inhaled nitric oxide (iNO) presages recurrence of clinically apparent (and consequential) pulmonary hypertension. Although the figure provided (Fig 1) suggests no overlap between the ranges of BNP levels after iNO discontinuation,

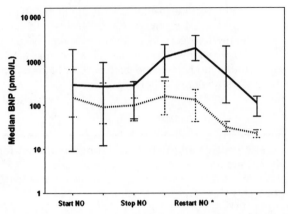

**FIGURE 1.**—Line plot representing median changes in BNP (pmol/L) during PPHN treatment. The *continuous line* represents the patients with rebound PPHN; the *interrupted line* represents the PPHN patients without rebound. The *error bars* represent the range. *Only in rebound patients. (Reprinted from Journal of Pediatrics, Vijlbrief DC, Benders MJNL, Kemperman H, et al. B-type natriuretic peptide and rebound during treatment for persistent pulmonary hypertension. *J Pediatr.* 2012;160:111-115. Copyright 2012 with permission from Elsevier Inc.)

the text reports ranges of 7 to 448 pmol/L in infants who did not go on to have recurrent pulmonary hypertension of the newborn (PPHN) and 430 to 2339 pmol/L in those who did. Although these overlapping ranges indicate that the performance of this test will not be perfect (100% sensitivity and specificity), it appears likely that it will be quite good. BNP may therefore prove useful in monitoring the course and treatment of PPHN, particularly as a predictor of recrudescent PPHN, potentially allowing adjustment of treatment (such as resumption of iNO therapy) in anticipation of rather than in response to clinical deterioration. Additional experience in more infants is needed to confirm these intriguing observations.

**W. E. Benitz, MD**

---

## Effect of persistent patent ductus arteriosus on mortality and morbidity in very low-birthweight infants

Tauzin L, Joubert C, Noel A-C, et al (Territorial Hosp Centre, New Caledonia, France; Univ Hosp Centre, Reims, France; et al)
*Acta Paediatr* 101:419-423, 2012

---

*Aim.*—Because New Caledonia is geographically isolated from the nearest cardiac surgical centre, surgical closure of ductus arteriosus is not performed in very low-birthweight (VLBW) infants who have a persistent patent ductus in spite of having undergone treatment with ibuprofen. This study aimed at investigating the possible effect of persistent patent ductus in VLBW infants.

*Methods.*—The study included 177 VLBW infants born at 25—31 weeks of gestation from January 2006 to May 2011. Mortality and major morbidities were compared between infants with a persistent patent ductus ($n = 33$) and those without it ($n = 104$). Statistical associations between potential neonatal risk factors and significant morbidities were identified using multivariate regression analyses.

*Results.*—Rates of mortality and major morbidities, including the rate of bronchopulmonary dysplasia, necrotizing enterocolitis, intraventricular haemorrhage grades I–II and III–IV, periventricular leucomalacia, late-onset infections and failure of hearing screening, were insignificantly higher in VLBW infants with a persistent patent ductus than in those without it.

*Conclusion.*—This study adds further evidence that persistent patent ductus arteriosus has no significant effect on mortality and morbidity in VLBW infants born at $\geq 25$ weeks' gestational age.

▶ Evidence continues to accumulate that aggressive management to induce closure of the persistently patent ductus arteriosus (pPDA) in very low birth weight (VLBW) infants is neither necessary nor helpful. In this cohort of 177 VLBW infants born between 25 and 31 weeks' gestation at a facility without ready access to surgical ligation, 51 had a significant PDA beyond 3 days of age. Of these, 43 received ibuprofen and 4 received indomethacin. A total of 33 infants, including 24 who had been treated with ibuprofen, had pPDA beyond 6 days of age and were managed without further cyclo-oxygenase (COX) inhibitor treatment or surgical ligation. Outcomes for those infants were compared with those of 104 infants in whom ductal closure was confirmed by echocardiography. Infants with pPDA were not significantly more likely to have adverse outcomes, including necrotizing enterocolitis, intraventricular hemorrhage, periventricular leukomalacia, and late-onset infection. In univariate analysis, bronchopulmonary dysplasia (BPD) was more common in infants with persistent PDA (42% vs 18%; $P = .04$), but this difference was not significant after risk adjustment (adjusted odds ratio for BPD in presence of pPDA 1.55; 95% confidence interval, 0.43–5.59). Although this difference might have been significant with a larger sample size, regression analysis suggested that BPD risk was primarily related to the severity of respiratory distress. Notably, only 3 infants had pPDA at 36 weeks' postmenstrual age, and it was hemodynamically significant in only 1. These observations strongly indicate that the ductus is very likely to close in VLBW infants before hospital discharge and that the consequences of ductal patency can be managed effectively while awaiting closure without major adverse sequelae. These data should support equipoise and encourage enrollment in clinical trials designed to compare 2 well-defined approaches to management of pPDA. Development of evidence from such trials is long overdue.

**W. E. Benitz, MD**

**Selective serotonin reuptake inhibitors during pregnancy and risk of persistent pulmonary hypertension in the newborn: population based cohort study from the five Nordic countries**
Kieler H, Artama M, Engeland A, et al (Karolinska Univ Hosp, Stockholm, Sweden; THL Natl Inst for Health and Welfare, Helsinki, Finland; Norwegian Inst of Public Health, Oslo, Norway; et al)
*BMJ* 344:d8012, 2012

*Objective.*—To assess whether maternal use of selective serotonin reuptake inhibitors (SSRIs) increases the risk of persistent pulmonary hypertension in the newborn, and whether such an effect might differ between specific SSRIs.
*Design.*—Population based cohort study using data from the national health registers.
*Setting.*—Denmark, Finland, Iceland, Norway, and Sweden, 1996-2007.
*Participants.*—More than 1.6 million infants born after gestational week 33.
*Main Outcome Measures.*—Risks of persistent pulmonary hypertension of the newborn associated with early and late exposure to SSRIs during pregnancy and adjusted for important maternal and pregnancy characteristics. Comparisons were made between infants exposed and not exposed to SSRIs.
*Results.*—Around 30 000 women had used SSRIs during pregnancy and 11 014 had been dispensed an SSRI later than gestational week 20. Exposure to SSRIs in late pregnancy was associated with an increased risk of persistent pulmonary hypertension in the newborn: 33 of 11 014 exposed infants (absolute risk 3 per 1000 liveborn infants compared with the background incidence of 1.2 per 1000); adjusted odds ratio 2.1 (95% confidence interval 1.5 to 3.0). The increased risks of persistent pulmonary hypertension in the newborn for each of the specific SSRIs (sertraline, citalopram, paroxetine, and fluoxetine) were of similar magnitude. Filling a prescription with SSRIs before gestational week 8 yielded slightly increased risks: adjusted odds ratio 1.4 (95% confidence interval 1.0 to 2.0).
*Conclusions.*—The risk of persistent pulmonary hypertension of the newborn is low, but use of SSRIs in late pregnancy increases that risk more than twofold. The increased risk seems to be a class effect.

▶ Since Chambers et al reported a putative association between persistent pulmonary hypertension of the newborn (PPHN) and antenatal exposure to selective serotonin-reuptake inhibitors (SSRI) in 2006,[1] there has been some uncertainty about the validity and clinical significance of that finding. Although they described a 6-fold increase in the odds of PPHN among infants exposed to SSRI after the 20th week of gestation, the implications at the bedside for an infant with PPHN or (more importantly) for pregnant women needing treatment for severe depression have not been clear. Drawing data covering 1 618 255 singleton births in national health care databases for Denmark, Finland, Iceland, Norway, and Sweden over a 12-year period, this report both confirms the association and places it in a population-based context. Like Chambers et al, these authors found an increased risk of PPHN with SSRI exposure, which appeared to be a class effect, as the risk estimates for different SSRIs were similar. The size of the effect was not as large, however, with an adjusted odds ratio of 2.1 (95% CI, 1.5—3.0) for infants exposed after 20 weeks of gestation. They also found that risk was increased slightly among infants of women with a previous psychiatric hospital admission for whom SSRI had not been prescribed from 3 months before pregnancy until birth; their data did not permit exclusion of the possibility that there has been SSRI exposure from drugs prescribed earlier and taken during pregnancy, however. Analysis using more specific subcodes available in Denmark, Finland, and Sweden did not support a relationship between PPHN and psychiatric admissions, however (odds ratio, 1.0; 95% CI, 0.6—1.6), implying that the risk is associated with this class of drugs and not the condition for which they are prescribed.

Nonetheless, the contribution of antenatal SSRI exposure to the incidence of PPHN is quite small. For the mother-to-be considering SSRI use in late pregnancy, the incremental risk of PPHN for her baby is about 1.8 per 1000 (unadjusted) to 2.6 per 1000 (adjusted)—modest but perhaps nontrivial. For the clinician seeking an etiology at the bedside of an infant with PPHN, the prior probability that it is attributable to SSRI exposure is low: only 33 of the 1932 cases (1.7%) of PPHN observed in this population survey were associated with SSRI exposure in the last half of pregnancy.

**W. E. Benitz, MD**

*Reference*

1. Chambers CD, Hernandez-Diaz S, Van Marter LJ, et al. Selective serotonin-reuptake inhibitors and risk of persistent pulmonary hypertension of the newborn. *N Engl J Med.* 2006;354:579-587.

---

## Isolated Atrioventricular Block in the Fetus: A Retrospective, Multinational, Multicenter Study of 175 Patients

Eliasson H, for the Fetal Working Group of the European Association of Pediatric Cardiology (Karolinska Univ Hosp, Stockholm, Sweden)
*Circulation* 124:1919-1926, 2011

---

*Background.*—Isolated complete atrioventricular block in the fetus is a rare but potentially lethal condition in which the effect of steroid treatment on outcome is unclear. The objective of this work was to study risk factors associated with death and the influence of steroid treatment on outcome.

*Methods and Results.*—We studied 175 fetuses diagnosed with second- or third-degree atrioventricular block (2000—2007) retrospectively in a multinational, multicenter setting. In 80% of 162 pregnancies with documented antibody status, atrioventricular block was associated with maternal anti-Ro/SSA antibodies. Sixty-seven cases (38%) were treated with fluorinated corticosteroids for a median of 10 weeks (1−21 weeks). Ninety-one percent were alive at birth, and survival in the neonatal period was 93%, similar in steroid-treated and untreated fetuses, regardless of degree of block and/or presence of anti-Ro/SSA. Variables associated with death were gestational age <20 weeks, ventricular rate ≤50 bpm, fetal hydrops, and impaired left ventricular function at diagnosis. The presence of ≥1 of these variables was associated with a 10-fold increase in mortality before birth and a 6-fold increase in the neonatal period independently of treatment. Except for a lower gestational age at diagnosis in treated than untreated (23.4 ± 2.9 versus 24.9 ± 4.9 weeks; $P = 0.02$), risk factors were distributed equally between treatment groups. Two-thirds of survivors had a pacemaker by 1 year of age; 8 children developed cardiomyopathy.

*Conclusions.*—Risk factors associated with a poor outcome were gestation <20 weeks, ventricular rate ≤50 bpm, hydrops, and impaired left ventricular function. No significant effect of treatment with fluorinated corticosteroids was seen (Fig 1).

▶ When complete atrioventricular block without associated cardiac structural anomalies is recognized in the course of prenatal care, it arouses great concern in the affected mother and her care providers. Once second- or third-degree heart block develops, fetal bradycardia is often progressive, and affected infants may develop endocardial fibroelastosis. These conditions often result in fetal hydrops and/or intrauterine fetal demise. Because this process is frequently mediated by anti-Ro/SSA autoantibodies associated with maternal autoimmune disorders such as systemic lupus erythematosus, transplacental treatment of fetal immune-mediated cardiac injury by administration of potent steroids to the mother seems like a logical choice. Although some retrospective reports suggested that this may be an effective strategy,[1] more recent prospective data have failed to support that hypothesis.[2] Accordingly, fetal cardiologists, high-risk obstetricians, and neonatologists have not found consensus on whether, when, or how antenatal corticosteroids should be used.

From a multicenter collaboration among 28 centers in Europe and Brazil, these authors report outcomes for 175 affected fetuses. Rates of antenatal steroid treatment at different centers ranged from 0% to 100% (0% to 83% among centers that enrolled 10 or more subjects; see Fig 1). Remarkably, there was no correlation between treatment and severity of fetal heart rhythm or function. Even though treated and untreated cases did not differ with respect to identified factors associated with mortality, treatment was not associated with any survival advantage. Even among fetuses with multiple risk factors, steroids did not improve survival. Maternal steroid therapy, at least after heart block has already developed, therefore appears to be ineffective, but retrospective study design and heterogeneity in criteria for and particulars of steroid therapy make it difficult to reach definitive conclusions. In the absence of clear evidence of benefit, however, the known hazards of repeated or prolonged intrauterine exposure, for both the mother and fetus, should be carefully considered before embarking on such interventions. For the moment, management may have to hinge on intensive antepartum monitoring and selection of the optimal time of delivery. That is a daunting task

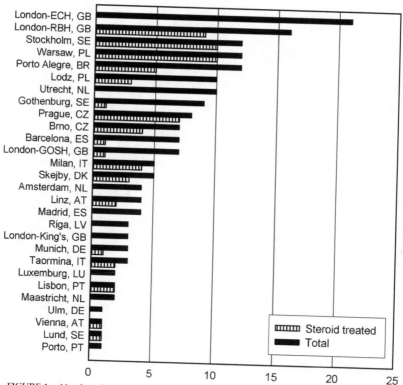

FIGURE 1.—Number of patients (total and steroid treated) from each participating center. (Reprinted from Eliasson H, for the Fetal Working Group of the European Association of Pediatric Cardiology. Isolated atrioventricular block in the fetus: a retrospective, multinational, multicenter study of 175 patients. *Circulation.* 2011;124:1919-1926. © American Heart Association Inc.)

because premature birth is associated with increased mortality (perhaps because more severely affected fetuses are more likely to be delivered earlier), yet transplacental transfer of the injurious antibodies and the opportunity for disease progression ends only at birth.

**W. E. Benitz, MD**

*References*

1. Jaeggi ET, Fouron JC, Silverman ED, Ryan G, Smallhorn J, Hornberger LK. Transplacental fetal treatment improves the outcome of prenatally diagnosed complete atrioventricular block without structural heart disease. *Circulation.* 2004;110: 1542-1548.

2. Friedman DM, Kim MY, Copel JA, Llanos C, Davis C, Buyon JP. Prospective evaluation of fetuses with autoimmune-associated congenital heart block followed in the PR Interval and Dexamethasone Evaluation (PRIDE) Study. *Am J Cardiol.* 2009;103:1102-1106.

**Early postnatal hypotension and developmental delay at 24 months of age among extremely low gestational age newborns**
Logan JW, for the ELGAN Study Investigators (New Hanover Regional Med Ctr, Wilmington, NC; et al)
*Arch Dis Child Fetal Neonatal Ed* 96:F321-F328, 2011

*Objectives.*—To evaluate in extremely low gestational age newborns, relationships between indicators of hypotension during the first 24 postnatal hours and developmental delay at 24 months of age.

*Methods.*—The 945 infants in this prospective study were born at <28 weeks, were assessed for three indicators of hypotension in the first 24 postnatal hours, and were evaluated with the Bayley Mental Development Index (MDI) and Psychomotor Development Index (PDI) at 24 months corrected age. Indicators of hypotension included: (1) mean arterial pressure in the lowest quartile for gestational age; (2) treatment with a vasopressor; and (3) blood pressure lability, defined as the upper quartile for the difference between the lowest and highest mean arterial pressure. Logistic regression was used to evaluate relationships between hypotension and developmental outcomes, adjusting for potential confounders.

*Results.*—78% of infants in this cohort received volume expansion or vasopressor; all who received a vasopressor were treated with volume expansion. 26% had an MDI <70 and 32% had a PDI <70. Low MDI and PDI were associated with low gestational age, which in turn, was associated with receipt of vasopressor treatment. Blood pressure in the lowest quartile for gestational age was associated with vasopressor treatment and labile blood pressure. After adjusting for potential confounders, none of the indicators of hypotension were associated with MDI <70 or PDI <70.

*Conclusions.*—In this large cohort of extremely low gestational age newborns, we found little evidence that early postnatal hypotension indicators are associated with developmental delay at 24 months corrected gestational age.

▶ Infants contributing to this analysis were enrolled in the large multicenter prospective observational Extremely Low Gestational Age Newborn (ELGAN) study, an endeavor designed to assess biomarkers and other characteristics and exposures potentially influencing neurodevelopmental outcomes of extremely low gestational age newborns. The current analysis assessed 945 infants (a subset of the initial cohort of 1506) for hypotension in the first 24 postnatal hours who were seen for follow-up neurodevelopmental assessments, via Bayley Scales of Infant Development-II (BSID-II) Mental Development Index (MDI) and Psychomotor Development Index (PDI), at 24 months' corrected age. Blood pressures and interventions (eg, vasopressor medications and volume expansion) were evaluated. Analyses were adjusted for potential confounding factors and showed no association between 24-month BSID-II MDI less than 70 or PDI less than 70 and measures of hypotension, including lowest quartile mean arterial pressure for gestational age, vasopressor treatment, or labile mean arterial pressure. Noteworthy limitations of the study included the fact that a high proportion (75%) of the study infants received volume expansion in the first 24 postnatal hours, possibly limiting generalizability of study results. No consistent method was used to assess blood pressure. This study adds to existing literature citing a lack of evidence among preterm infants that treating numerically low blood pressure improves outcomes. In the excellent accompanying editorial, Barrington[1] points out the limitations of many prior studies that have linked hypotension and neurodevelopmental outcomes—specifically, low study power and small sample sizes—that did not allow multivariate modeling. He further discusses the challenges of ascertaining the relation between blood pressure, end-organ perfusion, and the benefits, if any, of interventions for hypotension. Several clinical trials now launching should contribute information that will lead to a firmer evidence base for management of neonatal hypotension.

**L. J. Van Marter, MD, MPH**

*Reference*

1. Barrington KJ. Low blood pressure in extremely preterm infants: does treatment affect outcome? *Arch Dis Child Fetal Neonatal Ed.* 2011;96:F316-F317.

## The right ventricular systolic to diastolic duration ratio: a simple prognostic marker in congenital diaphragmatic hernia?

Aggarwal S, Stockman PT, Klein MD, et al (Children's Hosp of Michigan, Detroit)
*Acta Paediatr* 100:1315-1318, 2011

*Aims.*—(i) To compare the ratio of right ventricular systolic to diastolic duration (SD/DD) in infants with congenital diaphragmatic hernia (CDH) and normal controls and (ii) to examine its association, if any, with outcomes in CDH.

*Methods.*—Retrospective chart and echocardiographic review of consecutive neonates (<1 month old) with CDH and term controls without structural heart defects. Right ventricular SD/DD was calculated by a single reader.

*Results.*—Infants with CDH (n = 29) were comparable to controls (n = 27) in their mean (SD) age [2.2 (3.3) vs. 2 (4.0) days], birthweight [3 (0.67) vs. 3 (0.69) kg] and proportion of males (48.2% vs. 72.4%). The DD and SD/DD were significantly abnormal in the CDH group, compared to controls. Among infants with CDH, those who died (n = 15) and those who died or required ECMO (n = 17) had significantly shorter DD and higher SD/DD ratio. At a cut-off of 1.3, SD/DD ratio had a sensitivity of 92.8 (95% CI 64–99%) and specificity of 61.5 (32–85%) for prediction of mortality. Significant independent associations with mortality were observed with antenatal diagnosis ($p = 0.003$) and higher SD/DD ratio ($p = 0.04$).

*Conclusion.*—The right ventricular SD/DD ratio is a sensitive objective prognostic marker in infants with CDH. Further studies incorporating SD/DD ratio as a guide to intervention are warranted.

▶ In this study involving infants with congenital diaphragmatic hernia (CDH), the investigators appear to be seeking the Holy Grail of diagnostic tests: a test with the ability to accurately predict mortality. Simply put, the proper question is: "In infants with CDH does a positive test accurately predict mortality?"

This study asks and answers a different question. The question examined here is "Do patients with CDH who die have different test results than those who don't?" Although not as clinically important as the first question, the latter is easier to study and is a logical question to ask first because if the answer to it is "no," then one need go no further.

Depending on the population selected to study, it can be relatively easy to discriminate survivors from nonsurvivors. The 36-hour-old crying "slightly dusky CDH baby" found in the nursery is probably going to do well, whereas ashen gray acidotic babies on multiple vasopressors are not likely to do well. The populations many are interested in testing are those for which there is the most clinical uncertainty. In general, when populations are selected for testing on the basis of signs or symptoms (referral bias), such selection usually raises sensitivity, reduces specificity, and decreases the likelihood ratio for both negative and positive results. In other words, the diagnostic accuracy of tests is often "used up" with referral of patients. The population these investigators should examine next should be restricted to those who appear very ill. That is the population that clinicians seek diagnostic help in discriminating mortality rates.

The investigators select an optimal cut point value of 1.3. This value is presumably chosen as the "best cut point" in this sample of patients. Because this is a sample of CDH patients, it is likely that all future samples will have indices that approach but do not exactly match those presented here. Using 1.3 as a cut point in a different sample will not have the same diagnostic accuracy. Every population studied has its own optimal cut point value. When applying it to another population, one will never achieve the same predictive accuracy. A prospective study of a large population would help refine estimates of accuracy.

How much diagnostic accuracy is required of such a test? The authors opine that such tests will be used to "optimize" patient outcomes. Certainly this is a truism, but it begs the question what does "optimize patient outcomes" mean? If one were to use it as a means for withholding treatment in fatal cases, the accuracy of such a test must be very high indeed. Under such a scenario, patients with false positives (predicted to die but don't) may have treatment withheld inappropriately. With the accuracy presented here, the false-positive rate is probably too high to use the indices as a justification for withholding treatment. The test might be useful in determining which patients to offer earlier treatment with therapies that have intrinsic risk such as extracorporeal membrane oxygen (ECMO), here the cost of a false positive would be unnecessary ECMO, which seems more palatable. In a similar vein, the false-negative rate (babies who are not predicted to die but do) must be considered in clinical terms. A false negative could mean delay in withholding a treatment that might save them (perhaps early ECMO) or could prolong dying, with all of its attendant pain and suffering. In the end, the question boils down to the proper selection of the relative utility of the ratio of false positives to false negatives (eg, in the case of using ECMO, it might be how many unnecessary ECMOs is prolonging a death worth). The proper way to do this is to determine the relative consequences and then select the sensitivity and specificity that is required to achieve this end.

One should take the authors' conclusions that the test holds promise as being true, but not use these results to treat patients until the diagnostic accuracy in the proper population can be refined.

**R. E. Schumacher, MD**

---

**Which inotrope and when in neonatal and paediatric intensive care?**
Turner MA, Baines P (Univ of Liverpool, UK; Alder Hey Hosp, Liverpool, UK)
*Arch Dis Child Educ Pract Ed* 96:216-222, 2011

---

*Background.*—Inotropes increase the force of cardiac muscle contraction, improve cardiac output, and increase oxygen delivery to the tissues. It can be difficult to determine which inotrope to use and when to use it, since the evidence base for these medications is incomplete. Mistakes made when patients are being treated for sepsis include a lack of appropriate fluid supplementation, delay in beginning inotrope use even with clear evidence of poor circulation, and lack of attention to other parameters, such as electrolytes. Shock may result from abnormal rhythms and afterload; these two may require manipulation to increase cardiac output. The therapeutic strategies appropriate for initial stabilization using inotropes in pediatric and neonatal intensive care unit (PICU and NICU) patients were outlined.

*PICU Guidelines.*—For pediatric patients with sepsis, the clinician must determine fluid levels and cardiac output. Status can be determined using invasive monitoring, functional echocardiography, blood pressure (BP) levels, or other methods of assessing circulation. The goal is to identify the underlying physiologic status and design appropriate treatments. If the child does not improve with specific treatment, the diagnosis may be in error. Initial treatment of septic shock involves the liberal use of fluids until heart rate, peripheral perfusion, and other clinical parameters return to normal. A central venous line allows the reliable delivery of inotrope and permits measurement of the adequacy of fluid resuscitation. Central venous pressure should be between 10 and 15 cm $H_2O$. If inotropes are delivered via peripheral access, more dilute concentrations should be given so they can run at higher infusion rates.

Most children must be sedated, intubated, and ventilated. If the shock is refractory to fluid resuscitation, dopamine can be given, or dobutamine in cases of preexisting cardiac dysfunction. Cold shock (low cardiac output) is managed with epinephrine, whereas warm shock (high cardiac output and low systemic vascular resistance) is treated with norepinephrine.

Other medications that can be used in children include phosphodiesterase inhibitors, steroids, vasopressin, and calcium.

*NICU Guidelines.*—For neonates, the clinician must first determine if the child is in a transitional circulation or not; a transitional circulation includes the ductus arteriosus. Once the duct closes, hemodynamics change. Other important factors are developmental stage and disease presence. Echocardiography may help assess neonates but requires a high level of skill and continuous supervision by pediatric cardiologists. It is not yet associated with an improved outcome clinically.

Circulatory insufficiency just after birth can be managed by targeting the post-ductal systemic circulation or the brain circulation. BP and systemic signs are used to assess these infants if the systemic circulation is targeted. Dopamine affects BP more than dobutamine does, but the latter is important if vasoconstriction may complicate the situation of an immature myocardium. Epinephrine has effects comparable to those of dopamine. If the brain circulation is targeted, some data indicate dobutamine should be used first, the dopamine, and finally epinephrine. Hydrocortisone can be a useful subclinical adrenal insufficiency rescue medication, but safety concerns arise should it be used as a first-line inotrope. Persistent fetal circulation/pulmonary hypertension (PHT), renal dopamine, high-frequency oscillatory ventilation, patent ductus arteriosus (PDA), and congenital heart disease can complicate cases of neonates with sepsis.

Once the neonate has a post-transitional circulation, a low threshold is needed for fluid resuscitation. Inotropes with vasoconstriction can be useful because systemic vasodilatation is an important factor. Dobutamine can be used to target contractility, or the combination of dopamine first, dobutamine, then epinephrine can address a wider target. Should a duct persist, diuretics can be used because of the risk of heart failure.

*Conclusions.*—"Aggressive" inotrope therapy may save lives. This approach consists of steps to carefully assess the child's hemodynamic status, intervene early, titrate judiciously, and be aware of other factors that can alter cardiovascular function.

▶ Turner and Baines discuss the use of inotropes in neonatal and pediatric patients. Although the article helps us to understand the principles of management, there are many uncertainties reflected through varying clinical practices from assessment to the choice of inotrope. This is further compounded by the emerging use of functional echocardiography for treating sick infants.

Assessment and management of perfusion in sick infants is debated routinely on every neonatal intensive care unit. The clinical markers of perfusion, such as capillary refill time and core-peripheral temperature differences, have poor sensitivity and predictive values.[1] Measurement of blood pressure is widely practiced for assessing perfusion, but there are conflicting views regarding treatment decisions based on mean blood pressure (BP)[2] or systolic BP.[3] Other markers, such as serum lactate and mixed venous saturation, are also used for decision making in conjunction with other parameters. Functional echocardiography and noninvasive cardiac output monitoring are now increasingly used for assessment but limited by lack of expertise or technology. Using BP values to decide when to start inotropes is currently advocated but might be inappropriate treatment in many babies.

In newborn infants, the value of echocardiographic assessment is becoming increasingly important before deciding on an intervention. The value of such assessment is mentioned, but the authors fail to provide a management plan for common hypotension scenarios, including how ventilation strategy can affect circulation by ventilation-perfusion mismatch and impaired venous return to the heart. The authors recognize the risk of low BP with the use of high-frequency ventilation but do not provide guidance. This is one example in which unnecessary and injudicious use of inotropes can be averted.

The choice of inotropes and titration of the dose need special attention. In extremely premature babies, clinicians try to target a reference BP while adding the recommended drug, dopamine, as the first inotrope. Though dopamine increases the inotropic effect on the heart, it also increases the peripheral resistance. This could lead to further exhaustion of the immature myocardium and reduce cardiac output. Phosphodiesterase inhibitor drugs, such as milrinone, reduce afterload while improving cardiac contractility, but a clinical trial failed to demonstrate any benefit.[4] Trials are now underway to assess dobutamine, which has effects similar to milrinone. Similarly, in pulmonary hypertension, maintaining systemic vascular tone and cardiac inotropy is important, and dopamine or epinephrine might be more effective.

The pharmacokinetics of inotropes at different gestational and postnatal ages are complex and poorly understood. Because of this, the current practice of titrating infusion rates to response and the selection of a maximum dose are guided by personal practice rather than evidence.

The authors correctly criticize the injudicious use of fluid boluses in preterm infants and highlight that excessive fluid and sodium intake in first few days can be associated with increased oxygen dependency. On the other hand, they seem to advocate fluid resuscitation in pediatric patients as the gold standard first-line therapy citing a study in which 80% of patients with septic shock who did not respond to fluids had low cardiac output and needed inotropes.[5] This is further supported by a recent study in which the trial was stopped prematurely because of higher mortality in fluid-resuscitated patients.[6] A cautious approach to fluid resuscitation and incorporating objective assessments of cardiac output and central venous pressure might help in limiting unnecessary fluids.

Management of perfusion still remains an area of uncertainty in neonatal medicine, where the approach is still based more on practice than on evidence. Clinicians need to agree on the definition of hypotension or poor perfusion and search for clinical parameters with good sensitivity and predictive values. Functional echocardiography looks promising but calls for uniform standards and accreditation of clinicians before routine incorporation into clinical practice. Further more, the selection of an inotrope should be based on the underlying pathophysiology, and future trials should include pharmacokinetic analyses and meaningful long-term outcomes.

**S. Gupta, DM, MRCP, MD, FRCPCH, FRCPI**

*References*

1. Kluckow M, Evans N, Leslie G, Rowe J. Prostacyclin concentrations and transitional circulation in preterm infants requiring mechanical ventilation. *Arch Dis Child Fetal Neonatal Ed.* 1999;80:F34-F47.
2. Cunningham S, Symon AG, Elton RA, Zhu C, McIntosh N. Intra-arterial blood pressure reference ranges, death and morbidity in very low birthweight infants during the first seven days of life. *Early Hum Dev.* 1999;56:151-165.
3. Randomised trial of prophylactic early fresh-frozen plasma or gelatin or glucose in preterm babies: outcome at 2 years. Northern Neonatal Nursing Initiative Trial Group. *Lancet.* 1996;348:229-232.
4. Paradisis M, Evans N, Kluckow M, Osborn D. Randomized trial of milrinone versus placebo for prevention of low systemic blood flow in very preterm infants. *J Pediatr.* 2009;154:189-195.
5. Cineviva G, Paschall JA, Maffei F, Carcillo JA. Hemodynamic support in fluid refractory pediatric septic shock. *Pediatrics.* 1998;102:e19.
6. Maitland K, Kiguli S, Opoka RO, et al. Mortality after fluid bolus in African children with severe infection. *N Engl J Med.* 2011;364:2483-2495.

---

**Very low-birth-weight infants with congenital cardiac lesions: Is there merit in delaying intervention to permit growth and maturation?**
Hickey EJ, Nosikova Y, Zhang H, et al (Univ of Toronto, Ontario, Canada)
*J Thorac Cardiovasc Surg* 143:126-136, 2012

---

*Background.*—Low birth weight and prematurity are known risks for mortality in congenital heart lesions. It is not known whether risks of delayed intervention are offset by benefits of growth and maturation. We explored this question.

*Methods.*—All 1618 infants admitted to our institution within 30 days after birth for a congenital heart defect since 2000 were analyzed. Birth details and admission progress notes were detailed on all. For infants requiring cardiac interventions, clinical conference records and progress notes enabled their management to be classified as either USUAL (normal timing and mode of intervention) or DELAYED (intentional delay for growth/maturation). The survival implications of birth weight and prematurity were examined via parametric multiphase methodology with bootstrap resampling. Subsequently, the impact of DELAYED management was sought in propensity-adjusted and multivariable time-related models.

*Results.*—Low birth weight is a strong, robust and independent predictor of death within the first year of life ($P < .0001$; 99.6% bootstrap resamples). The relationship is nonlinear with an inflection point at approximately 2.0 kg, below which decrements in survival are increasingly pronounced. Prematurity is also associated with poor outcome but less reliably so ($P < .0001$; 53% resamples); its variance appears partially mitigated by colinearity with multiple factors including diagnosis and chromosomal aneuploidy. Of the 149 infants with birth weight less than 2.0 kg (highest risk and most likely to receive delayed care in this cohort), care was USUAL in 34 and DELAYED in 46. The remaining children received comfort care only (27), were not considered for intervention owing to severe noncardiac problems (12) or were routinely observed for nonurgent lesions (30). Survival between the children weighing less than 2.0 kg and receiving USUAL or DELAYED care was identical (78% ± 2% at 1 year; $P=.88$), even when adjusted via propensity score ($P=0.65$) or multivariable analysis ($P=0.55$). Major determinants of death in this very low-birth-weight population were antenatal diagnosis ($P=.01$), presence of congenital gastrointestinal defects ($P=.07$), or lesion type (all higher risk: anomalous pulmonary venous drainage, $P=.03$; pulmonary atresia and intact septum, $P=.05$; and truncus, $P=.01$).

*Conclusions.*—For very low-birth-weight neonates (<2.0 kg) with congenital heart defects, imposed delays in intervention neither compromise nor improve survival. Other factors instead appear to account for survival differences, including lesion type, associated noncardiac congenital defects, and antenatal diagnosis.

▶ For very low birth weight infants with serious congenital heart disease, a clinical dilemma exists: whether to pursue early and presumably higher-risk therapeutic intervention or to wait until the infant is more mature and heavier before performing a presumably lower-risk therapeutic intervention. This retrospective observational study suggests there is no advantage to delaying therapeutic intervention, because the survival rates for the early and delayed approach were not significantly different. In fact, the article contains additional data suggesting that there may be a disadvantage to delaying surgery. Prior to surgical intervention, 38% of the delayed cohort experienced a medical complication. After surgical intervention, the rates of medical complications were 33% and 50% for the usual and delayed intervention cohorts, respectively. Thus, although the overall survival for infants managed by the delayed strategy was not compromised, these infants experienced a significantly greater burden of medical morbidity and probably a higher rate of neurodevelopmental problems.

**L. A. Papile, MD**

---

**Complications After the Norwood Operation: An Analysis of the Society of Thoracic Surgeons Congenital Heart Surgery Database**
Hornik CP, He X, Jacobs JP, et al (Duke Univ School of Medicine, Durham, NC; Duke Univ Med Ctr, Durham, NC; Univ of South Florida College of Medicine, Tampa, FL; et al)
*Ann Thorac Surg* 92:1734-1741, 2011

---

*Background.*—Limited multicenter data exist regarding the prevalence of postoperative complications after the Norwood operation and their associated mortality risk.

*Methods.*—We evaluated infants in The Society of Thoracic Surgeons Congenital Heart Surgery Database who underwent the Norwood operation from 2000 to 2009. The prevalence of postoperative complications after the Norwood operation and associated in-hospital mortality were described. Patient factors associated with complications were evaluated in multivariable analyses.

*Results.*—A total of 2,557 patients from 53 centers were included. Median age at operation was 6 days (interquartile range, 4 to 9 days) and 90% had a right dominant ventricle. Overall mortality was 22%, and 75% had 1 complication or more. Mortality increased with increasing number of complications: 1 complication, 17%; 2 complications, 21%; 3 complications, 26%; 4 complications, 33%; and 5 or more complications, 45%. Renal and cardiovascular complications carried the greatest mortality risk. Patient factors associated with 1 complication or more included weight less than 2.5 kg (odds ratio [OR], 1.6; 95% confidence interval [CI], 1.2 to 2.1), single right versus single left ventricle (OR, 1.4; 95% CI, 1.01 to 2.0), preoperative shock (OR, 1.5; 95% CI, 1.1 to 2.1), non−cardiac/genetic abnormality (OR, 1.5; 95% CI, 1.2 to 1.9), and preoperative mechanical ventilatory (OR, 1.3; 95% CI, 1.03 to 1.6) or circulatory (OR 4.0; 95% CI, 1.6 to 10.2) support.

*Conclusions.*—Complications after the Norwood operation are common, carry significant mortality risk, and are associated with several preoperative patient characteristics. These data may aid in providing prognostic information to families and in guiding quality improvement initiatives.

▶ Improving survival and decreasing morbidity following surgical palliation for hypoplastic left heart syndrome (HLHS) over the past 2 to 3 decades have resulted in more favorable attitudes toward palliation and increasing reluctance to consider comfort care alone, particularly in the United States. In 2011, Murtuza and Elliott[1] reported results of a survey of 16 mostly European pediatric heart surgeons who were asked about their personal choices for management of HLHS if it were diagnosed in one of their own offspring. Remarkably, 75% indicated that they would opt for termination of pregnancy or comfort care after birth if the condition was recognized prenatally, and 50% would opt for comfort care if the diagnosis became apparent only after birth. By bringing quantitation to the subjective impressions of physicians who are closest to the realities of the Norwood palliation surgery, this analysis of outcomes reported to the Society of Thoracic Surgeons (STS) Congenital Heart Surgery Database (which includes results from nearly three-quarters of the centers in the United States where surgery for congenital heart disease is performed) may provide some explanation for this pessimistic assessment. Reviewing data for 2557 infants who had the Norwood procedure performed between 2000 and 2009, these authors document that complications after first-stage palliation are very common: 1906 infants (75%) had at least 1 complication; 584 (23%) had 1 complication, 388 (15%) had 2 complications, 310 (12%) had 3 complications, 212 (9%) had 4 complications, and 412 (16%) had 5 or more complications. Complications were strongly associated with the risk of death, with 27% of infants with any complication dying versus only 7% of those who did not have a complication (*P* < .0001). Thus, an uneventful postoperative course is the exception rather than the rule for these infants, and the postoperative period is likely to be difficult for both the infant and the parents. It is essential to communicate this to parents as they contemplate how to best care for an affected infant. Even with these data, the challenges of fully informing families about what they can expect in these very complex and challenging circumstances still seem nearly insurmountable.

**W. E. Benitz, MD**

*Reference*

1. Murtuza B, Elliott MJ. Changing attitudes to the management of hypoplastic left heart syndrome: a European perspective. *Cardiol Young.* 2011;21:148-158.

# 7 Respiratory Disorders

## Randomized Controlled Trial of Restrictive Fluid Management in Transient Tachypnea of the Newborn

Stroustrup A, Trasande L, Holzman IR (Kravis Children's Hosp, NY; Mount Sinai School of Medicine, NY)
*J Pediatr* 160:38-43.e1, 2012

*Objective.*—To determine the effect of mild fluid restriction on the hospital course of neonates with transient tachypnea of the newborn (TTN).

*Study Design.*—In this pilot prospective randomized controlled trial of 64 late preterm and term neonates diagnosed with TTN at a single tertiary care hospital in the United States, patients were randomized to receive standard fluid management or mild fluid restriction. The primary outcome was duration of respiratory support. Secondary outcomes were duration of admission to the intensive care unit, time to first enteral feed, and total and composite hospital costs. Results were analyzed by *t*-test, $\chi^2$ test, Kaplan-Meier estimation, and proportional hazards regression.

*Results.*—Fluid restriction did not cause adverse events or unsafe dehydration. Fluid management strategy did not affect primary or secondary outcomes in the total study population. Fluid restriction significantly reduced the duration of respiratory support ($P = .008$) and hospitalization costs ($P = .017$) in neonates with severe TTN.

*Conclusion.*—Mild fluid restriction appears to be safe in late preterm and term neonates with uncomplicated TTN. Fluid restriction may be of benefit in decreasing the duration of respiratory support and reducing hospitalization costs in term and late preterm neonates with uncomplicated severe TTN.

▶ Our understanding of the etiopathogenesis of transient tachypnea of the newborn (TTN) has improved substantially in the last 25 years. It is indeed more complex than what many of us were taught as medical students, that it resulted from an inadequate thoracic squeeze during delivery and was thus more common in infants delivered by cesarean section. Retention of fetal lung fluid occurs primarily as a consequence of delayed or inadequate ion channel clearance. Thus, these investigators hypothesized that restriction of fluid intake might promote faster resorption of lung fluid and speed resolution of the disease process. They designed a small, single-center trial to test their hypothesis and found a signal in infants deemed to have severe TTN. They related this to cost of care, and not surprisingly, they found differences favoring fluid restriction in this subset.

A closer look at the study, however, raises a number of questions. From an enrollment standpoint, it was unclear why tachypnea was not considered an element of respiratory distress. Hypoxia was defined as an oxygen saturation less than 95% of room air. The mode of respiratory support (and how it was managed) was determined by personal preference, rather than by protocol, and importantly, the study was not blinded, and thus the element of investigator bias cannot be excluded. This is especially important in evaluating the duration of treatments and the computation of cost analysis. The sample size calculated for this study was based on a presumed difference in the duration of respiratory support of 8 hours. Many would argue the lack of clinical significance in this difference, and the smaller the difference, the greater the likelihood of investigator bias.

The authors also proposed a classification system, based on their findings. However, these were based not on the actual severity of the respiratory distress, but rather were defined by the degree and duration of respiratory support, which was determined by physician preference. Thus, there is some circular logic involved.

The study is somewhat problematic.

It is reassuring that there were no apparent adverse events associated with the fluid restriction. Yet looking at the data, it is hard to find a biologic plausibility for the results.

**S. M. Donn, MD**

---

### Surfactant Deficiency in Transient Tachypnea of the Newborn

MacHado LU, Fiori HH, Baldisserotto M, et al (Centro Universitário Feevale, Novo Hamburgo, Brazil; Pontifícia Universidade Católica do Rio Grande do Sul, Porto Alegre, Brazil)
J Pediatr 159:750-754, 2011

---

*Objective.*—To evaluate surfactant production and function in term neonates with transient tachypnea of the newborn (TTN).

*Study Design.*—Samples of gastric aspirates collected within 30 minutes of birth from 42 term newborns with gestational age $\geq 37$ weeks (21 patients with TTN and 21 control subjects), delivered via elective cesarean delivery, were analyzed with lamellar body count and stable microbubble test.

*Results.*—Results of lamellar body counts and stable microbubble tests were significantly lower in the TTN group than in control subjects ($P = .004$ and .013, respectively). Lamellar body counts were significantly lower in infants with TTN requiring oxygen for $\geq 24$ hours after birth than in infants requiring oxygen for $< 24$ hours ($P = .029$). When the cutoff point was 48 hours, the stable microbubble count was significantly lower in the group requiring oxygen for $\geq 48$ hours than in the group requiring oxygen for $< 48$ hours ($P = .047$).

*Conclusions.*—Term infants with TTN had low lamellar body counts associated with decreased surfactant function, suggesting that prolonged disease is associated with surfactant abnormalities.

▶ Pulmonary surfactant replacement therapy seems to be good for what ails you. In addition to its use in treating respiratory distress syndrome, surfactant has been given to infants with meconium aspiration syndrome, pneumonia, congenital diaphragmatic hernia, pulmonary edema, bronchopulmonary dysplasia, and transient tachypnea of the newborn. From a theoretical standpoint, these conditions may be characterized by either surfactant deficiency or surfactant inhibition or inactivation, so repletion is logical, even if evidence may be lacking.

This study examined the role of surfactant deficiency in the pathogenesis of transient tachypnea of the newborn (TTN). Forty-two infants delivered by elective cesarean section at term were included in the analysis; 21 had clinical and radiologic signs consistent with TTN and were compared with a matched group of 21 controls without TTN. Surfactant deficiency was determined by lamellar body counts and a stable microbubble test performed on gastric aspirate samples. The results suggest that surfactant deficiency or dysfunction is indeed associated with TTN, especially in prolonged disease.

Before we all rush to replete our patients with exogenous surfactant, it would be nice to see a randomized trial performed to test the hypothesis generated by this interesting observation.

**S. M. Donn, MD**

## Randomized Trial Comparing 3 Approaches to the Initial Respiratory Management of Preterm Neonates

Dunn MS, for the Vermont Oxford Network DRM Study Group (Univ of Toronto, Ontario, Canada; et al)
*Pediatrics* 128:e1069-e1076, 2011

*Objective.*—We designed a multicenter randomized trial to compare 3 approaches to the initial respiratory management of preterm neonates: prophylactic surfactant followed by a period of mechanical ventilation (prophylactic surfactant [PS]); prophylactic surfactant with rapid extubation to bubble nasal continuous positive airway pressure (intubate-surfactant-extubate [ISX]) or initial management with bubble continuous positive airway pressure and selective surfactant treatment (nCPAP).

*Designs/Methods.*—Neonates born at $26 0/7$ to $29 6/7$ weeks' gestation were enrolled at participating Vermont Oxford Network centers and randomly assigned to PS, ISX, or nCPAP groups before delivery. Primary outcome was the incidence of death or bronchopulmonary dysplasia (BPD) at 36 weeks' postmenstrual age.

*Results.*—648 infants enrolled at 27 centers. The study was halted before the desired sample size was reached because of declining enrollment. When compared with the PS group, the relative risk of BPD or death was 0.78

(95% confidence interval: 0.59–1.03) for the ISX group and 0.83 (95% confidence interval: 0.64–1.09) for the nCPAP group. There were no statistically significant differences in mortality or other complications of prematurity. In the nCPAP group, 48% were managed without intubation and ventilation, and 54% without surfactant treatment.

Conclusions.—Preterm neonates were initially managed with either nCPAP or PS with rapid extubation to nCPAP had similar clinical outcomes to those treated with PS followed by a period of mechanical ventilation. An approach that uses early nCPAP leads to a reduction in the number of infants who are intubated and given surfactant.

▶ Unlike pharmacotherapeutic trials for preterm infants, comparative studies using various ventilatory strategies have been difficult, if not impossible, to blind. This is a big challenge in interpreting the results of such studies, as idiosyncratic ventilator strategies vary widely and clearly impact outcome. It is therefore very reassuring that there is great consistency in the results of recent studies comparing initial prophylactic surfactant versus initial continuous positive airway pressure (CPAP)–based strategies for very low birth weight infants. The most recent trial, conducted by the Vermont-Oxford Network Study Group led by Michael Dunn from Toronto, provides confirmation that an early elective CPAP-based approach provides comparable outcome, defined as a composite of bronchopulmonary dysplasia and death, to prophylactic early surfactant followed by rapid extubation.[1] Such an approach eliminates the need for subsequent intubation in approximately 50% of infants at 26 0/7 to 29 6/7 weeks' gestation, with an accompanying reduction in surfactant use and presumptive cost saving.

These findings certainly represent a shift from the widespread strategy of a decade earlier when prophylactic early surfactant therapy was widely practiced, and any delay in surfactant administration was frowned upon.[1] Unfortunately, there is still a subpopulation of preterm infants who will benefit maximally from early surfactant, and we do not yet have a good biomarker (clinical, physiologic, or biochemical) to identify this group. In other words, some high risk neonates will need exogenous surfactant therapy; significant delay in its administration may do them a disservice. It is always unfortunate when a trial such as this one is prematurely terminated for declining enrollment. However, given prior and concurrent studies, it is unlikely that group differences in major outcomes would have emerged. It is of interest that bubble CPAP was consistently used as the initial CPAP-based strategy. With the proliferation of CPAP-based strategies in neonatal care, it becomes all the more imperative to identify which mode of CPAP delivery is optimal in this population.

**R. J. Martin, MD**

*Reference*

1. Soll RF, Morley CJ. Prophylactic versus selective use of surfactant in preventing morbidity and mortality in preterm infants. *Cochrane Database Syst Rev.* 2001; (2):CD000510.

Randomized Trial Comparing 3 Approaches to the Initial Respiratory Management of Preterm Neonates

Dunn MS, for the Vermont Oxford Network DRM Study Group (Univ of Toronto, Ontario, Canada; et al)

*Pediatrics* 128:e1069-e1076, 2011

*Objective.*—We designed a multicenter randomized trial to compare 3 approaches to the initial respiratory management of preterm neonates: prophylactic surfactant followed by a period of mechanical ventilation (prophylactic surfactant [PS]); prophylactic surfactant with rapid extubation to bubble nasal continuous positive airway pressure (intubate-surfactant-extubate [ISX]) or initial management with bubble continuous positive airway pressure and selective surfactant treatment (nCPAP).

*Design/Methods.*—Neonates born at 26 0/7 to 29 6/7 weeks' gestation were enrolled at participating Vermont Oxford Network centers and randomly assigned to PS, ISX, or nCPAP groups before delivery. Primary outcome was the incidence of death or bronchopulmonary dysplasia (BPD) at 36 weeks' postmenstrual age.

*Results.*—648 infants enrolled at 27 centers. The study was halted before the desired sample size was reached because of declining enrollment. When compared with the PS group, the relative risk of BPD or death was 0.78 (95% confidence interval: 0.59–1.03) for the ISX group and 0.83 (95% confidence interval: 0.64–1.09) for the nCPAP group. There were no statistically significant differences in mortality or other complications of prematurity. In the nCPAP group, 48% were managed without intubation and ventilation, and 54% without surfactant treatment.

*Conclusions.*—Preterm neonates were initially managed with either nCPAP or PS with rapid extubation to nCPAP had similar clinical outcomes to those treated with PS followed by a period of mechanical ventilation. An approach that uses early nCPAP leads to a reduction in the number of infants who are intubated and given surfactant.

▶ Most neonates less than 30 weeks' gestational age require some form of respiratory support. This article, like the recently published SUPPORT trial,[1] shows that early nasal continuous positive airway pressure (CPAP) with selective surfactant use, compared with management with early intubation, surfactant administration, and continuous positive pressure ventilation, results in fewer infants ever receiving surfactant or requiring mechanical ventilation. Both of these randomized controlled trials also demonstrated no differences in morbidity or mortality rates between these strategies. This article adds another strategy not evaluated in the SUPPORT trial: intubation, surfactant, and rapid extubation if the infant remained clinically stable. In this group, surfactant use, but not use of mechanical ventilation, was more frequent than in the early CPAP group. The morbidity and mortality rates were generally not different. However, fewer infants in the intubate-surfactant-extubate group had a patent ductus arteriosus (PDA) as compared with both other groups (odds ratio [OR] 0.62; 95% confidence interval [CI] 0.42–0.92 vs early CPAP and OR 0.66; 95% CI, 0.44–0.97

vs early surfactant, respectively). There also were significantly lower rates of severe retinopathy of prematurity (ROP) compared to the early CPAP group (OR 0.31; 95% CI, 0.11–0.93). However, despite its potential significance, the authors do not present an analysis or comment on this difference in PDA and ROP rates.

There were several limitations to this study. First, although the study was randomized, it was not blinded, possibly leading to bias in decision making around surfactant use. Second, 55% of infants came from 3 of the 27 contributing centers; if these 3 centers also happened to be those with the most (or least) CPAP experience, then study results might be significantly skewed. Third, the study was stopped after 74% of the desired sample size was recruited due to difficulty with enrollment, although the specifics of these difficulties are unknown.

Despite these shortcomings, this study clearly supports the current trend toward initially trialing infants on nasal CPAP with surfactant administration only if clinically indicated. In addition, trials such as reported in this article and the SUPPORT trial demonstrate the feasibility of studies designed to address the complex question of how to manage respiratory support in infants less than 30 weeks' gestational age.

**W. E. Benitz, MD**

*Reference*

1. SUPPORT Study Group of the Eunice Kennedy Shriver NICHD Neonatal Research Network, Finer NN, Carlo WA, Walsh MC, et al. Early CPAP versus surfactant in extremely preterm infants. *N Engl J Med.* 2010;362:1970-1979.

**Avoidance of mechanical ventilation by surfactant treatment of spontaneously breathing preterm infants (AMV): an open-label, randomised, controlled trial**
Göpel W, on behalf of the German Neonatal Network (Univ of Lübeck, Germany; et al)
*Lancet* 378:1627-1634, 2011

*Background.*—Surfactant is usually given to mechanically ventilated preterm infants via an endotracheal tube to treat respiratory distress syndrome. We tested a new method of surfactant application to spontaneously breathing preterm infants to avoid mechanical ventilation.

*Method.*—In a parallel-group, randomised controlled trial, 220 preterm infants with a gestational age between 26 and 28 weeks and a birthweight less than 1·5 kg were enrolled in 12 German neonatal intensive care units. Infants were independently randomised in a 1:1 ratio with variable block sizes, to standard treatment or intervention, and randomisation was stratified according to centre and multiple birth status. Masking was not possible. Infants were stabilised with continuous positive airway pressure and received rescue intubation if necessary. In the intervention group, infants received surfactant treatment during spontaneous breathing via a thin catheter inserted into the trachea by laryngoscopy if they needed a fraction of inspired oxygen more than 0·30. The primary endpoint was need for any mechanical ventilation, or being not ventilated but having a partial pressure of carbon dioxide more than 65 mm Hg (8·6 kPa) or a fraction of inspired oxygen more than 0·60, or both, for more than 2 h between 25 h and 72 h of age. Analysis was by intention to treat. This study is registered, number ISRCTN05025922.

*Findings.*—108 infants were assigned to the intervention group and 112 infants to the standard treatment group. All infants were analysed. On day 2 or 3 after birth, 30 (28%) infants in the intervention group were mechanically ventilated versus 51 (46%) in the standard treatment group (number needed to treat 6, 95% CI 3—20, absolute risk reduction 0·18, 95% CI 0·30—0·05, $p = 0·008$). 36 (33%) infants in the intervention group were mechanically ventilated during their stay in the hospital compared with 82 (73%) in the standard treatment group (number needed to treat: 3, 95% CI 2—4, $p < 0·0001$). The intervention group had significantly fewer median days on mechanical ventilation, (0 days. IQR 0—3 *vs* 2 days, 0—5) and a lower need for oxygen therapy at 28 days (30 infants [30%] *vs* 49 infants [45%], $p = 0·032$) compared with the standard treatment group. We recorded no differences between groups for mortality (seven deaths in the intervention group vs five in the standard treatment group) and serious adverse events (21 *vs* 28).

*Interpretation.*—The application of surfactant via a thin catheter to spontaneously breathing preterm infants receiving continuous positive airway pressure reduces the need for mechanical ventilation.

▶ Surfactant therapy has been an integral component of neonatal intensive care for more than 20 years. In addition to reducing mortality, ongoing studies confirm that surfactant replacement therapy reduces oxygen and mechanical ventilation requirements as well as the severity of respiratory distress syndrome (RDS). It also reduces pulmonary air leaks and interstitial pulmonary emphysema. It has been administered successfully to both preterm infants with RDS as well as term infants with pneumonia, meconium aspiration syndrome, and congenital diaphragmatic hernia. The search for better surfactants and means of delivery of surfactant without the need for intubation continues. It is thus encouraging to note that the German multicenter trial led by Göpel demonstrated the ability to successfully deliver surfactant through a small tube into infants breathing spontaneously on continuous positive airway pressure (CPAP). Fewer infants treated this way ultimately required any mechanical ventilation. The switch in current practice to more liberal use of CPAP even for infants as young as 25 weeks' gestation makes such an application highly desirable.[1] Of course, validation of this technique in larger trials is necessary before this approach becomes more widely used.

Intrapartum pharyngeal instillation of surfactant before the first breath may result in surfactant administration to the infant lung, with the potential benefit of avoiding endotracheal intubation and ventilation, ventilator-induced lung injury, and bronchopulmonary dysplasia. To date, there are only observational human studies that suggest that the technique is feasible and safe. But there have been no randomized trials. Well-designed trials are needed.[2] Other means of surfactant administration, including aerosolized products, have yet to be proven effective.

On the new surfactant front, the US Food and Drug Administration has approved SURFAXIN (lucinactant) for the prevention of RDS in premature infants at high risk for RDS. SURFAXIN is the first synthetic, peptide-containing surfactant approved for use in neonatal medicine. It contains a peptide that mimics the action of surfactant protein B. Its role will have to be established.

**A. A. Fanaroff, MBBCh, FRCPE**

*References*

1. SUPPORT Study Group of the Eunice Kennedy Shriver NICHD Neonatal Research Network, Finer NN, Carlo WA, Walsh MC, et al. Early CPAP versus surfactant in extremely preterm infants. *N Engl J Med.* 2010;362:1970-1979.
2. Abdel-Latif ME, Osborn DA. Pharyngeal instillation of surfactant before the first breath for prevention of morbidity and mortality in preterm infants at risk of respiratory distress syndrome. *Cochrane Database Syst Rev.* 2011;(3):CD008311.

---

**Mortality in preterm infants with respiratory distress syndrome treated with poractant alfa, calfactant or beractant: a retrospective study**
Ramanathan R, Bhatia JJ, Sekar K, et al (LAC+USC Med Ctr and Children's Hosp Los Angeles, CA; Georgia Health Sciences Univ, Augusta; Univ of Oklahoma Health Sciences Center; et al)
*J Perinatol* 1-7, 2011

---

*Objective.*—The objective of this study is to compare all-cause in-hospital mortality in preterm infants with respiratory distress syndrome (RDS) treated with poractant alfa, calfactant or beractant.

*Study Design.*—A retrospective cohort study of 14 173 preterm infants with RDS, treated with one of three surfactants between 2005 and 2009, using the Premier Database was done. Multilevel, multivariable logistic regression modeling, adjusting for patient- and hospital-level factors was performed.

*Result.*—Calfactant treatment was associated with a 49.6% greater likelihood of death than poractant alfa (odds ratio (OR): 1.496, 95% confidence interval (CI): 1.014–2.209, $P = 0.043$). Beractant treatment was associated with a non-significant 37% increase in mortality, compared with poractant alfa (OR: 1.370, 95% CI: 0.996–1.885, $P = 0.053$). No differences in mortality were observed between calfactant and beractant treatment (OR: 1.092, 95% CI: 0.765–1.559, $P = 0.626$).

*Conclusion.*—Poractant alfa treatment for RDS was associated with a significantly reduced likelihood of death when compared with calfactant and a trend toward reduced mortality when compared with beractant.

▶ In the late 1980s, surfactant therapy for the prevention and treatment of neonatal respiratory disorders was available only for subjects participating in rigorous randomized trials. Only then was surfactant available for general use with immediate reduction noted in mortality and air leak syndromes. As noted by Moya, there are now a variety of surfactants available for use, but the comparative trials of these agents have not been as well-controlled, nor is there compelling evidence that 1 product is superior to the others. Indeed the outcomes are very similar.

The US Food and Drug Administration finally approved SURFAXIN (lucinactant) in March 2012 for the prevention of respiratory distress syndrome in premature infants at high risk for this disease. It is the first synthetic, peptide-containing surfactant approved for use in neonatal medicine and is expected to be commercially available in the United States in late 2012. It remains to be proven that the synthetic surfactant is superior to the animal-based products currently in vogue.

**A. A. Fanaroff, MBBCh, FRCPE**

---

## Preliminary evaluation of a new technique of minimally invasive surfactant therapy

Dargaville PA, Aiyappan A, Cornelius A, et al (Royal Hobart Hosp and Univ of Tasmania, Australia)
*Arch Dis Child Fetal Neonatal Ed* 96:F243-F248, 2011

---

*Objective.*—To investigate a method of minimally invasive surfactant therapy (MIST) to be used in spontaneously breathing preterm infants on continuous positive airway pressure (CPAP), evaluating the feasibility of the technique and the therapeutic benefit after MIST.

*Design.*—Non-randomised feasibility study.

*Setting.*—Tertiary neonatal intensive care unit.

*Patients and Interventions.*—Study subjects were preterm infants with respiratory distress supported with CPAP, with early enrolment of 25–28-week infants (n = 11) at any CPAP pressure and fractional inspired $O_2$ concentration ($FiO_2$), and enrolment of 29–34-week infants (n = 14) at CPAP pressure $\geq 7$ cm $H_2O$ and $FiO_2 \geq 0.35$. Without premedication, a 16 gauge vascular catheter was inserted through the vocal cords under direct vision. Porcine surfactant ($\sim 100$ mg/kg) was then instilled, followed by reinstitution of CPAP.

*Measurements and Results.*—Respiratory indices were documented for 4 h following MIST, and neonatal outcomes ascertained. In all cases, surfactant was successfully administered and CPAP re-established. Coughing (32%) and bradycardia (44%) were transiently noted, and 44% received positive pressure inflations. There was a clear surfactant effect, with lower $FiO_2$ after MIST (pre-MIST: $0.39 \pm 0.092$ (mean $\pm$ SD); 4 h: $0.26 \pm 0.093$; $p < 0.01$), and a modest reduction in CPAP pressure. Adverse outcomes were few: intubation within 72 h (n = 3), pneumothorax (n = 1), chronic lung disease (n = 3) and death (n = 1), all in the 25–28-week group. Outcome was otherwise favourable in both gestation groups, with a trend towards reduction in intubation in the first 72 h in the 25—28-week infants compared with historical controls.

*Conclusions.*—Surfactant can be effectively delivered via a vascular catheter, and this method of MIST deserves further investigation.

▶ Dargaville and colleagues report the results of a feasibility trial in which preterm infants with respiratory distress syndrome, managed with continuous positive airway pressure (CPAP), were given surfactant through a 16-gauge vascular catheter inserted into the trachea under direct laryngoscopy. After instillation of surfactant, the infants were returned to CPAP therapy. Complications of surfactant administration included coughing or gagging, reflux of surfactant, bradycardia, and need for positive pressure mask ventilation. Infants demonstrated a response to treatment similar to what occurs with surfactant administration by endotracheal intubation, with a reduction in the fraction of inspired oxygen and the ability to wean mean airway pressure (CPAP).

The authors named this method MIST (minimally invasive surfactant therapy). This should not, however, be confused with administration of aerosolized surfactant, given by nasal CPAP and reported by Finer et al.[1] Moreover, laryngoscopy and intubation with the catheter were electively performed without pretreatment with sedative or analgesic agents.

Although the catheter is smaller than a standard endotracheal tube, labeling it as minimally invasive may be an overstatement. Certainly, endotracheal intubation has been associated with the release of inflammatory mediators, so it would have been a nice addition to this pilot trial to have obtained such data. In essence, the trial design mimics the INSURE protocol that is widely in use in which infants are transiently intubated, given surfactant, and extubated. Are we merely trying to build a better mousetrap?

**S. M. Donn, MD**

*Reference*

1. Finer NN, Merritt TA, Bernstein G, Job L, Mazela J, Segal R. An open label, pilot study of Aerosurf® combined with nCPAP to prevent RDS in preterm neonates. *J Aerosol Med Pulm Drug Deliv.* 2010;23:303-309.

---

**Mortality in preterm infants with respiratory distress syndrome treated with poractant alfa, calfactant or beractant: a retrospective study**
Ramanathan R, Bhatia JJ, Sekar K, et al (LAC+USC Med Ctr and Children's Hosp Los Angeles, CA; Georgia Health Sciences Univ, Augusta; Univ of Oklahoma Health Sciences Ctr; et al)
*J Perinatol* 1-7, 2011

*Objective.*—The objective of this study is to compare all-cause in-hospital mortality in preterm infants with respiratory distress syndrome (RDS) treated with poractant alfa, calfactant or beractant.

*Study Design.*—A retrospective cohort study of 14 173 preterm infants with RDS, treated with one of three surfactants between 2005 and 2009, using the Premier Database was done. Multilevel, multivariable logistic regression modeling, adjusting for patient- and hospital-level factors was performed.

*Result.*—Calfactant treatment was associated with a 49.6% greater likelihood of death than poractant alfa (odds ratio (OR): 1.496, 95% confidence interval (CI): 1.014−2.209, *P* = 0.043). Beractant treatment was associated with a non-significant 37% increase in mortality, compared with poractant alfa (OR: 1.370, 95% CI: 0.996−1.885, *P* = 0.053). No differences in mortality were observed between calfactant and beractant treatment (OR: 1.092, 95% CI: 0.765−1.559, *P* = 0.626).

*Conclusion.*—Poractant alfa treatment for RDS was associated with a significantly reduced likelihood of death when compared with calfactant and a trend toward reduced mortality when compared with beractant.

▶ All commercially available surfactants improve the outcome of preterm infants although differing in composition and administration method. The quest for which of these surfactants is better is ongoing. Ramanathan et al report interesting data, but with major shortcomings, primarily from its retrospective nature and potential selection bias. It is unclear why data from only 236 hospitals out of 600 reporting to the Premier Database were selected for study. Moreover, even though the authors attempted to control for certain characteristics, too many variables that have been shown in randomized trials or systematic reviews to markedly influence survival and morbidity were omitted, including the use of antenatal steroids, inborn/outborn status, prophylactic versus later administration, and the number of doses used, among others.[1]

To date there are no published randomized trials comparing poractant and calfactant. The study by Ramanathan does not add any relevant information regarding this comparison. Fortunately, there are several published randomized comparisons of poractant and beractant. A recent systematic review examined 5 of those trials and concluded that administering the higher dose of poractant (200 mg phospholipid/kg) significantly reduced death and the need for redosing compared with beractant, which is given at a lower dose (100 mg/kg).[2] Another study that did not show any major outcome differences and was larger than most of the included studies was not incorporated in the systematic review since it used quasi-randomization.[3] A recently published trial comparing poractant and beractant reported differences in oxygenation, but not in mortality.[4] This notwithstanding, it appears that a higher phospholipid dose may have important clinical benefits, because a randomized trial of the new-generation synthetic surfactant lucinactant, which provides 175 mg phospholipid/kg per dose in addition to a synthetic peptide that mimics surfactant protein B (SP-B), also reported a survival advantage over beractant.[5] This biologic plausibility needs to be tempered by the fact that the amount of SP-B, a key determinant of surfactant action, is quite different among surfactants including lucinactant. Among animal-derived surfactants, calfactant contains the highest amount of SP-B.

Whether any of these differences between surfactants are relevant when the care of preterm infants with respiratory distress syndrome is becoming less invasive is unclear. Nonetheless, as we move forward, improvements in neonatal care need to remain true to the principle that the best available evidence still comes from well-designed randomized trials and not from retrospective studies.

**F. Moya, MD**

*References*

1. Soll R. Early versus delayed selective surfactant treatment for neonatal respiratory distress syndrome. *Cochrane Database Syst Rev.* 1999;(4):CD001456.
2. Singh N, Hawley KL, Viswanathan K. Efficacy of porcine versus bovine surfactants for preterm newborns with respiratory distress syndrome: systematic review and meta-analysis. *Pediatrics.* 2011;128:e1588-e1595.
3. Gharehbaghi MM, Sakha SH, Ghojazadeh M, Firoozi F. Complications among premature neonates treated with beractant and poractant alfa. *Indian J Pediatr.* 2010;77:751-754.
4. Dizdar EA, Sari FN, Aydemir C, et al. A randomized, controlled trial of poractant alfa versus beractant in the treatment of preterm infants with respiratory distress syndrome. *Am J Perinatol.* 2012;29:95-100.
5. Moya FR, Gadzinowski J, Bancalari E, et al. A multicenter, randomized, masked, comparison trial of lucinactant, colfosceril palmitate, and beractant for the prevention of respiratory distress syndrome among very preterm infants. *Pediatrics.* 2005; 115:1018-1029.

---

## Nasal Continuous Positive Airway Pressure With Heliox in Preterm Infants With Respiratory Distress Syndrome

Colnaghi M, Pierro M, Migliori C, et al (Universitá degli Studi di Milano, Italy; Spedali Civili Hosp, Brescia, Italy; et al)
*Pediatrics* 129:e333-e338, 2012

*Objective.*—To assess the therapeutic effects of breathing a low-density helium and oxygen mixture (heliox, 80% helium and 20% oxygen) in premature infants with respiratory distress syndrome (RDS) treated with nasal continuous positive airway pressure (NCPAP).

*Methods.*—Infants born between 28 and 32 weeks of gestational age with radiologic findings and clinical symptoms of RDS and requiring respiratory support with NCPAP within the first hour of life were included. These infants were randomly assigned to receive either standard medical air (control group) or a 4:1 helium and oxygen mixture (heliox group) during the first 12 hours of enrollment, followed by medical air until NCPAP was no longer needed.

*Results.*—From February 2008 to September 2010, 51 newborn infants were randomly assigned to two groups, 24 in the control group and 27 in the heliox group. NCPAP with heliox significantly decreased the risk of mechanical ventilation in comparison with NCPAP with medical air (14.8% vs 45.8%).

*Conclusions.*—Heliox increases the effectiveness of NCPAP in the treatment of RDS in premature infants.

▶ In this small pilot trial, 51 infants between 28 and 32 weeks' gestation with respiratory distress syndrome (RDS) were randomly selected to receive nasal continuous positive airway pressure (NCPAP) using either standard medical gas or heliox (20% oxygen/80% helium) for 12 hours "to test the efficacy, safety, and feasibility of using heliox to reduce the need for mechanical ventilation." Unfortunately, the study design does not enable me to be convinced that heliox treatment does any of these.

The sample size was chosen on the premise that 65% of enrolled infants would not respond to CPAP and require mechanical ventilation. This figure is much higher than that reported in the literature. Infants were selected for enrollment based on the antiquated Silverman score, a need for greater than 25% oxygen to maintain $SpO_2$ from 88% to 95%, and positive radiologic findings. Objective data to assess the degree of respiratory dysfunction are not provided, and this is a major weakness. Because the authors wrote that "helium decreases the pressure required to move gases to the periphery of the lung and enhances gas exchange in the distal airways," it is important to know the degree of impaired gas exchange at the outset, and thus some measure of gas exchange (A-aDO2 or A/a ratio) should have been included. On the whole, the babies in this trial do not appear to be particularly ill.

Randomization was stratified by gestational age, but data analyses were not. Although randomization was blinded, it is not clear how the actual administration of gas was blinded, since heliox was contained in large cylinders. This is critical, since the decision to intubate and ventilate was the primary outcome measure. Treatment lasted 12 hours, but need for mechanical ventilation was assessed for 7 days. Is there a biological plausibility for some immediate effect of heliox in preventing a later need for mechanical ventilation?

The authors do address the considerable expense involved. The 12-hour treatment cost is approximately $1000 per patient. Thus, a longer course would ensure it to be the most expensive respiratory therapy in the neonatal intensive care unit.

Interpretation of the data was also a bit fuzzy; no statistically significant differences were found in $FiO_2$, $SpO_2$, or blood pressure, yet the investigators saw a positive trend. They cite a total duration of NCPAP of $26 \pm 37$ days in the heliox group, versus $33 \pm 6$ days in the control group, but the data for the heliox group are not normally distributed, and the $P$ value was .681. Does this convince you? Additionally, almost 20% of infants assigned to heliox were small-for-gestational age versus 8% of controls.

Pilot trials of new drugs or devices do play an important role in the evolution of care. However, they need to be done meticulously and have a limited focus, and care needs to be taken to avoid overstatement of the results.

**S. M. Donn, MD**

---

**Positive effects of early continuous positive airway pressure on pulmonary function in extremely premature infants: results of a subgroup analysis of the COIN trial**

Roehr CC, Proquitté H, Hammer H, et al (Charité Universitätsmedizin Berlin, Germany; et al)

*Arch Dis Child Fetal Neonatal Ed* 96:F371-F373, 2011

---

*Objective.*—Early continuous positive airway pressure (CPAP) may reduce lung injury in preterm infants.

*Patients and Methods.*—Spontaneously breathing preterm infants were randomised immediately after birth to nasal CPAP or intubation, surfactant treatment and mechanical ventilation. Pulmonary function tests approximately 8 weeks post-term determined tidal breathing parameters, respiratory mechanics and functional residual capacity (FRC).

*Results.*—Seventeen infants received CPAP and 22 mechanical ventilation. Infants with early CPAP had less mechanical ventilation (4 vs 7.5 days; $p = 0.004$) and less total respiratory support (30 vs 47 days; $p = 0.017$). Postterm the CPAP group had lower respiratory rate (41 vs 48/min; $p = 0.007$), lower minute ventilation (223 vs 265 ml/min/kg; $p = 0.009$), better respiratory compliance (0.99 vs 0.82 ml/cm $H_2O$/kg; $p = 0.008$) and improved elastic work of breathing ($p = 0.004$). No differences in FRC were found.

*Conclusions.*—Early CPAP is feasible, shortens the duration of respiratory support and results in improved lung mechanics and decreased work of breathing.

▶ This article reports on a subgroup analysis of 39 of the 610 infants enrolled in the Continuous Positive Airway Pressure or Intubation at Birth (COIN) randomized clinical trial of nasal continuous positive airway pressure (nCPAP) versus mechanical ventilation for respiratory failure in very preterm infants[1] who underwent pulmonary function testing at approximately 8 weeks' postterm. Comparison of 17 infants randomized to nCPAP and 22 who were treated with mechanical ventilation showed among nCPAP-treated infants, in addition to shorter duration of mechanical and total respiratory support, improved markers of pulmonary function, including respiratory compliance and elastic work of breathing. The observation of a statistically significant effect in such a small sample of subjects suggests the population benefits in improved pulmonary function associated with early nCPAP are likely to be substantial. The COIN trial investigated the impact of nCPAP on bronchopulmonary dysplasia (BPD), a disorder with multifactorial origins and a continuum of severity. Pulmonary benefits of various proposed preventive therapies are likely to be incremental with none offering "silver bullet" potential to eradicate BPD. Some readers and clinicians dismissed the COIN study results published in 2008[1] as indicating "early nCPAP does not work." This secondary study of a subset of COIN study subjects underscores the importance of looking beyond the primary outcomes of large randomized clinical trials and using secondary analyses and linked research initiatives to gain better understanding of the benefits, risks, and variability in response associated with a particular therapeutic approach.

**L. J. Van Marter, MD, MPH**

*Reference*

1. Morley CJ, Davis PG, Doyle LW, Brion LP, Hascoet JM, Carlin JB. Nasal CPAP or intubation at birth for very preterm infants. *N Engl J Med.* 2008;358:700-708.

**Predictors of early nasal CPAP failure and effects of various intubation criteria on the rate of mechanical ventilation in preterm infants of <29 weeks gestational age**

Fuchs H, Lindner W, Leiprecht A, et al (Univ Children's Hosp, Ulm, Germany)
*Arch Dis Child Fetal Neonatal Ed* 96:F343-F347, 2011

*Introduction.*—Delivery room management using early nasal continuous positive airway pressure (nCPAP) may delay surfactant therapy. *Objective.*—To identify factors associated with early nCPAP failure and effects of various intubation criteria on rate and time of intubation. *Design.*—Retrospective analysis of the first 48 h in infants of 23–28 weeks gestational age (GA) treated with sustained inflations followed by early nCPAP.

*Results.*—Of 225 infants (GA 26.2 ± 1.6 weeks) 140 (62%) could be stabilised with nCPAP in the delivery room, of whom 68 (49%; GA 26.9 ± 1.5 weeks) succeeded on nCPAP with favourable outcome and 72 infants (51%; GA 26.3 ± 1.4 weeks) failed nCPAP within 48 h at a median (IQR) age of 5.6 (3.3–19.3) h. History or initial blood gases were poor predictors of subsequent nCPAP failure. Intubation at fraction of inspired oxygen (FiO$_2$)≥0.35 versus 0.4 versus 0.45 instead of ≥0.6 would have resulted in unnecessary intubations of 16% versus 9% versus 6% of infants with nCPAP success but decreased the age at intubation of infants with nCPAP failure to 3.1 (2.2–5.2) versus 3.8 (2.5–8.7) versus 4.4 (2.7–10.9) h. *Conclusions.*—Medical history or initial blood gas values are poor predictors of subsequent nCPAP failure. A threshold FiO$_2$ of ≥0.35–0.45 compared to ≥0.6 for intubation would shorten the time to surfactant delivery without a relevant increase in intubation rate. An individualised approach with a trial of early nCPAP and prompt intubation and surfactant treatment at low thresholds may be the best approach in very low birthweight infants.

▶ Clinical decision making in neonatology, as much as or more than many fields of medicine, involves assessing the risk/benefit ratios of competing therapeutic options. This report by Fuchs and colleagues addresses the challenge of achieving optimal balance between offering an extremely preterm infant the benefits of noninvasive respiratory support versus the downsides of delaying surfactant treatment or needed mechanical support. In this study population, 140 of 225 infants born before 29 weeks' gestation could be stabilized with delivery room (DR) nasal continuous positive airway pressure (nCPAP) administered after several sustained inflations; 49% required no intubation with favorable outcome. Although the success rate was inversely proportional to gestational age, even the youngest babies had greater success with nCPAP when nCPAP was initiated in the DR. The authors found that medical history and initial blood gases did not predict respiratory failure. On the other hand, intubation and surfactant administration were delayed in those who ultimately did not respond to nCPAP and required intubation. The authors note that decreasing the fraction of inspired oxygen limit at which the infant qualifies for intubation from 0.45 to 0.35 would result in a 16% increase in unnecessary intubations yet would reduce the delay in mechanical ventilation and surfactant treatment by approximately 1 hour (from 4 to 3 hours of age). These data will be useful to neonatal caregivers seeking to establish programs that expand the population of infants eligible for initiation of nCPAP in the DR and simultaneously ensure that needed intubations occur without undue delay.

**L. J. Van Marter, MD, MPH**

---

### Early prediction of nasal continuous positive airway pressure failure in preterm infants less than 30 weeks gestation

De Jaegere AP, van der Lee JH, Canté C, et al (Emma Children's Hosp AMC, Amsterdam, The Netherlands)
*Acta Paediatr* 101:374-379, 2012

---

*Aim.*—To predict early nasal continuous positive airway pressure failure within the first 2 h after birth in preterm infants.

*Methods.*—Patient and respiratory support variables significantly associated with continuous positive airway pressure failure in the first 72 h after birth were identified in a cohort of preterm infants < 30 weeks gestation. Using multivariable logistic regression analysis, risk estimates for early nasal continuous positive airway pressure failure were calculated.

*Results.*—From 182 infants included, 62 (34%) failed early nasal continuous positive airway pressure. Birth weight $\leq 800$ g, male gender and a fraction of inspired oxygen $> 0.25$ at 1 and 2 h of age were significantly associated with early nasal continuous positive airway pressure failure. Combining these variables in a logistic regression model provided a minimal risk estimate for failure of 0.04 [0.01−0.23] (female >800 g, $FiO_2 \leq 0.25$ at 1, and 2 h) and maximal estimate of 0.92 [0.44−0.99] (male $\leq 800$ g, $FiO_2$ $> 0.25$ at 1 and 2 h).

*Conclusion.*—Combining gender, birth weight and the fraction of inspired oxygen at 1 and 2 h of age allows for a better and more individualized prediction of early nasal continuous positive airway pressure failure in preterm infants less than 30 weeks gestation.

▶ This study addresses a very important—and controversial—area of neonatal respiratory care: the ability to predict which babies less than 30 weeks' gestation will fail an initial attempt of nasal continuous positive airway pressure (CPAP) to treat respiratory distress syndrome (RDS). Since more clinicians are embracing a noninvasive approach to the treatment of RDS, this must be balanced against the advantages of early versus later surfactant administration. In this historical cohort study, which included 182 infants, 34% failed CPAP. Birth weight of less than 800 g, male gender, and fraction of inspired oxygen ($FiO_2$) greater than 0.25 at 1 and 2 hours of age were significant in the univariate logistic regression. In the subsequent multivariable model, minimal risk of failure was found for female infants greater than 800 g with $FiO_2$ less than or equal to 0.25 at 1 and 2 hours and maximal risk of failure for male infants less than 800 g with $FiO_2$ 0.25 at 1 and 2 hours.

The authors concluded that a more individualized approach to management is possible using gender, birth weight, and $FiO_2$ at 1 and 2 hours as the determinant variables. As others have found, lower birth weight and gestational age do predict early CPAP failure.

As a cautionary note, before we all embrace this model, we must realize that (1) this was a retrospective study and thus may have had a selection bias, and (2) the population studied is very homogeneous, and all were managed under a relatively rigorous protocol. Whether the conclusion will be exportable to a heterogeneous population subjected to different schemes of management remains to be seen. Nevertheless, the importance of this article is to remind us that we need to continuously assess our own care practices to ensure that our patients are getting the best possible care, and to modify the practices when our data tell us to.

**S. M. Donn, MD**

---

**Prediction of Bronchopulmonary Dysplasia by Postnatal Age in Extremely Premature Infants**

Laughon MM, for the Eunice Kennedy Shriver National Institute of Child Health and Human Development Neonatal Research Network (Univ of North Carolina, Chapel Hill; et al)

*Am J Respir Crit Care Med* 183:1715-1722, 2011

---

*Rationale.*—Benefits of identifying risk factors for bronchopulmonary dysplasia in extremely premature infants include providing prognostic information, identifying infants likely to benefit from preventive strategies, and stratifying infants for clinical trial enrollment.

*Objectives.*—To identify risk factors for bronchopulmonary dysplasia, and the competing outcome of death, by postnatal day; to identify which risk factors improve prediction; and to develop a Web-based estimator using readily available clinical information to predict risk of bronchopulmonary dysplasia or death.

*Methods.*—We assessed infants of 23–30 weeks' gestation born in 17 centers of the Eunice Kennedy Shriver National Institute of Child Health and Human Development Neonatal Research Network and enrolled in the Neonatal Research Network Benchmarking Trial from 2000–2004.

*Measurements and Main Results.*—Bronchopulmonary dysplasia was defined as a categorical variable (none, mild, moderate, or severe). We developed and validated models for bronchopulmonary dysplasia risk at six postnatal ages using gestational age, birth weight, race and ethnicity, sex, respiratory support, and $FIO_2$, and examined the models using a C statistic (area under the curve). A total of 3,636 infants were eligible for this study. Prediction improved with advancing postnatal age, increasing from a C statistic of 0.793 on Day 1 to a maximum of 0.854 on Day 28. On Postnatal Days 1 and 3, gestational age best improved outcome prediction; on Postnatal Days 7, 14, 21, and 28, type of respiratory support did so. A Web-based model providing predicted estimates for bronchopulmonary dysplasia by postnatal day is available at https://neonatal.rti.org.

*Conclusions.*—The probability of bronchopulmonary dysplasia in extremely premature infants can be determined accurately using a limited amount of readily available clinical information.

▶ The group of investigators of the Eunice Kennedy Shriver National Institutes of Health Neonatal Research Network developed and validated a predictive model for bronchopulmonary dysplasia (BPD) risk based on postnatal factors in extremely premature infants. These infants were participants in a prior trial by the Network, the Benchmarking Trial, that was conducted in 17 centers in the United States between 2000 and 2004. Using data from 3629 infants, the investigators determined that the risk factors that increased the predictive ability of the model were dependent on the infant's postnatal age. For postnatal days 1 and 3, gestational age improved the model's prediction the most, while for postnatal days 7, 14, 21, and 28, the type of respiratory support improved outcome prediction the most. This model was subsequently internally and externally validated, and a Web-based prediction tool, or "estimator," for BPD was reported. The tool (available at https://neonatal.rti.org/) provides individual predicted estimates of BPD and death based on 6 parameters: gestational age, birth weight, sex, race/ethnicity, type of respiratory support, and fractional inspired oxygen concentration.

This is an important contribution to neonatal care, analogous to the "preemie outcome calculator," also developed by the Neonatal Research Network, to predict extremely preterm birth outcomes. Given that the predictive ability of the model did not seem to be affected by clinical center, the tool's utility in guiding clinical practices and research efforts to prevent BPD is potentially substantial. Stratification by risk category may enhance both the efficacy as well as the risk/benefit ratio of interventions previously thought to be noneffective, marginally effective, or even harmful.

**H. Christou, MD**

## Clarithromycin in Preventing Bronchopulmonary Dysplasia in *Ureaplasma urealyticum*-Positive Preterm Infants

Ozdemir R, Erdeve O, Dizdar EA, et al (Zekai Tahir Burak Maternity Teaching Hosp, Ankara, Turkey; et al)

*Pediatrics* 128:e1496-e1501, 2011

*Objective.*—To evaluate the efficacy and safety of clarithromycin treatment in preventing bronchopulmonary dysplasia (BPD) in *Ureaplasma urealyticum*-positive preterm infants.

*Patients and Methods.*—Nasopharyngeal swabs for *U urealyticum* culture were taken from infants with a birth weight between 750 and 1250 g in the first 3 postnatal days. Infants with a positive culture for *U urealyticum* were randomly assigned to 1 of 2 groups to receive either intravenous clarithromycin or placebo. All the patients were followed at least up to the 36th postmenstrual week.

*Results.*—A total of 224 infants met the eligibility criteria of the study. Seventy-four (33%) infants had a positive culture for *U urealyticum* in the first 3 day cultures. The rate of BPD development was significantly higher in patients with *U urealyticum* positivity (15.9% vs 36.4%; $P < .01$). However, multivariate logistic regression analysis failed to reveal a significant association between the presence of *U urealyticum* and BPD development (odds ratio: 2.4 [95% confidence interval: 0.9–6.3]; $P = .06$). Clarithromycin treatment resulted in eradication of *U urealyticum* in 68.5% of the patients. The incidence of BPD was significantly lower in the clarithromycin group than in the placebo group (2.9% vs 36.4%; $P < .001$). Multivariate logistic regression analysis confirmed the independent preventive effect of clarithromycin for the development of BPD (odds ratio: 27.2 [95% confidence interval: 2.5–296.1]; $P = .007$).

*Conclusions.*—Clarithromycin treatment prevents development of BPD in preterm infants who are born at 750 to 1250 g and colonized with *U urealyticum*.

▶ Bronchopulmonary dysplasia (BPD) and necrotizing enterocolitis continue to contribute to the morbidity and mortality of extremely premature infants (birth weight ≤1 kg; gestational age ≤28 weeks). Whereas there is indisputable evidence that almost 40% of these infants are colonized with *Ureaplasma*, controversy persists over whether *Ureaplasma* colonization or infection of the respiratory tract contributes to the development of BPD. Schelonka et al[1] sought to evaluate and critique the current medical literature and to document the reported association between *Ureaplasma* and BPD. They reported that "Ureaplasma colonization is associated with higher reported rates of BPD, but as the greatest reported effect is seen in small studies; reporting bias may be partially responsible for this effect."[1] More recently, Kasper et al[2] confirmed the association between *Ureaplasma* species and BPD as well as all grades of intraventricular hemorrhage after adjustment for multiple risk factors. Inatomi et al.[3] concluded that antenatal exposure to *Ureaplasma* species induces lung injury before birth and synergistically contributes to the development of BPD in infants requiring prolonged mechanical ventilation, defined as greater than 2 weeks. In their experience, colonization alone without prolonged mechanical ventilation was not associated with BPD.

Most clinicians accept that many of these extremely premature infants are colonized with *Ureaplasma* but don't know what to do about it. A survey of the recent literature unfortunately does not provide enough evidence to move one way or the other. As noted above, Ozdemir et al conclude that "Clarithromycin treatment prevents development of BPD in preterm infants who are born at 750 to 1250 g and colonized with *U urealyticum*." However, Ballard et al[4] randomly assigned 220 infants with birth weight less than 1250 g to azithromycin or placebo and found no benefit with extraordinary high rates of BPD. The incidence of BPD was 76% for the azithromycin group versus 84% for the placebo group ($P = .2$).In contrast to Ozdemir, who only enrolled colonized infants, Ballard's assignment was based on birth weight, and cultures were done subsequently. Subgroup analysis of the colonized infants showed that the incidence of BPD in the *Ureaplasma* subgroup was 73% in the azithromycin group versus 94% in the placebo group ($P = .03$). Further analysis of patients in the *Ureaplasma* subgroup only, using the exact logistic model, demonstrated a significant decrease in BPD or death in the azithromycin group. They concluded that "routine use of azithromycin therapy for the prevention of BPD cannot be recommended. The early treatment of *Ureaplasma* colonized/infected patients might be beneficial, but a larger multi-centered trial is required to assess this more definitively."[4]

There is never any argument when it comes to doing large prospective, randomized trials until it is time to organize and finance these trials. The logistics can become overbearing. So given the current available evidence, it would appear reasonable to use clarithromycin or azithromycin in extremely preterm infants know to be colonized with *Ureaplasma* species. This clearly begs the question as to whether every extremely preterm infant should be evaluated for *Ureaplasma* species and if so, by culture, polymerase chain reaction, or both methods.

A. A. Fanaroff, MBBCh, FRCPE

*References*

1. Schelonka RL, Katz B, Waites KB, Benjamin DK Jr. Critical appraisal of the role of Ureaplasma in the development of bronchopulmonary dysplasia with metaanalytic techniques. *Pediatr Infect Dis J.* 2005;24:1033-1039.
2. Kasper DC, Mechtler TP, Böhm J, et al. In utero exposure to Ureaplasma spp. is associated with increased rate of bronchopulmonary dysplasia and intraventricular hemorrhage in preterm infants. *J Perinat Med.* 2011;39:331-336.
3. Inatomi T, Oue S, Ogihara T, et al. Antenatal exposure to Ureaplasma species exacerbates bronchopulmonary dysplasia synergistically with subsequent prolonged mechanical ventilation in preterm infants. *Pediatr Res.* 2012;71:268-273.
4. Ballard HO, Shook LA, Bernard P, et al. Use of azithromycin for the prevention of bronchopulmonary dysplasia in preterm infants: a randomized, double-blind, placebo controlled trial. *Pediatr Pulmonol.* 2011;46:111-118.

## Clarithromycin in Preventing Bronchopulmonary Dysplasia in *Ureaplasma urealyticum*–Positive Preterm Infants

Ozdemir R, Erdeve O, Dizdar EA, et al (Zekai Tahir Burak Maternity Teaching Hosp, Ankara, Turkey; et al)
*Pediatrics* 128:e1496-e1501, 2011

*Objective.*—To evaluate the efficacy and safety of clarithromycin treatment in preventing bronchopulmonary dysplasia (BPD) in *Ureaplasma urealyticum*–positive preterm infants.

*Patients and Methods.*—Nasopharyngeal swabs for *U urealyticum* culture were taken from infants with a birth weight between 750 and 1250 g in the first 3 postnatal days. Infants with a positive culture for *U urealyticum* were randomly assigned to 1 of 2 groups to receive either intravenous clarithromycin or placebo. All the patients were followed at least up to the 36th postmenstrual week.

*Results.*—A total of 224 infants met the eligibility criteria of the study. Seventy-four (33%) infants had a positive culture for *U urealyticum* in the first 3 day cultures. The rate of BPD development was significantly higher in patients with *U urealyticum* positivity (15.9% vs 36.4%; $P < .01$). However, multivariate logistic regression analysis failed to reveal a significant association between the presence of *U urealyticum* and BPD development (odds ratio: 2.4 [95% confidence interval: 0.9–6.3]; $P = .06$). Clarithromycin treatment resulted in eradication of *U urealyticum* in 68.5% of the patients. The incidence of BPD was significantly lower in the clarithromycin group than in the placebo group (2.9% vs 36.4%; $P < .001$). Multivariate logistic regression analysis confirmed the independent preventive effect of clarithromycin for the development of BPD (odds ratio: 27.2 [95% confidence interval: 2.5–296.1]; $P = .007$).

*Conclusions.*—Clarithromycin treatment prevents development of BPD in preterm infants who are born at 750 to 1250 g and colonized with *U urealyticum*.

▶ A strong relationship between airway colonization by *Ureaplasma urealyticum* in preterm infants and an increased risk of bronchopulmonary dysplasia (BPD) has been recognized for many years, but numerous barriers have blocked translation of that observation into an effective strategy for BPD prevention. *Ureaplasma* is quite fastidious, so culture requires careful sample collection, special transport media, and specific culture techniques. Few hospitals have in-house capability for *Ureaplasma* culture, so specimens typically must be sent to reference laboratories. Turnaround times of several days preclude early treatment, compromising the opportunity to affect inflammatory sequelae of infection. The low solubility of intravenous erythromycin preparations requires large volumes of fluid, impinging nutritional intake. Most importantly, early trials failed to show reduction in BPD in preterm infants treated with erythromycin, suggesting that even early postnatal treatment might come too late to alter an inflammatory cascade triggered by intra-uterine *Ureaplasma* infection. It is not clear whether these negative results reflect absence of efficacy, lack of statistical power, or other defects in trial design.

This article helps clarify those issues. In this trial, nasopharyngeal cultures were obtained from infants with birth weights between 750 and 1250 g in the first 3 days after birth; infants with positive cultures were randomly assigned to treatment with intravenous clarithromycin or placebo. The age at which treatment was initiated was not reported. Clarithromycin was associated with a 92% reduction in the risk of BPD, significant by both univariate (odds ratio [OR] for BPD, 0.051; 95% confidence interval [CI], 0.008–0.34; $P = 0.0005$) and multivariate analyses (OR, 0.037; 95% CI, 0.003–0.40; $P = 0.007$; adjusted for birth weight, pneumonia, patent ductus arteriosus, caffeine, mechanical ventilation, and continuous positive airway pressure). One infant in each group died before assessment of oxygen need at 36 weeks; analysis of the combined outcome of death or BPD did not change the conclusion (OR, 0.093; 95% CI, 0.022–0.42; $P = 0.001$). The authors speculate that differences from results obtained with erythromycin may reflect greater in vitro activity against *Ureaplasma* or better penetration of clarithromycin into respiratory tissues and secretions. These results cannot be immediately applied in the United States, however, because the intravenous formulation of clarithromycin is not currently approved by the US Food and Drug Administration.

Azithromycin, which has in vitro efficacy intermediate between clarithromycin and erythromycin and tissue penetration comparable to that of clarithromycin, may be an alternative. Ballard et al[1] randomly assigned infants to treatment with intravenous azithromycin or placebo before *Ureaplasma* colonization was ascertained. Although there was no statistically significant effect on rates of death or BPD, secondary multiple logistic regression analysis of subjects with positive *Ureaplasma* cultures showed a substantially decreased risk of death or BPD (OR, 0.026; 95% CI, 0.001–0.62). Clinical trials to determine whether rapid ascertainment of *Ureaplasma* using rapid polymerase chain reaction (now commercially available on a platform suitable for most hospital laboratories) followed by early treatment with azithromycin can reproduce these effects on BPD rates are urgently needed.

**W. E. Benitz, MD**

*Reference*

1. Ballard HO, Shook LA, Bernard P, et al. Use of azithromycin for the prevention of bronchopulmonary dysplasia in preterm infants: a randomized, double-blind, placebo controlled trial. *Pediatr Pulmonol.* 2011;46:111-118.

**Molecular Identification of Bacteria in Tracheal Aspirate Fluid from Mechanically Ventilated Preterm Infants**
Mourani PM, Harris JK, Sontag MK, et al (Univ of Colorado Denver, Aurora; et al)
*PLoS One* 6:e25959, 2011

*Background.*—Despite strong evidence linking infections to the pathogenesis of bronchopulmonary dysplasia (BPD), limitations of bacterial culture methods have precluded systematic studies of airway organisms relative to disease outcomes. Application of molecular bacterial identification strategies may provide new insight into the role of bacterial acquisition in the airways of preterm infants at risk for BPD.

*Methods.*—Serial (within 72 hours, 7, 14, and 21 days of life) tracheal aspirate samples were collected from 10 preterm infants with gestational age ≤34 weeks at birth, and birth weight of 500–1250 g who required mechanical ventilation for at least 21 days. Samples were analyzed by quantitative real time PCR assays for total bacterial load and by pyrosequencing for bacterial identification.

*Results.*—Subjects were diagnosed with mild (1), moderate (3), or severe (5) BPD. One patient died prior to determination of disease severity. 107,487 sequences were analyzed, with mean of 3,359 (range 1,724–4,915) per sample. 2 of 10 samples collected <72 hours of life contained adequate bacterial DNA for successful sequence analysis, one of which was from a subject exposed to chorioamnionitis. All other samples exhibited bacterial loads >70 copies/reaction. 72 organisms were observed in total. Seven organisms represented the dominant organism (>50% of total sequences) in 31/32 samples with positive sequences. A dominant organism represented >90% of total sequences in 13 samples. *Staphylococcus, Ureaplasmaparvum,* and *Ureaplasmaurealyticum* were the most frequently identified dominant organisms, but *Pseudomonas, Enterococcus,* and *Escherichia* were also identified.

*Conclusions.*—Early bacterial colonization with diverse species occurs after the first 3 days of life in the airways of intubated preterm infants, and can be characterized by bacterial load and marked species diversity. Molecular identification of bacteria in the lower airways of preterm infants has the potential to yield further insight into the pathogenesis of BPD.

▶ The human microbiome roadmap initiative, based on novel technologies that allow for the delineation of microbial DNA sequences, has spurred studies primarily in the human gastrointestinal tract. This study, based on preliminary work suggesting that the lungs of healthy older children and adults are rich with microbes, hypothesized that early colonization with diverse microbial agents occurs early after birth in ventilated preterm infants and that these microorganisms might help better define risk for chronic lung disease. *Ureaplasma* was found to be the dominant organism for at least 6 of the 10 infants in the study. It was suspected that some of these infections were acquired postnatally and may have been associated with antibiotic usage. The importance of this article is that it shows that microbes are detectable in even the distal airways postnatally. Whether the organisms detected actually play a role in disease pathogenesis is not addressed in this study. However, this is a nice start in applying these new technologies to the neonatal lung and should mature to additional studies using functional metagenomics—much more sophisticated technology that may actually be used to evaluate pathogenesis.

**J. Neu, MD**

**A new method for continuous monitoring of chest wall movement to characterize hypoxemic episodes during HFOV**

Waisman D, Levy C, Faingersh A, et al (Carmel Med Ctr and Faculty of Medicine, Haifa, Israel; Technion-Israel Inst of Technology, Haifa)

*Intensive Care Med* 37:1174-1181, 2011

*Introduction.*—Monitoring ventilated infants is difficult during high-frequency oscillatory ventilation (HFOV). This study tested the possible causes of hypoxemic episodes using a new method for monitoring chest wall movement during HFOV in newborn infants.

*Methods.*—Three miniature motion sensors were attached to both sides of the chest and to the epigastrium to measure the local tidal displacement (TDi) at each site. A >20% change in TDi was defined as deviation from baseline.

*Results.*—Eight premature infants (postmenstrual age 30.6 ± 2.6 weeks) were monitored during 10 sessions (32.6 h) that included 21 hypoxemic events. Three types of such events were recognized: decrease in TDi that preceded hypoxemia ($n = 11$), simultaneous decrease in TDi and $SpO_2$ ($n = 6$), and decrease in $SpO_2$ without changes in TDi ($n = 4$). In the first group, decreases in TDi were detected 22.4 ± 18.7 min before hypoxemia, and were due to airway obstruction by secretions or decline in lung compliance. The second group resulted from apnea or severe abdominal contractions. In the third group, hypoxia appeared following a decrease in $FiO_2$.

*Conclusions.*—Monitoring TDi may enable early recognition of deteriorating ventilation during HFOV that eventually leads to hypoxemia. In about half of cases, hypoxemia is not due to slowly deteriorating ventilation.

▶ High-frequency oscillatory ventilation (HFOV) plays a major role as both a primary and rescue strategy for babies with respiratory failure. Perhaps its 1 drawback is our inability to monitor babies as extensively as we can with conventional ventilation, especially with respect to lung mechanics. I have often wondered about the subjectivity of the chest wiggle factor as well as the radiographic assessment of lung volume.

This article describes a relatively new technique for objectively measuring chest wall movement during HFOV using miniature motion sensors affixed to the left and right hemithoraces and the epigastrium. The method was conducted on 8 babies (10 sessions) receiving HFOV for respiratory failure. The investigation revealed hypoxemic events, which the authors categorized as early detection (slow deterioration) related to obstruction, inadequate ventilation, or unresolved; paroxysmal, secondary to apnea or abdominal contractions; or desaturation without decreased ventilation from either a decrease in the fraction of inspired oxygen or unknown.

The numbers are far too small to really validate the conclusions, but they do suggest that there are different patterns of chest wall displacement during HFOV that might be helpful in monitoring patients and guiding adjustments in ventilator settings. However, no data on ventilation were provided, and it seems that the greater impact from changes in tidal volume will be on carbon dioxide removal than on oxygenation. The latter could be impacted by determination of functional residual capacity or total lung capacity, so developing a correlation between these volumes and this technique could be a laudable accomplishment. Additionally, these measurements were obtained from babies ventilated with the SLE 2000 or SLE 500 ventilators. It would certainly be of interest to neonatologists in the United States to see how the technique works with the SensorMedics 3100A, a much more powerful oscillatory device.

**S. M. Donn, MD**

---

**Airway obstruction and gas leak during mask ventilation of preterm infants in the delivery room**

Schmölzer GM, Dawson JA, Kamlin CO, et al (The Royal Women's Hosp, Melbourne, Australia; et al)
*Arch Dis Child Fetal Neonatal Ed* 96:F254-F257, 2011

*Introduction.*—Preterm infants with inadequate breathing receive positive pressure ventilation (PPV) by mask with variable success. The authors examined recordings of PPV given to preterm infants in the delivery room for prevalence of mask leak and airway obstruction.

*Methods and patients.*—The authors reviewed recordings of infants at <32 weeks' gestation born between February 2006 and March 2009. PPV was delivered with a T-piece or self-inflating bag and a round silicone face mask. Airway pressures and gas flow were recorded with a respiratory function monitor (RFM). Videos recorded from a web camera were used to review the resuscitation. The first 2 min of PPV were analysed for each infant. Obstruction was arbitrarily defined as a 75% reduction in delivered expired tidal volume ($V_{Te}$) and significant face-mask leak as >75%.

*Results.*—The authors analysed recordings of 56 preterm infants. Obstruction occurred in 14 (26%) recordings and leaks in 27 (51%). Both obstruction and mask leaks were seen in eight (14%) recordings, and neither was seen in 15 (27%). Obstruction occurred at a median (IQR) of 48 (24—60) s after the start of PPV. A median (range) of 22 (3—83) consecutive obstructed inflations were delivered. Face-mask leaks occurred from the first inflation in 19/27 (70%) and in the remaining eight at a median (IQR) of 30 (24—46) s after the start of PPV. A median (range) of 10 (3—117) consecutive inflations with a leak >75% were delivered.

*Conclusion.*—Airway obstruction and face-mask leak are common during the first 2 min of PPV. An RFM enables detection of important airway obstruction and mask leak.

▶ It will come as a surprise to no one who has administered mask positive pressure ventilation (PPV) to an infant that the skill is more challenging than it appears. This is especially true when the recipient of the intervention is a newly delivered preterm infant. This study of the first 2 minutes of resuscitation of 56 infants born at less than 32 weeks' gestation who received PPV in the delivery room, showed high rates of airway obstruction (26%), facemask air leak (51%), or both (17%), with only 27% of subjects experiencing neither obstruction nor mask air leak. Many instances of obstruction or mask air leak occurred before the heart rate or oxygen saturation was recorded. Both issues occurred regardless of the type of mask or mode of administration (T-piece resuscitator or self-inflating bag; anesthesia bags were not used in this study). In some instances, the problems were prolonged (eg, as many as 83 obstructed breaths and 117 breaths accompanied by facemask air leak were delivered), suggesting the resuscitation team might have been unaware of the issues—probably a more common occurrence than we appreciate. This study was conducted by combining video recording to assess interventions and the use of a respiratory function monitor (RFM) that recorded ventilation pressure, gas flow, and tidal volume. Perhaps future iterations of neonatal resuscitation will move beyond measures of inflating pressure and exhaled carbon dioxide to incorporate immediate RFM feedback on such important aspects of mask ventilation, with the goal of decreasing response time to instituting corrections for airway obstruction or mask leak and enhancing safety and effectiveness of mask ventilation.

**L. J. Van Marter, MD, MPH**

---

**Mask leak in one-person mask ventilation compared to two-person in newborn infant manikin study**
Tracy M, Klimek J, Coughtrey H, et al (Nepean Hosp Sydney West Area Health Service, New South Wales, Australia; et al)
*Arch Dis Child Fetal Neonatal Ed* 96:F195-F200, 2011

---

*Aim.*—To compare a new two-person method (four hands) of delivering mask ventilation with a standard one-person method using the Laerdal self-inflating bag (SIB) and the Neopuff (NP) infant resuscitator in a manikin model.

*Background.*—Recent studies of simulated neonatal resuscitation using bag and mask ventilation techniques have shown facemask leak levels of 55–57% in expert hands.

*Methods.*—48 participants were randomly paired and instructed to give mask ventilation for a 2-min period as single-person resuscitators, then as two-person paired resuscitators at set pressures for NP and set parameters for SIB. Airway pressure, flow, inspiratory tidal volume, expiratory tidal volume and mask leak were recorded.

*Results.*—A total of 21 578 inflations were recorded and analysed. For SIB, mask leak was greater (11.5%) with single-person compared to two-person (5.4%; mean difference 6.1%, 95% CI 1.5 to 10.7, $p < 0.01$). For NP, mask leak was greater for single-person (22.2%) compared to two-person (9.1%; mean difference 13.1%, 95% CI 3.6 to 22.6, $p < 0.01$). For single-person mask ventilation, mask leak was greater with NP (22.2%) compared to SIB (11.5%; mean difference 10.7%, 95% CI 1.4 to 19.7, $p < 0.01$). For two-person mask ventilation, mask leak was greater for NP (9.1%) compared to SIB (5.4%; mean difference 3.7%, 95% CI 0.1 to 6.4, $p < 0.05$).

*Conclusions.*—Two-person mask ventilation technique reduces mask leak by approximately 50% compared to the standard one-person mask ventilation method. NP mask ventilation has higher mask leak than Laerdal SIB for both single- and two-person technique mask ventilation.

▶ In the last 6 years, research groups have used manikins to simulate newborn resuscitation in order to evaluate manual ventilation devices,[1,2] face masks,[1,3] mask-hold techniques,[4] and technique training.[4-6]

Importantly, this article is the first to formally evaluate the effectiveness of a 2-person airway control method for neonatal mask ventilation. Evidence is provided to support the view that newborn face mask ventilation may be much easier with 2 people.[7,8] The use of both self-inflating bags and T-piece devices in the study broadens its applicability.

The only apparent modification to the Laerdal ALST manikin has been to block the esophageal tube, resulting in compliance comparable to that of a term newborn with healthy lungs. Other researchers[1,3-6,9] have chosen to replace the internal lung system favoring nondistensible tubing and reusable test lungs for their resilience to use over time; lung compliance is then comparable to a diseased lung state (eg, respiratory distress syndrome).

While the majority of newborns have normal lungs, those born prematurely or in difficulty may not. During transition, the fluid-filled lungs need to be aerated, and lung compliance during this time may be initially poor. Choosing an appropriate lung model for resuscitation research is difficult, and manikins with a static compliance may be too limiting.

Manikin studies are valuable in that they allow robust, standardized, and reproducible studies of techniques, training strategies, and devices to be undertaken. Simulations can be used to answer important research questions and generate new hypotheses to enhance the quality of clinical trials.

The most obvious limitations of manikin studies relate to their clinical applicability. Manikins cannot replicate the dynamic changes that occur at birth, nor the variability between infants of the same or differing gestational ages. The design and modifications made to manikins for research purposes may affect the results observed, hindering the comparison of work from different research centers. Information regarding equipment modifications, accuracy of measurements, and the target population or disease state the simulation is intended to approximate must therefore be provided.

Caution needs to be exercised when considering how this work may apply to our everyday practice until confirmatory clinical evidence is established. The authors have shown that the 2-person mask ventilation technique halved mask leak compared with the single-person method in a manikin with a compliant lung system. Mask leak is common in both manikin and delivery room studies; however, the degree of leak that is important has yet to be defined. We can reasonably conclude that where a single resuscitator is experiencing difficulty in airway control and mask ventilation related to mask leak, by adopting a 2-person mask ventilation technique, some improvement in mask seal would be anticipated. This research provides evidence to justify current practice[8,10] and also to promote change.

**F. E. Wood, MD**

References

1. O'Donnell CP, Davis PG, Lau R, Dargaville PA, Doyle LW, Morley CJ. Neonatal resuscitation 2: an evaluation of manual ventilation devices and face masks. *Arch Dis Child Fetal Neonatal Ed.* 2005;90:F392-F396.
2. Tracy MB, Klimek J, Coughtrey H, et al. Ventilator-delivered mask ventilation compared with three standard methods of mask ventilation in a manikin model. *Arch Dis Child Fetal Neonatal Ed.* 2011;96:F201-F205.
3. Wood FE, Morley CJ, Dawson JA, et al. Assessing the effectiveness of two round neonatal resuscitation masks: study 1. *Arch Dis Child Fetal Neonatal Ed.* 2008; 93:F235-F237.
4. Wood FE, Morley CJ, Dawson JA, et al. Improved techniques reduce face mask leak during simulated neonatal resuscitation: study 2. *Arch Dis Child Fetal Neonatal Ed.* 2008;93:F230-F234.
5. Wood FE, Morley CJ, Dawson JA, Davis PG. A respiratory function monitor improves mask ventilation. *Arch Dis Child Fetal Neonatal Ed.* 2008;93:F380-F381.
6. Schilleman K, Witlox RS, Lopriore E, Morley CJ, Walther FJ, te Pas AB. Leak and obstruction with mask ventilation during simulated neonatal resuscitation. *Arch Dis Child Fetal Neonatal Ed.* 2010;95:F398-F402.
7. Resuscitation Council (UK). *Resuscitation at Birth. Newborn Life Support Provider Course Manual.* 2nd ed. London, UK: Resuscitation Council (UK); 2006.
8. Resuscitation Council (UK). *Resuscitation at Birth. Newborn Life Support Provider Course Manual.* 3rd ed. London, UK: Resuscitation Council (UK); 2011.
9. O'Donnell CP, Kamlin CO, Davis PG, Morley CJ. Neonatal resuscitation 1: a model to measure inspired and expired tidal volumes and assess leakage at the face mask. *Arch Dis Child Fetal Neonatal Ed.* 2005;90:F388-F391.
10. Richmond S, Wyllie J. European Resuscitation Council Guidelines for Resuscitation 2010 Section 7. Resuscitation of babies at birth. *Resuscitation.* 2010;81: 1389-1399.

**Hospital Variation in Nitric Oxide Use for Premature Infants**
Stenger MR, Slaughter JL, Kelleher K, et al (The Ohio State Univ College of Medicine and Nationwide Children's Hosp, Columbus; et al)
*Pediatrics* 129:e945-e951, 2012

*Objective.*—To describe inter-center hospital variation in inhaled nitric oxide (iNO) administration to infants born prior to 34 weeks' gestation at US children's hospitals.
*Methods.*—This was a retrospective cohort study using the Pediatric Health Information System to determine the frequency, age at first administration, and length of iNO use among 22 699 consecutive first admissions of unique <34 weeks' gestation infants admitted to 37 children's hospitals from January 1, 2007, through December 31, 2010.
*Results.*—A total of 1644 (7.2%) infants received iNO during their hospitalization, with substantial variation in iNO use between hospitals (range across hospitals: 0.5%−26.2%; $P < .001$). The age at which iNO was started varied by hospital (mean: 20.0 days; range: 6.0−65.1 days,

$P < .001$), as did the duration of therapy (mean: 13.1 days; range: 1.0–31.1 days; $P < .001$). Preterm infants who received iNO were less likely to survive (36.3% mortality vs 8.3%; odds ratio: 6.27; $P < .001$). The association between the use of iNO and mortality persists in propensity score–adjusted analyses controlling for demographic factors and diagnoses associated with the use of iNO (odds ratio: 3.79; $P < .0001$).

*Conclusions.*—iNO practice patterns in preterm infants varied widely among institutions. Infants who received iNO were less likely to survive, suggesting that iNO is used in infants already at high risk of death. Adherence to National Institutes of Health consensus guidelines may decrease variation in iNO use.

▶ Here we have a cautionary tale. Although a handful of clinical trials suggest potential benefit from administration of inhaled nitric oxide (iNO) to preterm infants with respiratory disease, reported favorable effects are limited to results of post hoc analyses or remain unreplicated. The critical questions of which infants, for what indications, at what age, at which dose, for what duration, and to what end remain unresolved. Recent consensus guidelines and systematic reviews suggest that iNO use in this population should be limited to infants enrolled in controlled trials to facilitate resolution of these issues. Nonetheless, these data from 37 children's hospitals across the United States demonstrate both extensive iNO use and enormous practice variation. Rates of iNO administration to infants under 34 weeks' gestation varied more than 17-fold among hospitals; there was a 10-fold range in the age at initiation and a 20-fold range in the average number of days of use. This lack of standardization reflects the paucity of evidence to guide use of this treatment in preterm infants. It is worrisome that iNO use was associated with a substantial increase in mortality rates (35.6% compared with 8.3% among the infants not receiving iNO; odds ratio 6.13; 95% confidence interval, 5.48–6.85; $P < .001$), even after heroic statistical efforts to adjust for possible selective iNO use in the most severely ill infants. Randomized trials may still demonstrate benefit in some subgroup of preterm infants, but this article is a firm reminder that those infants have not yet been identified. The observation that there was a small (and probably not statistically significant) decrease in the overall rate of iNO use in the first half of 2010, following yearly increases in 2008 and 2009, is hopeful. Perhaps publication of the Agency for Healthcare Research and Quality evidence assessment late in 2010 and the National Institutes of Health consensus conference statement and Cochrane review in 2011 have led to more circumspect application of this unproven therapy. These authors correctly conclude that "there is a need for adherence to and further development of evidence-based protocols to standardize care to avoid unnecessary and costly treatment."

**W. E. Benitz, MD**

## Inhaled Nitric Oxide in Preterm Infants: An Individual-Patient Data Meta-analysis of Randomized Trials

Askie LM, on behalf of the Meta-analysis of Preterm Patients on Inhaled Nitric Oxide (MAPPiNO) Collaboration (Univ of Sydney, New South Wales, Australia; et al)
*Pediatrics* 128:729-739, 2011

*Background.*—Inhaled nitric oxide (iNO) is an effective therapy for pulmonary hypertension and hypoxic respiratory failure in term infants. Fourteen randomized controlled trials ($n = 3430$ infants) have been conducted on preterm infants at risk for chronic lung disease (CLD). The study results seem contradictory.

*Design/Methods.*—Individual-patient data meta-analysis included randomized controlled trials of preterm infants (<37 weeks' gestation). Outcomes were adjusted for trial differences and correlation between siblings.

*Results.*—Data from 3298 infants in 12 trials (96%) were analyzed. There was no statistically significant effect of iNO on death or CLD (59% vs 61%: relative risk [RR]: 0.96 [95% confidence interval (CI): 0.92–1.01]; $P = .11$) or severe neurologic events on imaging (25% vs 23%: RR: 1.12 [95% CI: 0.98–1.28]; $P = .09$). There were no statistically significant differences in iNO effect according to any of the patient-level characteristics tested. In trials that used a starting iNO dose of >5 vs ≤5 ppm there was evidence of improved outcome (interaction $P = .02$); however, these differences were not observed at other levels of exposure to iNO. This result was driven primarily by 1 trial, which also differed according to overall dose, duration, timing, and indication for treatment; a significant reduction in death or CLD (RR: 0.85 [95% CI: 0.74–0.98]) was found.

*Conclusions.*—Routine use of iNO for treatment of respiratory failure in preterm infants cannot be recommended. The use of a higher starting dose might be associated with improved outcome, but because there were differences in the designs of these trials, it requires further examination.

▶ An extensive body of work in animal models suggests that inhaled nitric oxide (iNO) should have beneficial effects in preterm human infants at risk of developing chronic lung disease. In preterm baboon and lamb models, for example, provision of iNO yields more normal lung growth, angiogenesis, and alveolar development, significantly ameliorating the pathology associated with new bronchopulmonary dysplasia. These observations have inspired 14 randomized controlled trials that have had somewhat inconsistent and generally disappointing results. The remarkable collaborative effort reported in this article pools individual patient data from 11 of those trials in an effort to elucidate the effects of iNO that no single study—or even group-based meta-analyses, such as the Cochrane reviews—has had sufficient power to demonstrate. Despite this more robust approach, no effects on the primary outcomes (death or bronchopulmonary dysplasia, severe neurological events after enrollment) were identified. Notably, benefits in certain subgroups (such as infants > 1000 g or with lower pretreatment oxygenation indices, as suggested by some individual trials) also were not evident. Subgroup analyses did suggest lower rates of death or chronic lung disease (CLD) in infants who were multiples (relative risk [RR] 0.88; 95% confidence interval [CI], 0.79—0.98), had not received antepartum steroids (RR 0.87; 95% CI, 0.79—0.96), were older than 3 or 7 days at enrollment (RR 0.89 and 0.87; 95% CI, 0.79—1.00 and 0.76—0.99, respectively), had patent ductus arteriosus (RR 0.87; 95% CI, 0.76—0.99), or had not received postnatal steroids (RR 0.91; 95% CI, 0.84—0.98). None of these conditions were associated with significant treatment-condition interaction coefficients in logistic regressions, however, so the implications of those observations remain speculative. Along with the observation that the rate of death or CLD was lower if the initial iNO dose was greater than 5 ppm, these findings leave open the possibility that some infants might benefit from some iNO regimen. This magnificent effort therefore leaves unresolved the critical questions of which babies might benefit and how, and when, at what dose, and for what duration they should be treated. We must hope that the 3 trials currently ongoing can help resolve this uncertainty. Until then, we should resist the impulse to extrapolate favorable findings in animal models into our nurseries.

**W. E. Benitz, MD**

---

**Protocolized management of infants with congenital diaphragmatic hernia: effect on survival**
Antonoff MB, Hustead VA, Groth SS, et al (Univ of Minnesota, Minneapolis; Children's Hosps and Clinics of Minnesota, Minneapolis)
*J Pediatr Surg* 46:39-46, 2011

---

*Background/Purpose.*—In 2006, we introduced a new protocol for congenital diaphragmatic hernia (CDH) management featuring nitric oxide in the delivery room, gentle ventilation, lower criteria for extracorporeal membrane oxygenation (ECMO), and appropriately timed operative repair on ECMO. Our goals were to assess outcomes after institution of this protocol and to compare results with historical controls.

*Methods.*—Charts were reviewed of all newborns admitted to a large metropolitan children's hospital from 2002 to 2009 with a diagnosis of CDH. Data were recorded regarding delivery, ECMO, operative repair, length of stay, comorbidities/anomalies, complications, and survival. Postprotocol outcomes were compared to those from the preprotocol era and to data from the international CDH Registry.

*Results.*—Comparison of the protocolized group (n = 43) to the historical group (n = 51) revealed no significant differences in gestational age, birth weight, Apgar scores, or comorbidities. New treatment strategies substantially improved survival to discharge (67% preprotocol, 88% postprotocol; $P = .015$). Among ECMO patients, survival increased to 82% (20% preprotocol; $P = .002$).

*Conclusions.*—Our new protocol significantly improved survival to discharge for newborns with CDH. Institution of such a protocol is valuable in improving outcomes for patients with CDH and merits consideration for widespread adoption.

▶ Antonoff and colleagues demonstrate significant improvement in survival to discharge among neonates with congenital diaphragmatic hernia (CDH) compared with both historical controls and contemporaneous data from the CDH Study Group database after the initiation of a detailed management protocol in a single high-volume center. Previous single-center studies have similarly found a survival benefit after institution of detailed management protocols based heavily on the principles of gentle ventilation and the avoidance of barotrauma.[1-4] This protocol is distinct in including the standard use of inhaled nitric oxide (iNO) in the delivery room, permissive criteria for the use of extracorporeal membrane oxygenation (ECMO), and repair of the CDH on ECMO, in addition to gentle ventilation strategies. In keeping with the protocol design, the percentage of infants receiving iNO (88% vs 60.8%, $P = .04$) and infants receiving ECMO (51.2% vs 19.6%, $P = .002$) were significantly higher in the postprotocol group. The use of ECMO in the postprotocol group was higher than that in patients in the CDH registry during the same time period (35%). Of note, there was a trend toward shorter duration of ECMO postprotocol as well as significantly improved survival in those treated with ECMO (81.8% vs 20.0%, $P = .02$). Importantly, survival also trended up in those not receiving ECMO (95.2% vs 78.1%, $P = .143$), such that the increased use of ECMO alone does not completely explain the improved survival. As in all complex protocols for management of complicated conditions, it is difficult to tease out which changes contributed to the most improvement in survival, but it is clear that those infants born during the protocol era had improved survival, even when controlling for ECMO status, birth weight, gestational age, sex, and 5-minute Apgar score.

It is of interest that similar improvements in survival to discharge with institution of protocolized management have been demonstrated by other groups with far less use of iNO and ECMO.[1-4] While it appears clear that protocols based on the principles of gentle ventilation improve survival, the specific therapies utilized are possibly less important than adoption of uniform practice, regular audit, and a multidisciplinary team philosophy. Only large multicenter, randomized, controlled trials are likely to ultimately tease out the effects of specific therapies in the management of this complicated disease process. In the meantime, this article further supports the role of detailed management protocols in improving outcomes in infants born with congenital diaphragmatic hernia.

**R. L. Chapman, MD**

*References*

1. Tracy ET, Mears SE, Smith PB, et al. Protocolized approach to the management of congenital diaphragmatic hernia: benefits of reducing variability in care. *J Pediatr Surg.* 2010;45:1343-1348.
2. Boloker J, Bateman DA, Wung JT, Stolar CJ. Congenital diaphragmatic hernia in 120 infants treated consecutively with permissive hypercapnea/spontaneous respiration/elective repair. *J Pediatr Surg.* 2002;37:357-366.

3. Bagolan P, Casaccia G, Crescenzi F, Nahom A, Trucchi A, Giorlandino C. Impact of a current treatment protocol on outcome of high-risk congenital diaphragmatic hernia. *J Pediatr Surg.* 2004;39:313-318.
4. Finer NN, Tierney A, Etches PC, Peliowski A, Ainsworth W. Congenital diaphragmatic hernia: developing a protocolized approach. *J Pediatr Surg.* 1998;33: 1331-1337.

# 8 Central Nervous System and Special Senses

**Application of Criteria Developed by the Task Force on Neonatal Encephalopathy and Cerebral Palsy to Acutely Asphyxiated Neonates**

Phelan JP, Korst LM, Martin GI (Citrus Valley Med Ctr, West Covina, CA; Childbirth Injury Prevention Foundation, City of Industry, CA; Univ of Southern California Keck School of Medicine, Los Angeles, CA)
*Obstet Gynecol* 118:824-830, 2011

*Objective.*—To estimate whether term neonates with acute intrapartum hypoxic ischemic encephalopathy and permanent brain injury satisfied the criteria for causation of cerebral palsy developed by the Task Force on Neonatal Encephalopathy and Cerebral Palsy.

*Methods.*—In this descriptive study, patients in the case group were obtained from a registry of singleton, liveborn, term, neurologically impaired neonates. Entry criteria included a reactive intrapartum fetal heart rate pattern followed by a sudden, rapid, and sustained deterioration of the fetal heart rate that lasted until delivery and an umbilical artery cord pH. All patients in the case group were then assessed to determine if they met the criteria developed by the Task Force on Neonatal Encephalopathy and Cerebral Palsy.

*Results.*—Thirty-nine neonates met the entry criteria, and the proportion meeting each essential criterion was as follows: 38 of 39 (97.4%) had umbilical artery pH of less than 7.00 and 30 of 30 (100%) had a base deficit of 12 mmol/L or higher; 33 of 34 (97%) had either moderate or severe encephalopathy; 34 of 36 (94%) had spastic quadriplegia or dyskinetic cerebral palsy or death attributable to brain injury; and 39 of 39 (100%) had no identifiable reason for exclusion.

*Conclusion.*—Fetuses that underwent a sudden and sustained deterioration of the fetal heart rate and that subsequently were found to have cerebral palsy demonstrated characteristics consistent with criteria developed by the Task Force on Neonatal Encephalopathy and Cerebral Palsy for intrapartum asphyxial injury.

*Level of Evidence.—*III.

▶ This descriptive study attempted to validate the criteria developed by the 2003 Task Force on Neonatal Encephalopathy and Cerebral Palsy by examining concordance in a specifically chosen cohort of babies. The authors selected a sudden, rapid, and sustained decrease in the fetal heart rate lasting until delivery as the marker of an intrauterine sentinel event. Thirty-nine such infants, who developed long-term neurological sequelae compatible with intrapartum hypoxic-ischemic encephalopathy were found from a 25-year registry database. All 39 infants met the base deficit criterion, none had exclusionary reasons, 97% had severe or moderate encephalopathy, 97.4% had an umbilical cord arterial pH greater than 7.00, and 94% had cerebral palsy or death attributable to brain injury (the other 2 had hemiplegia and ataxia, respectively).

It is difficult to argue with the conclusion that this type of intrauterine event is capable of producing neonatal encephalopathy and subsequent cerebral palsy, and it does validate the Task Force Criteria in this population of babies. However, it also raises the question of injury threshold for fetuses undergoing a similar but less severe insult. In this study, the duration of the deceleration could be determined in 36 fetuses and lasted a mean of 32 minutes, with a range of 16 to 57. Presumably, these were all neurologically intact fetuses before the fall in the heart rate. Will the case be the same for fetuses who sustain "multiple hits" or who have comorbidities, such as anemia or growth restriction?

There are obvious medicolegal implications. Arguing causation seldom involves cases in which there is relatively strong evidence of an intrapartum sentinel event, such as occurred in the 39 selected infants in this study. The arguments emanate from the more subtle cases.

**S. M. Donn, MD**

---

**Childhood Outcomes after Hypothermia for Neonatal Encephalopathy**
Shankaran S, for the Eunice Kennedy Shriver NICHD Neonatal Research Network (Wayne State Univ, Detroit, MI; et al)
*N Engl J Med* 366:2085-2092, 2012

---

*Background.—*We previously reported early results of a randomized trial of whole-body hypothermia for neonatal hypoxic—ischemic encephalopathy showing a significant reduction in the rate of death or moderate or severe disability at 18 to 22 months of age. Long-term outcomes are now available.

*Methods.—*In the original trial, we assigned infants with moderate or severe encephalopathy to usual care (the control group) or whole-body cooling to an esophageal temperature of 33.5°C for 72 hours, followed by slow rewarming (the hypothermia group). We evaluated cognitive, attention and executive, and visuospatial function; neurologic outcomes; and physical and psychosocial health among participants at 6 to 7 years of age. The primary outcome of the present analyses was death or an IQ score below 70.

*Results.*—Of the 208 trial participants, primary outcome data were available for 190. Of the 97 children in the hypothermia group and the 93 children in the control group, death or an IQ score below 70 occurred in 46 (47%) and 58 (62%), respectively ($P = 0.06$); death occurred in 27 (28%) and 41 (44%) ($P = 0.04$); and death or severe disability occurred in 38 (41%) and 53 (60%) ($P = 0.03$). Other outcome data were available for the 122 surviving children, 70 in the hypothermia group and 52 in the control group. Moderate or severe disability occurred in 24 of 69 children (35%) and 19 of 50 children (38%), respectively ($P = 0.87$). Attention–executive dysfunction occurred in 4% and 13%, respectively, of children receiving hypothermia and those receiving usual care ($P = 0.19$), and visuo-spatial dysfunction occurred in 4% and 3% ($P = 0.80$).

*Conclusions.*—The rate of the combined end point of death or an IQ score of less than 70 at 6 to 7 years of age was lower among children undergoing whole-body hypothermia than among those undergoing usual care, but the differences were not significant. However, hypothermia resulted in lower death rates and did not increase rates of severe disability among survivors. (Funded by the National Institutes of Health and the Eunice Kennedy Shriver NICHD Neonatal Research Network; ClinicalTrials.gov number, NCT00005772.)

▶ The search for effective therapies for perinatal hypoxic-ischemic encephalopathy (HIE) proved elusive—at least until cranial or whole-body cooling was evaluated. Earlier studies[1-4] of cranial or whole-body therapeutic hypothermia (TH) have shown improved outcomes among infants with HIE randomized to hypothermia (eg, reduced mortality and moderate to severe neurodevelopmental outcomes). This article summarizes the results of outcomes at 6 to 7 years of age; 91% of the 208 trial participants contributed outcome data. The primary study outcome was death or IQ less than 70, observed in 47% of hypothermia-treated and 62% of control subjects; the *P*-value detected in analyses of this outcome was .06. Nevertheless, many other outcomes at 6 to 7 years were significantly ($P < .05$) improved among the hypothermia group, including death (28% vs 44%), death or severe disability (41% vs 60%), death or IQ less than 55 (41% vs 55%), or death or cerebral palsy (41% vs 60%). Furthermore, stratification of outcomes by severity of HIE at study entry revealed trends in the direction of more likely benefit in primary outcome among those with moderately severe (33% vs 47%) rather than severe (80% vs 82%) HIE, providing support for ongoing studies of TH for HIE among infants with moderately severe, and perhaps even milder forms, of HIE. The bottom line is: in neonatal HIE, TH shows no evidence of worsening outcomes, improves selected outcomes, and appears most likely to benefit infants with moderately severe HIE. Perhaps the next steps will include efforts to combine TH with other therapies in search for synergistic benefit in treating neonatal HIE.

**L. J. Van Marter, MD, MPH**

*References*

1. Shankaran S, Laptook AR, Ehrenkranz RA, et al. Whole body hypothermia for neonates with hypoxic-ischemic encephalopathy. *N Engl J Med.* 2005;353:1574-1584.

2. Shankaran S, Laptook AR, Ehrenkranz RA, et al. Whole-body hypothermia for term and near-term newborns with hypoxic-ischemic encephalopathy: a randomized controlled trial. *Arch Pediatr Adolesc Med.* 2011;165:692-700.
3. Simbruner G, Mittal RA, Rohlmann F, Muche R. Systemic hypothermia after neonatal encephalopathy: outcomes of neo.nEURO.network RCT. *Pediatrics.* 2010;126:e771-e778.
4. Zhou WH, Cheng GQ, Shao XM, et al. Selective head cooling with mild systemic hypothermia after neonatal hypoxic-ischemic encephalopathy: a multicenter randomized controlled trial in China. *J Pediatr.* 2010;157:367-372.

---

## Childhood Outcomes after Hypothermia for Neonatal Encephalopathy

Shankaran S, for the Eunice Kennedy Shriver NICHD Neonatal Research Network (Wayne State Univ, Detroit, MI; et al)

*N Engl J Med* 366:2085-2092, 2012

---

*Background.*—We previously reported early results of a randomized trial of whole-body hypothermia for neonatal hypoxic—ischemic encephalopathy showing a significant reduction in the rate of death or moderate or severe disability at 18 to 22 months of age. Long-term outcomes are now available.

*Methods.*—In the original trial, we randomly assigned infants with moderate or severe encephalopathy to usual care (the control group) or whole-body cooling to an esophageal temperature of 33.5°C for 72 hours, followed by slow rewarming (the hypothermia group). We evaluated cognitive, attention and executive, and visuospatial function; neurologic outcomes; and physical and psychosocial health among participants at 6 to 7 years of age. The primary outcome of the present analyses was death or an IQ score below 70.

*Results.*—Of the 208 trial participants, primary outcome data were available for 190. Of the 97 children in the hypothermia group and the 93 children in the control group, death or an IQ score below 70 occurred in 46 (47%) and 58 (62%), respectively ($P = 0.06$); death occurred in 27 (28%) and 41 (44%) ($P = 0.04$); and death or severe disability occurred in 38 (41%) and 53 (60%) ($P = 0.03$). Other outcome data were available for the 122 surviving children, 70 in the hypothermia group and 52 in the control group. Moderate or severe disability occurred in 24 of 69 children (35%) and 19 of 50 children (38%), respectively ($P = 0.87$). Attention—executive dysfunction occurred in 4% and 13%, respectively, of children receiving hypothermia and those receiving usual care ($P = 0.19$), and visuospatial dysfunction occurred in 4% and 3% ($P = 0.80$).

*Conclusions.*—The rate of the combined end point of death or an IQ score of less than 70 at 6 to 7 years of age was lower among children undergoing whole-body hypothermia than among those undergoing usual care, but the differences were not significant. However, hypothermia resulted in lower death rates and did not increase rates of severe disability among survivors. (Funded by the National Institutes of Health and the Eunice

Kennedy Shriver NICHD Neonatal Research Network; ClinicalTrials.gov number, NCT00005772.)

▶ The significant difference in the rate of the primary outcome of death or moderate to severe disability at 18 to 22 months of age between the hypothermia group and the control group that was noted in the National Institutes of Child Health and Human Development Neonatal Research Network's clinical trial of whole-body hypothermia was largely driven by deaths. Because developmental outcome in early childhood is a poor predictor of later neurodevelopment, it was uncertain whether the markedly reduced rate of death in the hypothermia group would result in an increase in the number of children who survive with disabilities, especially intellectual impairment. This study was designed to assess the rates of death and neurodevelopment impairment associated with whole-body hypothermia at 6 to 7 years of age, when outcomes of neonatal interventions are believed to be more definitive.

Data related to the primary outcome of the study, death or an IQ score below 70, were obtained for 91% of the original cohort. Among surviving infants, 93% of the hypothermia group and 80% of the control group were evaluated at a median age of 6.7 years and 6.8 years, respectively. A total of 27 children in the hypothermia group and 41 children in the control group had died, with only 6 deaths (hypothermia 3 deaths, control 3 deaths) occurring after the evaluation at 18 to 24 months of age. In contrast to the initial report demonstrating a beneficial effect of hypothermia in early childhood, there was no effect on outcome noted at 6 to 7 years of age. This was true even when the outcome of death or moderate to severe disability, the outcome analyzed in the article, was considered (relative risk 0.84; 95% confidence interval, 0.66−1.06). The lack of effect on the latter was primarily because of instability in the diagnosis of moderate to severe disability for children in the hypothermia group. At 6 to 7 years of age, an additional 7 children were noted to have moderate to severe disability.

The authors conclude that whole-body hypothermia does not increase the rate of severe disability among survivors. However, the lower death rate associated with hypothermia and the unchanged rate of moderate to severe disability among survivors most likely will result in an increase in the number of surviving children with severe disability.

**L. A. Papile, MD**

---

**Long-term neuroprotective effects of allopurinol after moderate perinatal asphyxia: follow-up of two randomised controlled trials**
Kaandorp JJ, van Bel F, Veen S, et al (Univ Med Ctr Utrecht, The Netherlands; Leiden Univ Med Ctr, The Netherlands; et al)
*Arch Dis Child Fetal Neonatal Ed* 97:F162-F166, 2012

---

*Objective.*—Free-radical-induced reperfusion injury has been recognised as an important cause of brain tissue damage after birth asphyxia. Allopurinol reduces the formation of free radicals, thereby potentially limiting the amount of hypoxia—reperfusion damage. In this study the long-term outcome of neonatal allopurinol treatment after birth asphyxia was examined.

*Design.*—Follow-up of 4 to 8 years of two earlier performed randomised controlled trials.

*Setting.*—Leiden University Medical Center, University Medical Center Groningen and University Medical Center Utrecht, The Netherlands.

*Patients.*—Fifty-four term infants were included when suffering from moderate-to-severe birth asphyxia in two previously performed trials.

*Intervention.*—Infants either received 40 mg/kg allopurinol (with an interval of 12 h) starting within 4 h after birth or served as controls.

*Main Outcome Measures.*—Children, who survived, were assessed with the Wechsler Preschool and Primary Scales of Intelligence test or Wechsler Intelligence Scale for Children and underwent a neurological examination. The effect of allopurinol on severe adverse outcome (defined as mortality or severe disability at the age of 4—8 years) was examined in the total group of asphyxiated infants and in a predefined subgroup of moderately asphyxiated infants (based on the amplitude integrated electroencephalogram).

*Results.*—The mean age during follow-up (n = 23) was 5 years and 5 months (SD 1 year and 2 months). There were no differences in long-term outcome between the allopurinol-treated infants and controls. However, subgroup analysis of the moderately asphyxiated group showed significantly less severe adverse outcome in the allopurinol-treated infants compared with controls (25% vs 65%; RR 0.40, 95% CI 0.17 to 0.94).

*Conclusions.*—The reported data may suggest a (neuro) protective effect of neonatal allopurinol treatment in moderately asphyxiated infants.

▶ Investigators continue to seek therapies that will augment the long-term effectiveness of therapeutic hypothermia (TH). Kaandorp and colleagues report 4- to 8-year follow-up of 54 infants with moderate to severe hypoxic ischemic encephalopathy (HIE) randomly assigned to either a control group or treatment with high-dose allopurinol (40 mg/kg/d), 2 doses 12 hours apart, beginning within 4 hours of birth. Allopurinol is thought to reduce reperfusion injury by downregulating formation or scavenging of free radicals. Infants were evaluated at 4 to 8 years with a neurologic examination and the Weschler Preschool and Primary Scales of Intelligence test or Weschler Intelligence Scale. No differences in mortality or other outcomes were detected. Subgroup analyses, however, showed a reduction in severe neurodevelopmental outcome at age 4 to 8 years among allopurinol-treated infants whose HIE initially was designated moderately severe. Although the number of infants with HIE treated with allopurinol is modest and the data do not suggest it is a viable alternative to TH,[1] along with other proposed therapies, such as xenon, melatonin, erythropoietin, and N-acetylcysteine, allopurinol appears well worth considering in future studies of HIE-directed therapies potentially complementary to TH.

**L. J. Van Marter, MD, MPH**

*Reference*

1. Perrone S, Stazzoni G, Tataranno ML, Buonocore G. New pharmacologic and therapeutic approaches for hypoxic-ischemic encephalopathy in the newborn. *J Matern Fetal Neonatal Med.* 2012;25:83-88.

**Long-term neuroprotective effects of allopurinol after moderate perinatal asphyxia: follow-up of two randomised controlled trials**
Kaandorp JJ, van Bel F, Veen S, et al (Univ Med Ctr Utrecht, The Netherlands; Leiden Univ Med Ctr, The Netherlands; et al)
*Arch Dis Child Fetal Neonatal Ed* 97:F162-F166, 2012

*Objective.*—Free-radical-induced reperfusion injury has been recognised as an important cause of brain tissue damage after birth asphyxia. Allopurinol reduces the formation of free radicals, thereby potentially limiting the amount of hypoxia—reperfusion damage. In this study the long-term outcome of neonatal allopurinol treatment after birth asphyxia was examined.

*Design.*—Follow-up of 4 to 8 years of two earlier performed randomised controlled trials.

*Setting.*—Leiden University Medical Center, University Medical Center Groningen and University Medical Center Utrecht, The Netherlands.

*Patients.*—Fifty-four term infants were included when suffering from moderate-to-severe birth asphyxia in two previously performed trials.

*Intervention.*—Infants either received 40 mg/kg allopurinol (with an interval of 12 h) starting within 4 h after birth or served as controls.

*Main Outcome Measures.*—Children, who survived, were assessed with the Wechsler Preschool and Primary Scales of Intelligence test or Wechsler Intelligence Scale for Children and underwent a neurological examination. The effect of allopurinol on severe adverse outcome (defined as mortality or severe disability at the age of 4—8 years) was examined in the total group of asphyxiated infants and in a predefined subgroup of moderately asphyxiated infants (based on the amplitude integrated electroencephalogram).

*Results.*—The mean age during follow-up (n=23) was 5 years and 5 months (SD 1 year and 2 months). There were no differences in long-term outcome between the allopurinol-treated infants and controls. However, subgroup analysis of the moderately asphyxiated group showed significantly less severe adverse outcome in the allopurinol-treated infants compared with controls (25% vs 65%; RR 0.40, 95% CI 0.17 to 0.94).

*Conclusions.*—The reported data may suggest a (neuro) protective effect of neonatal allopurinol treatment in moderately asphyxiated infants.

▶ This study examined long-term follow-up of 23 of 54 infants who had participated in 2 randomized controlled trials of high-dose allopurinol to reduce the neurologic consequences of severe intrapartum asphyxia. The studies were originally performed in 3 Dutch neonatal intensive care units and published in 1998 and 2006, respectively. Entry criteria were similar to those used in the large cooling trials. At a mean age of 5 years, 5 months, there were no differences in long-term outcomes between those who had been treated and those who had not. When subgroup analysis was performed, using amplitude-integrated electroencephalogram (aEEG) to characterize the severity of the neonatal encephalopathy, moderately asphyxiated infants fared better than controls.

Before we rush to add xanthine oxidase inhibitors to our treatment regimen, a number of issues will have to be addressed. First, does the aEEG serve as an adequate marker of encephalopathy? We have advocated that it should not be used as an entry criterion for therapeutic hypothermia because of an alarmingly high rate of false-negative recordings.[1] Second, as in the hypothermia trials, we do not know the exact point at which hypoxia ischemia results in brain injury. Although most trials have attempted intervention by 6 hours of postnatal life, injury could well be underway and past the therapeutic window, so timing is indeed everything.

We are at an interesting point in dealing with hypoxic-ischemic encephalopathy. Hypothermia has produced modest improvement in moderately asphyxiated newborns. Work continues with pharmacologic agents, such as xenon and erythropoietin, and stem cell infusions. Most of these interventions target a single site of the neurotoxic cascade, so it seems logical that combining these interventions might yield a better result than using a single agent. Unfortunately, to do so in a prospective randomized trial will require thousands of patients, years of enrollment, and prohibitively high cost. It seems that we are going to have to rely on experimental animal models, or small clinical trials, where patient selection is going to be crucial.

**S. M. Donn, MD**

*Reference*

1. Sarkar S, Barks JD, Donn SM. Should amplitude-integrated electroencephalography be used to identify infants suitable for hypothermic neuroprotection? *J Perinatol.* 2008;28:117-122.

---

**Seven- to eight-year follow-up of the CoolCap trial of head cooling for neonatal encephalopathy**
Guillet R, on behalf of the CoolCap Trial Group (Univ of Rochester Med Ctr, NY; et al)
*Pediatr Res* 71:205-209, 2012

---

*Introduction.*—We sought to determine whether 18- to 22-mo neurodevelopmental outcomes predicted functional outcomes at 7–8 y for survivors of the CoolCap study of therapeutic hypothermia for neonates with hypoxic–ischemic encephalopathy.

*Results.*—WeeFIM ratings were completed at 7–8 y of age on 62 (32 cooled; 30 standard care) of 135 surviving children who had had neurodevelopmental assessment at 18 mo. There was 1 refusal, 58 lost to follow-up, and 14 children whose centers declined to participate. Disability status at 18 mo was strongly associated with WeeFIM ratings ($P < 0.001$); there was no significant effect of treatment ($P = 0.83$).

*Discussion.*—Functional outcome at 7—8 y of survivors of neonatal encephalopathy is associated with 18-mo neurodevelopmental assessment, supporting the long-term predictive value of a favorable outcome at 18 mo assessed by published trials of therapeutic hypothermia.

*Methods.*—All surviving children who participated in the CoolCap study and were assessed at 18 mo were eligible for reassessment using the WeeFIM instrument that qualitatively measures self-care, mobility, and cognitive function. Center investigators obtained consent from the families for a certified researcher to administer the WeeFIM instrument by phone.

▶ In 2005, the 18-month outcomes of the CoolCap trial[1] were published, indicating a trend in the direction of benefit in the primary outcome (death or severe disability) overall and no benefit among infants with the most severe amplitude-integrated electroencephalographic changes. The current study reports 7-year to 8-year outcomes among the CoolCap study population. The conclusions that can be drawn are limited for 2 reasons: the CoolCap study was not designed to have adequate power to evaluate outcomes beyond age 18 months and also because of the substantial decline in children who returned for 7-year to 8-year follow-up (46% of the available cohort). Nevertheless, the investigators were able to evaluate correlations between 18-month compared with 7-year to 8-year outcomes, detecting positive correlation between 18-month outcomes and 7-year to 8-year outcomes as assessed by the WeeFIM II (the Functional Independence Measure for Children), suggesting outcomes at 18 months are useful in predicting major school-age outcomes.

**L. J. Van Marter, MD, MPH**

*Reference*

1. Gluckman PD, Wyatt JS, Azzopardi D, et al. Selective head cooling with mild systemic hypothermia after neonatal encephalopathy: multicentre randomised trial. *Lancet.* 2005;365:663-670.

---

## Xenon Augmented Hypothermia Reduces Early Lactate/N-Acetylaspartate and Cell Death in Perinatal Asphyxia

Faulkner S, Bainbridge A, Kato T, et al (Univ College London, UK; Univ College London Hosps, UK)
*Ann Neurol* 70:133-150, 2011

---

*Objective.*—Additional treatments for therapeutic hypothermia are required to maximize neuroprotection for perinatal asphyxial encephalopathy. We assessed neuroprotective effects of combining inhaled xenon with therapeutic hypothermia after transient cerebral hypoxia—ischemia in a piglet model of perinatal asphyxia using magnetic resonance spectroscopy (MRS) biomarkers supported by immunohistochemistry.

*Methods.*—Thirty-six newborn piglets were randomized (all groups n = 9), with intervention from 2 to 26 hours, to: (1) normothermia; (2) normothermia + 24 hours 50% inhaled xenon; (3) 24 hours hypothermia (33.5°C); or (4) 24 hours hypothermia (33.5°C) + 24 hours 50% inhaled xenon. Serial MRS was acquired before, during, and up to 48 hours after hypoxia—ischemia.

*Results.*—Mean arterial blood pressure was lower in all treatment groups compared with normothermia ($p < 0.01$) (although >40 mmHg); the combined therapy group required more fluid boluses ($p < 0.05$) and inotropes ($p < 0.001$). Compared with no intervention, both hypothermia and xenon-augmented hypothermia reduced the temporal regression slope magnitudes for phosphorus-MRS inorganic phosphate/exchangeable phosphate pool (EPP) and phosphocreatine/EPP (both $p < 0.05$); for lactate/N-acetylaspartate (NAA), only xenon-augmented hypothermia reduced the slope ($p < 0.01$). Xenon-augmented hypothermia also reduced transferase-mediated deoxyuridine triphosphate nick-end labeling (TUNEL)[+] nuclei and caspase 3 immunoreactive cells in parasagittal cortex and putamen and increased microglial ramification in midtemporal cortex compared with the no treatment group ($p < 0.05$). Compared with hypothermia, however, combination treatment did not reach statistical significance for any measure. Lactate/NAA showed a strong positive correlation with TUNEL; nucleotide triphosphate/EPP showed a strong negative correlation with microglial ramification (both $p < 0.01$).

*Interpretation.*—Compared with no treatment, xenon-augmented hypothermia reduced cerebral MRS abnormalities and cell death markers in some brain regions. Compared with hypothermia, xenon-augmented hypothermia did not reach statistical significance for any measure. The safety and possible improved efficacy support phase II trials.

▶ There is substantial evidence from multiple randomized, controlled trials that therapeutic hypothermia reduces death and disability in infants 36 weeks' gestation or greater with moderate to severe perinatal hypoxic—ischemic encephalopathy, but in all trials there was still a substantial minority of children in the hypothermia groups with a poor outcome. Thus, there is great interest in strategies to improve on the beneficial effects of hypothermia. One approach is to study combinations of pharmacotherapy with hypothermia. One of the best-studied combinations in the experimental literature, which is now moving to early-phase clinical trials in the United Kingdom, is xenon plus hypothermia.

The noble gas xenon, which has multiple reported mechanisms of action on neurons, is approved for use as an inhalational anesthetic in the United Kingdom. It is expensive, but cost can be limited through use of special closed ventilator circuits. Experimental studies in a rodent model of perinatal cerebral hypoxia ischemia demonstrated dose-dependent neuroprotection by xenon and additive or synergistic neuroprotective effects when xenon and hypothermia were combined in various regimens.[1-4] More recently, in a piglet model of global cerebral (and systemic) hypoxia—ischemia, xenon enhanced the therapeutic benefit of hypothermia on brain injury and function.[5]

The report of Faulkner et al sought to extend the body of work by evaluating the effect of xenon plus hypothermia on early proton and phosphorus magnetic resonance spectroscopy (MRS) biomarkers of brain injury in another piglet global cerebral hypoxia—ischemia model, compared with groups with normothermic recovery or treatment with hypothermia or xenon alone, with 9 animals in each of the 4 groups. This is of great translational relevance to early-phase clinical studies of xenon plus hypothermia, in which noninvasive evaluation of MRS biomarkers might be used to determine whether the combination showed sufficient preliminary evidence of efficacy to justify testing in a larger randomized trial. The primary outcome biomarker was the slope of the change in the ratio of lactate to N-acetyl aspartate (Lac/NAA) over 48 hours after insult. This ratio was selected because it is a good predictor of later adverse developmental outcome in infants with hypoxic—ischemic encephalopathy.[6] Complementary histochemical and immunohistochemical indices of brain injury were used to evaluate tissue damage 48 hours after hypoxia—ischemia.

In both dorsal subcortical white matter and deep gray matter in the normothermia control group, the mean slope of the Lac/NAA ratio was positive; that is, the ratio increased over time. In contrast, the Lac/NAA slope was significantly lower in the xenon plus hypothermia group. Results in the hypothermia-alone and xenon-alone groups were intermediate and were not statistically different from either the normothermia or the combined treatment groups. Both hypothermia alone and xenon plus hypothermia attenuated the loss of high-energy phosphate relative to normothermia controls, but there was no statistical difference between the 2 treatment groups. Neuropathologic measures of cell death and microglial activation revealed similar trends: a beneficial effect of combined treatment relative to normothermia with intermediate values for either hypothermia or xenon alone. Moderate correlations between the primary MRS biomarker and tissue injury measures were observed.

Although the authors were not able to show an incremental benefit of the addition of xenon to hypothermia, review of the trends in their Fig 1 in the original article and comparison with the sample sizes in the earlier piglet study of Chakkarapani et al[5] suggests that this study may simply have been underpowered. Thus, the results of this study should not be interpreted as casting doubt on plans for early-phase clinical trials of xenon plus hypothermia, nor should they cast doubt on plans to evaluate MRS biomarkers in those trials at selected centers. Further evaluation of biomarkers in experimental models, with larger sample sizes and focused on fewer but more clinically relevant treatment groups (eg, hypothermia vs xenon plus hypothermia) could continue in parallel with the early-phase clinical trials. Yet the findings of Faulkner et al remind us that it may prove to be more challenging to demonstrate enhancement of the beneficial effects of hypothermia in the next wave of "hypothermia plus" trials for hypoxic—ischemic encephalopathy than it was to demonstrate that hypothermia was superior to conventional neonatal intensive care at normothermia.

**J. D. E. Barks, MD**

*References*

1. Ma D, Hossain M, Chow A, et al. Xenon and hypothermia combine to provide neuroprotection from neonatal asphyxia. *Ann Neurol.* 2005;58:182-193.

2. Martin JL, Ma D, Hossain M, et al. Asynchronous administration of xenon and hypothermia significantly reduces brain infarction in the neonatal rat. *Br J Anaesth.* 2007; 98:236-240.
3. Hobbs C, Thoresen M, Tucker A, Aquilina K, Chakkarapani E, Dingley J. Xenon and hypothermia combine additively, offering long-term functional and histopathologic neuroprotection after neonatal hypoxia/ischemia. *Stroke.* 2008;39:1307-1313.
4. Thoresen M, Hobbs CE, Wood T, Chakkarapani E, Dingley J. Cooling combined with immediate or delayed xenon inhalation provides equivalent long-term neuroprotection after neonatal hypoxia–ischemia. *J Cereb Blood Flow Metab.* 2009;29: 707-714.
5. Chakkarapani E, Dingley J, Liu X, et al. Xenon enhances hypothermic neuroprotection in asphyxiated newborn pigs. *Ann Neurol.* 2010;68:330-341.
6. Thayyil S, Chandrasekaran M, Taylor A, et al. Cerebral magnetic resonance biomarkers in neonatal encephalopathy: a meta-analysis. *Pediatrics.* 2010;125: e382-e395.

## The effect of whole-body cooling on brain metabolism following perinatal hypoxic–ischemic injury

Corbo ET, Bartnik-Olson BL, Machado S, et al (Loma Linda Univ Med Ctr, CA)
*Pediatr Res* 71:85-92, 2012

*Introduction.*—Magnetic resonance imaging (MRI) and spectroscopy (MRS) have proven valuable in evaluating neonatal hypoxic–ischemic injury (HII).

*Results.*—MRI scores in the basal ganglia of HII/HT$^+$ neonates were significantly lower than HII/HT$^-$ neonates, indicating less severe injury and were associated with lower discharge encephalopathy severity scores in the HII/HT$^+$ group ($P = 0.01$). Lactate (Lac) was detected in the occipital gray matter (OGM) and thalamus (TH) of significantly more HII/HT$^-$ neonates (31.6 and 35.3%) as compared to the HII/HT$^+$ group (10.5 and 15.8%). In contrast, the N-acetylaspartate (NAA)-based ratios in the OGM and TH did not differ between the HII groups.

*Discussion.*—Our data show that the HT was associated with a decrease in the number of HII neonates with detectable cortical and subcortical Lac as well as a decrease in the number of MRI-detectable subcortical lesions.

*Methods.*—We retrospectively compared the medical and neuroimaging data of 19 HII neonates who received 72 h of whole-body cooling (HII/HT$^+$) with those of 19 noncooled HII neonates (HII/HT$^-$) to determine whether hypothermia was associated with improved recovery from the injury as measured by MRI and MRS within the first 14 days of life. MRI scores and metabolite ratios of HII/HT$^+$ and HII/HT$^-$ neonates were also compared with nine healthy, nonasphyxiated "control" neonates.

▶ Therapeutic hypothermia has become established as a standard of care for encephalopathic newborns who have sustained hypoxic-ischemic brain injury in the intrapartum period. Although the exact mechanisms through which hypothermia modulates brain injury remain relatively speculative, it has been suggested that hypothermia may impact the neurotoxic cascade at several levels, especially during primary energy failure.

This retrospective study examines the effect of whole-body cooling (WBC) on brain structure (using MRI) and brain metabolism by utilizing magnetic resonance spectroscopy (MRS) to measure brain metabolites in 19 infants undergoing WBC following intrapartum hypoxic-ischemic encephalopathy (HIE). Their objective was to determine whether WBC decreases structural lesions or metabolic defects. The comparison groups comprised 19 noncooled neonates with HIE and 9 healthy neonates scanned for other reasons. Infants underwent MRI and MRS evaluations within the first 14 days of life.

Not surprisingly, infants undergoing WBC had less injury to the basal ganglia and lower encephalopathy scores at discharge than noncooled infants. WBC also resulted in lower lactate levels in the occipital gray matter and thalamus, but it did not affect *N*-acetylaspartate levels. The authors concluded that WBC was associated with fewer infants having detectable cortical and subcortical lactate and fewer subcortical structural lesions on MRI.

The results of the study certainly show an advantage of WBC and provide a plausible mechanism for its benefit. However, the study raises several questions, given its nonrandomized nature. Infants undergoing WBC were scanned at an average age of 5.6 days versus 8 and 14 days for the noncooled HIE babies and healthy controls, respectively. Infants chosen for inclusion in the study spanned nearly 11 years of clinical practice. No details regarding long-term outcomes were provided; thus, the significance of these short-term findings cannot be determined.

Still, this observation does provide some metabolic data to suggest that WBC might result in better balance between brain energy provision and consumption. We will probably not see a randomized controlled trial of MRS applied to cooled and noncooled infants, so further studies of this nature will need to do a very good job of avoiding a selection bias by carefully matching comparator groups.

**S. M. Donn, MD**

---

**Distribution and severity of hypoxic–ischaemic lesions on brain MRI following therapeutic cooling: selective head versus whole body cooling**
Sarkar S, Donn SM, Bapuraj JR, et al (Univ of Michigan Health System, Ann Arbor; et al)
*Arch Dis Child Fetal Neonatal Ed* 2012 [Epub ahead of print]

---

*Background.*—Whole body cooling (WBC) cools different parts of the brain uniformly, and selective head cooling (SHC) cools the superficial brain more than the deeper brain structures. In this study, the authors hypothesised that the hypoxic–ischaemic lesions on brain MRI following cooling would differ between modalities of cooling.

*Aim.*—To compare the frequency, distribution and severity of hypoxic–ischaemic lesions on brain MRI between SHC or WBC.

*Methods.*—In a single centre retrospective study, 83 infants consecutively cooled using either SHC (n=34) or WBC (n=49) underwent brain MRI. MRI images were evaluated by a neuroradiologist, who was masked to clinical parameters and outcomes, using a basal ganglia/watershed (BG/W) scoring system. Higher scores (on a scale of 0 to 4) were given for more extensive injury. The score has been reported to be predictive of neuromotor and cognitive outcome at 12 months.

*Results.*—The two groups were similar for severity of depression as assessed by a history of an intrapartum sentinel event, Apgar scores, initial blood pH and base deficit and early neurological examination. However, abnormal MRI was more frequent in the SHC group (SHC 25 of 34, 74% vs WBC 22 of 49, 45%; $p = 0.0132$, OR 3.4, 95% CI 1.3 to 8.8). Infants from the SHC group also had more severe hypoxic—ischaemic lesions (median BG/W score: SHC 2 vs WBC 0, $p = 0.0014$).

*Conclusions.*—Hypoxic—ischaemic lesions on brain MRI following therapeutic cooling were more frequent and more severe with SHC compared with WBC.

▶ Both whole body cooling (WBC) and selective head cooling (SHC) have proved to be effective therapies for neonatal encephalopathy thought to be due to hypoxia-ischemia (HIE) in the term and near-term infant. Because animal studies of induced hypothermia indicate there is a significant temperature gradient between the superficial and deep brain structures during SHC, in contrast to uniform brain cooling with WBC, it is speculated that the distribution of brain lesions following cooling will differ depending on the chosen modality of cooling.

The observation in this study that more frequent and severe brain lesions were noted with SHC compared with WBC may reflect limitations inherent in retrospective studies, rather than a true difference in the efficacy of the treatment modality. Because the SHC group was cooled in an epoch before the WBC group, it is possible that clinicians' willingness to refer infants for consideration of therapeutic hypothermia was different between the 2 time periods, favoring the inclusion of less severely affected infants in the WBC group. Moreover, the added criterion of amplitude electroencephalogram (EEG) abnormalities for SHC compared to clinical criteria alone for HBC may have resulted in the selection of infants with more severe HIE. As the authors aptly conclude, this study highlights the need for an individual patient data meta-analysis of the Cool Cap and TOBY trials,[1,2] both of which had similar clinical and amplitude integrated EEG criteria for enrollment, but used different cooling techniques, to determine if 1 method is more beneficial than the other.

**L. A. Papile, MD**

*References*

1. Gluckman PD, Wyatt JS, Azzopardi D, et al. Selective head cooling with mild systemic hypothermia after neonatal encephalopathy: multicentre randomised trial. *Lancet.* 2005;365:663-670.
2. Azzopardi D, Strohm B, Edwards AD, et al. Moderate hypothermia to treat perinatal asphyxial encephalopathy. *N Engl J Med.* 2009;361:1349-1358.

## Changes of Positron Emission Tomography in Newborn Infants at Different Gestational Ages, and Neonatal Hypoxic-Ischemic Encephalopathy

Shi Y, Zhao J-N, Liu L, et al (Third Military Med Univ, Chongqing, China)
*Pediatr Neurol* 46:116-123, 2012

Cerebral glucose metabolism was measured by [18]F-fluorodeoxyglucose position emission tomography in infants at different gestational ages and with neonatal hypoxic-ischemic encephalopathy. Thirty-six preterm and term infants at different gestational ages without brain injury were divided into four subgroups: ≤32 weeks (n = 4), 33-34 weeks (n = 5), 35-36 weeks (n = 12), and ≥37 weeks (n = 15). Twenty-four newborn infants with hypoxic-ischemic encephalopathy were divided into three subgroups: mild (n = 13), moderate (n = 7), and severe (n = 4). Cerebral glucose metabolism manifested a trend toward increase, and the structure of cranial [18]F-fluorodeoxyglucose positron emission tomography images became clear with increased gestational age, especially at ≥37 weeks. Uptakes of [18]F-fluorodeoxyglucose in the ≥37-week group were significantly higher than in the ≤32-week group ($P < 0.01$). Cerebral glucose metabolism changed significantly in neonatal hypoxic-ischemic encephalopathy, and was either unbalanced bilaterally or relatively low at all sites. Moreover, uptakes of [18]F-fluorodeoxyglucose were significantly lower in severe than in mild and medium hypoxic-ischemic encephalopathy ($P < 0.05$). Cerebral glucose metabolism, as measured by [18]F-fluorodeoxyglucose positron emission tomography, may prove useful for estimating brain development and injury in newborn infants, and its clinical values need further investigation.

▶ With the facilitation of modern imaging techniques, knowledge of the nature, prognosis, and ways to treat brain lesions in neonatal infants has increased remarkably. Neonatal hypoxic-ischemic encephalopathy (HIE) (newer terminology—neonatal encephalopathy) in term infants exhibits a progressive sequence of excito-oxidative events that unfold in the brain after an asphyxial insult. The ability to monitor these events in real time and observe the effects of neuroprotective therapies will result in the faster introduction of such therapies into the hands of the clinicians.

Traditionally, in the neonate, positron emission tomography (PET) scanning has been used in the evaluation of patients with hyperinsulinemic hypoglycemia (HI). Congenital hyperinsulinism is a leading cause of severe neonatal hypoglycemia. PET scans help distinguish between the diffuse and focal histologic subtypes of congenital hyperinsulinism. The diffuse form affects the entire pancreas and, if medically unresponsive, will require a near total (95%—98%) pancreatectomy. The focal form affects only a small region of the pancreas and only requires a limited pancreatectomy. Recent advances in Fluorine-18-L-dihydroxyphenylalanine PET ([18]F-DOPA PET/CT) have radically changed the clinical approach to patients with congenital hyperinsulinism. In most patients, this novel imaging technique is able to offer precise preoperative localization of the focal lesion, thus guiding the extent of surgical resection.

Shi et al show that the PET scan is of value in following the course and severity of babies with neonatal encephalopathy. It should come as no surprise that the infants with the most severe encephalopathy manifest the most diffuse changes, characterized by asymmetric or very low glucose uptake. Furthermore, the scans showed significant changes with advancing gestational age. The brain architecture became clearer when gestational age increased beyond 37 weeks' gestation. PET scans have been used extensively in the evaluation of brain disorders in adults. It remains to be seen whether they will prove to be equally important in the investigation of neurologic problems in the neonate. This set of data will act as an important first step.

A. A. Fanaroff, MBBCh, FRCPE

## Cytokines and Neurodevelopmental Outcomes in Extremely Low Birth Weight Infants

Carlo WA, for the *Eunice Kennedy Shriver* National Institute of Child Health and Human Development Neonatal Research Network (Univ of Alabama at Birmingham; et al)
*J Pediatr* 159:919-925, 2011

*Objective.*—To determine if selected pro-inflammatory and anti-inflammatory cytokines and/or mediators of inflammation reported to be related to the development of cerebral palsy (CP) predict neurodevelopmental outcome in extremely low birth weight infants.

*Study Design.*—Infants with birth weights ≤1000 g (n = 1067) had blood samples collected at birth and on days 3 ± 1, 7 ± 1, 14 ± 3, and 21 ± 3 to examine the association between cytokines and neurodevelopmental outcomes. The analyses were focused on 5 cytokines (interleukin [IL] 1β; IL-8; tumor necrosis factor-α; regulated upon activation, normal T-cell expressed, and secreted (RANTES); and IL-2) reported to be most predictive of CP in term and late preterm infants.

*Results.*—IL-8 was higher on days 0-4 and subsequently in infants who developed CP compared with infants who did not develop CP in both unadjusted and adjusted analyses. Other cytokines (IL-12, IL-17, tumor necrosis factor-β, soluble IL rα, macrophage inflammatory protein 1β) were found to be altered on days 0-4 in infants who developed CP.

*Conclusions.*—CP in former preterm infants may, in part, have a late perinatal and/or early neonatal inflammatory origin (Fig, Table 2).

▶ The finding that elevated inflammatory mediators in the preterm neonate are associated with cerebral palsy and other developmental problems is not surprising. Several studies have suggested a relationship between fetal inflammatory response syndrome (FIRS) and poor neurodevelopmental outcomes. Of interest is that the studies of FIRS have shown elevations of interleukin (IL)-6.[1] The study by Carlo et al primarily shows changes in IL-8, with some suggestions of differences in IL-1β and tumor necrosis factor alpha. Of interest is the fact that IL-8, a neutrophil chemoattractant, seems to increase over time,

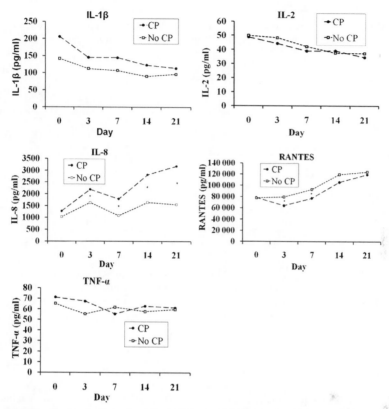

FIGURE.—Cytokine levels (median values) in infants with and without CP. Overall, IL-8 but not IL-1β, TNF-α, RANTES, or IL-2 differed on days 0-21 between the infants who went on to develop CP and those without CP. Statistical results of the comparison of cytokine levels at each time point are identified. (*P < .05 for comparison of infants with vs those without CP). (Reprinted from Journal of Pediatrics, Carlo WA, for the *Eunice Kennedy Shriver* National Institute of Child Health and Human Development Neonatal Research Network. Cytokines and neurodevelopmental outcomes in extremely low birth weight infants. *J Pediatr.* 2011;159:919-925. Copyright 2011, with permission from Elsevier.)

and the gradient in IL-8 in babies who subsequently develop cerebral palsy (CP) seems to become larger. On the other hand, IL-β, although not statistically different between CP and non-CP babies, appears to be high right at the time of birth, decreasing and converging over the first 21 days after birth (Fig). In this figure, it appears that the elevations of IL-8 at the time points after 0 to 4 days are the highest thus suggesting the greatest association with CP. However, Table 2 shows that IL-8 is significantly higher in the CP versus no CP groups from days 0 to 4. Furthermore, IL-1β is elevated at a *P* value of 0.06 and thus may also play a role. Several questions are raised here: why do some of the previous studies related to FIRS show elevations of IL-6 but these are not seen in this study? Is the early elevation of IL-1β of maternal origin and the IL-8 of fetal/neonatal origin? The timing of the elevations would suggest this. What is the source of the elevated cytokines in these preterm babies? Are

TABLE 2.—Unadjusted Comparison of Average Cytokine Levels in pg/mL on Days 0-4 in Infants with Moderate-Severe CP and in Infants with Any Degree of CP

|  | Moderate-Severe CP Median | IQR | No Moderate-Severe CP Median | IQR | P value* |
|---|---|---|---|---|---|
| IL-1β | 203 | 335 | 120 | 336 | .06 |
| IL-8 | 2363 | 3301 | 1652 | 2449 | .04 |
| TNF-α | 76 | 78 | 58 | 80 | .34 |
| RANTES | 59 772 | 89 680 | 80 059 | 70 707 | .20 |
| IL-2 | 46 | 48 | 50 | 64 | .53 |
|  | Any Degree of CP | | No CP | | |
| IL-1β | 163 | 351 | 119 | 332 | .06 |
| IL-8 | 2340 | 3732 | 1635 | 2273 | .01 |
| TNF-α | 69 | 89 | 58 | 76 | .32 |
| RANTES | 65 875 | 87 966 | 80 413 | 69 480 | .15 |
| IL-2 | 45 | 56 | 50 | 65 | .44 |

*Fran nonparametric 2-sample median test.

they of neonatal lung or intestinal origin? These organs would be exposed to a flux of amniotic fluid in utero and are highly immunoreactive. Are there methods by which this inflammatory response can be controlled? If these elevations in IL-8 in fact turn out to be causal for CP, means to control it could be preventative.

**J. Neu, MD**

*Reference*

1. Gotsch F, Romero R, Kusanovic JP, et al. The fetal inflammatory response syndrome. *Clin Obstet Gynecol.* 2007;50:652-683.

**Dendrimer-Based Postnatal Therapy for Neuroinflammation and Cerebral Palsy in a Rabbit Model**
Kannan S, Dai H, Navath RS, et al (Natl Insts of Health, Detroit, MI; et al)
*Sci Transl Med* 4:130ra46, 2012

Cerebral palsy (CP) is a chronic childhood disorder with no effective cure. Neuroinflammation, caused by activated microglia and astrocytes, plays a key role in the pathogenesis of CP and disorders such as Alzheimer's disease and multiple sclerosis. Targeting neuroinflammation can be a potent therapeutic strategy. However, delivering drugs across the blood-brain barrier to the target cells for treating diffuse brain injury is a major challenge. We show that systemically administered polyamidoamine dendrimers localize in activated microglia and astrocytes in the brain of newborn rabbits with CP, but not healthy controls. We further demonstrate that dendrimer-based N-acetyl-L-cysteine (NAC) therapy for brain injury suppresses neuroinflammation and leads to a marked improvement in motor function in the CP kits. The well-known and safe clinical profile for NAC, when combined with dendrimer-based targeting, provides opportunities for clinical translation in the treatment of neuroinflammatory disorders in humans. The effectiveness of the dendrimer-NAC treatment, administered in the postnatal period for a prenatal insult, suggests a window of opportunity for treatment of CP in humans after birth.

▶ A novel use of nanomaterials as vehicles for targeted drug delivery in perinatal brain injury is reported in this article. Intrauterine endotoxin administration in pregnant rabbits at 90% term gestation leads to neuroinflammation and cerebral palsy in the offspring. The authors intervened at 6 hours postnatally, with systemic (intravenous) administration of *N*-acetyl-L-cysteine (L-NAC) either alone or in conjunction with polyamidoamine dendrimers (PAMAM). Motor function and tone were videotaped and scored in the experimental animals. The dendrimers selectively localized to the activated microglia and astrocytes in animals exposed to endotoxin in utero. Dendrimer-conjugated L-NAC improved motor outcomes in the treated animals, whereas systemically administered L-NAC, even at 10 times higher dose, was significantly less effective in improving motor function. These results were associated with decreased markers of oxidative injury and inflammation, increased myelination, and amelioration of neuronal loss in the brains of the treated animals.

This is the first report of selective delivery of a neuroprotective agent to activated microglia and astrocytes using PAMAM as a vehicle. Given that studies of neuroprotective agents have so far yielded disappointing results, this approach has important translational implications after issues of safety, dose, and timing are further evaluated. In addition, to allow translation to human application, better methods of identifying infants at risk for cerebral palsy are needed in order to select the patient population likely to benefit the most from these novel postnatal interventions.

**H. Christou, MD**

---

### DTI reveals network injury in perinatal stroke

Dudink J, Counsell SJ, Lequin MH, et al (Sophia Children's Hosp, Rotterdam, The Netherlands; MRC Hammersmith/St Mary's Comprehensive Biomedical Res Centre, London, UK; ErasmusMC Sophia, Rotterdam, The Netherlands)
*Arch Dis Child Fetal Neonatal Ed* 2011 [Epub ahead of print]

---

*Background.*—Previous research showed acute diffusion-weighted imaging changes in pulvinar after extensive cortical injury from neonatal stroke. The authors used diffusion tensor imaging (DTI) to see how separate regions of ipsilateral thalamus are directly affected after a primary hit to their connected cortex in neonatal stroke.

*Methods.*—The authors analysed DTI images of three term infants with acute unilateral cortical arterial ischaemic stroke. Probabilistic tractography was used to define separate thalamic regions of interests (ROIs). The authors evaluated the three eigenvalues (EV) and apparent diffusion coefficient (ADC) values in the ROIs.

*Results.*—The ADC and EV in voxels of ROIs placed within the nuclei corresponding to ischaemic cortex were significantly lower than those in the unaffected contralesional thalamic nuclei.

*Conclusions.*—Our findings support the concept of acute network injury in neonatal stroke. ADC and EV were altered in specific thalamic regions that corresponded to the specific cortical areas affected by the primary ischaemic injury.

▶ The thalamus is a deep gray matter structure that relays sensory and motor signals received from diverse brain regions to the cerebral cortex. It can be considered a requisite 'last pit stop' for information going to the cortex. For many years neuropathologists have reported that primary cortical injury in the preterm infant is associated with cell loss in the thalamus. More recent studies have associated global thalamic shrinkage with preterm white matter injury and a disruption in thalamocortical connectivity with perinatal venous white matter infarction.

In this observational study, diffusion tensor imaging (DTI) was used to evaluate the acute effects of unilateral cortical neonatal arterial ischemic stroke (NAIS) on the thalamus. Significant changes in DTI values in the thalamus ipsilateral to an extensive NAIS were noted and are consistent with acute secondary injury after a primary injury to the connected cortex. Several possible mechanisms to explain this secondary neuronal cell death in the thalamus include excitotoxic injury from transmitted glutamateric signals from connected cortical neurons and neurodegeneration due to loss of trophic support from cortical targets.

These findings lend support to the concept of diffuse cortical injury occurring subsequent to a focal injury and show how deep gray matter is directly affected after a primary hit to its connected cortex. If the same mechanism is operative in preterm infants, it may help explain why white matter injury is associated with an increased risk of neuropsychological difficulties.

**L. A. Papile, MD**

---

**Symptomatic Neonatal Arterial Ischemic Stroke: The International Pediatric Stroke Study**
Kirton A, for the International Pediatric Stroke Study Investigators (Univ of Calgary and Alberta Children's Hosp, Canada; et al)
*Pediatrics* 128:e1402-e1410, 2011

---

*Background.*—Neonatal arterial ischemic stroke (AIS) has emerged as a leading cause of perinatal brain injury, cerebral palsy, and lifelong disability. The pathogenesis is poorly understood, which limits the development of treatment and prevention strategies. Multicenter studies must define epidemiology, risk factors, treatment practices, and outcomes to advance clinical trials and improve the adverse outcomes suffered by most survivors.

*Methods.*—The International Pediatric Stroke Study is a global research initiative of 149 coinvestigators (30 centers in 10 countries). Patients with clinical and neuroimaging confirmation of symptomatic neonatal AIS were enrolled (2003–2007). Standardized, Web-based data entry collected clinical presentations, risk factors, investigations, treatments, and early outcomes. We examined predictors of infarct characteristics and discharge outcome by using multivariate logistic regression.

*Results.*—Two hundred forty-eight neonates were studied (57% male, 10% premature). Most of them presented with seizure (72%) and nonfocal neurologic signs (63%). MRI was completed for 92% of the infants, although <50% had vascular imaging. Infarcts preferentially involved the anterior circulation and left hemisphere and were multifocal in 30%. Maternal health and pregnancies were usually normal. Neonates often required resuscitation (30%) and had systemic illnesses (23%). Cardiac and prothrombotic abnormalities were identified in <20% of the infants. Antithrombotic treatment was uncommon (21%) and varied internationally. Half (49%) of the infants had deficits at discharge, and data on their long-term outcomes are pending.

*Conclusions.*—Newborns with AIS are often systemically sick, whereas their mothers are usually healthy. Definitive causes for most neonatal AISs have not been established, and large-scale case-control studies are required to understand pathogenesis if outcomes are to be improved.

▶ This article highlights the value of including numerous medical investigators and centers in prospective registries of relatively uncommon diseases. Over a 54-month period of time, 149 physicians in 30 centers throughout the world who participated in the International Pediatric Stroke Study identified only 248 neonates with arterial ischemic stroke. The goal of the registry is to generate hypotheses in order to develop and execute international clinical trials.

The data in this article include several clinically relevant findings. More than 40% of infants had evidence of an acute neonatal illness and 30% received early neonatal resuscitation. This is in contrast to previous studies describing neonates with arterial ischemic stroke as otherwise normal infants who present at 1 to 2 days of age with seizures. Affected infants entered into the registry were unlikely to present with focal deficits, which emphasizes the need for a high index of clinical suspicion and prompt neuroimaging to diagnose stroke. Most infants (87%) presented in the first 7 days of age. Associated cardiac factors were identified in 18% of the infants, with the majority (88%) attributed to complex congenital heart disease. Although seizures were the most common presentation (72%), treatment with anticonvulsants was discontinued by the time of discharge for most patients.

**L. A. Papile, MD**

### Effects of Prone and Supine Position on Cerebral Blood Flow in Preterm Infants

Bembich S, Oretti C, Travan L, et al (Univ of Trieste, Italy; IRCCS "Burlo Garofolo" Children's Hosp, Italy; et al)
*J Pediatr* 60:162-164, 2012

We evaluated the effect of prone and supine position on cerebral blood flow (CBF) in stable preterm infants. CBF, $PO_2$, and $PCO_2$ were measured in the two positions. Peripheral oxygenation increased and CBF decreased in prone position. We speculate that CBF autoregulation may compensate for increased peripheral oxygenation, by decreasing CBF.

▶ In preterm infants, central apneas are less frequent in the prone position compared to the supine position.[1] Additionally, the prone position is associated with improved gas exchange and pulmonary function.[2] However, a recent observational study using near-infrared spectroscopy suggested that rotation of the head from midline reduced cerebral blood flow in extremely low gestational age infants (younger than 26 weeks).[3] Because head rotation is unavoidable with prone position, some neonatal intensive care units preclude placing preterm infants prone in an attempt to mitigate brain injury.

In this observational study, the investigators measured $PO_2$ and $PCO_2$ as well as cerebral blood flow in the prone and supine positions. In the supine position, the infant's head was held in midline by 2 small pillows placed on each side of the head. In the prone position, the head was rotated either to the left or the right. As was observed in the previous study,[2] cerebral blood flow was reduced in the prone position compared to the supine position. In contrast, $PO_2$ values were higher in the prone position compared to the supine position. The authors speculate that the differences observed in the 2 positions may reflect cerebral autoregulation. Oxygen delivery is determined by blood flow and the amount of oxygen in the blood. The decrease in cerebral blood flow noted in the previous study may merely reflect a compensatory mechanism rather than a compromised cerebral blood flow.

**L. A. Papile, MD**

*References*

1. Heimler R, Langlois J, Hodel DJ, Nelin LD, Sasidharan P. Effect of positioning on the breathing pattern of preterm infants. *Arch Dis Child.* 1992;67:312-314.
2. Wagaman MJ, Shutack JG, Moomjian AS, Schwartz JG, Shaffer TH, Fox WW. Improved oxygenation and lung compliance with prone positioning of neonates. *J Pediatr.* 1979;94:787-791.
3. Ancora G, Maranella E, Aceti A, et al. Effect of posture on brain hemodynamics in preterm newborns not mechanically ventilated. *Neonatology.* 2010;97:212-217.

**Recording conventional and amplitude-integrated EEG in neonatal intensive care unit**
Neubauer D, Osredkar D, Paro-Panjan D, et al (Univ Med Ctr Ljubljana, Slovenia)
*Eur J Paediatr Neurol* 15:405-416, 2011

Neonatal electroencephalography (EEG) presents a challenge due to its difficult interpretation that differs significantly from interpretation in older children and adolescents. Also, from the technological point of view, it is more difficult to perform and is not a standard procedure in all neonatal intensive care units (NICUs). During recent years, long-term cerebral function monitoring by the means of amplitude-integrated EEG (aEEG) has become popular in NICUs because it is easy to apply, allows real-time interpretation by the neonatologist treating the newborn, and has predictive value for outcome. On the other side, to record conventional EEG (cEEG), which is still considered the gold standard of neonatal EEG, the EEG technician should not only be well trained in performing neonatal EEG but also has to adapt to suboptimal working conditions. These issues need to be understood when approaching the neonatal cEEG in NICU and the main structure of the article is dedicated to this technique. The authors discuss the benefits of the digitalization and its positive effects on the improvement of NICU recording. The technical aspects as well as the standards for cEEG recording are described, and a section is dedicated to possible artifacts. Thereafter, alternative and concomitant use of aEEG and its benefits are briefly discussed. At the end there is a section that presents a review of our own cEEG and aEEG recordings that were chosen as the most frequently encountered patterns according to Consensus statement on the use of EEG in the intensive care unit.

▶ Neubauer et al present a review of important technical and interpretative aspects of neonatal electroencephalography (EEG). They highlight the major advantages of digital EEG technology as well as some of the most important pitfalls and review strategies for effectively recording conventional neonatal EEG. The authors focus on the need for repeated conventional EEG recordings to assess the evolution of background patterns. For EEG background evaluation, upon which prognosis is often estimated, this is an appropriate approach. However, for the detection of neonatal seizures, routine-length (60-minute) conventional EEG recording is insufficient, as outlined in the recent American Clinical Neurophysiology Guideline on neonatal EEG monitoring.[1]

Pattern recognition is pivotal for EEG interpretation. This article includes several sample conventional EEG figures, which show common abnormalities as well as normal graphoelements. The reader should carefully review the selected EEG montages, as local practice may use different configurations of EEG channels, resulting in slightly different display patterns.

Although this review highlights the stringent technical requirements that must be met for effective conventional neonatal EEG recordings, similar detail is not offered for amplitude-integrated EEG (aEEG). aEEG is increasingly used for long-term monitoring of at-risk neonates. Because of the compressed time-scale (6 cm/h), this is an ideal modality for observing background trends over time. Although this technology is touted as simple, there is a significant learning curve, both for effective application of electrodes to minimize artifact and for accurate interpretation of the data. Whitelaw and White highlighted some of the most important aspects of training for technical staff.[2]

One often-overlooked aspect of aEEG interpretation is that the "unprocessed" aEEG trace is subject to the same processing as the aEEG (filtering frequencies lower than 2 Hz and higher than 15 Hz, smoothing, and rectifying the signal), which is quite different from conventional EEG recording. This results in the "raw" aEEG tracing appearing dissimilar from that to which conventional EEG interpreters are accustomed.

In the initial paragraph on aEEG, the authors present an excessively optimistic perspective on this modality's sensitivity for neonatal seizure detection, citing sensitivity of 92% and higher. Most studies of seizure detection by aEEG have demonstrated significantly lower sensitivity.[3-5] A more sober perspective is subsequently presented, highlighting the fact that a 60-second neonatal seizure would result in, at best, a 1-mm deflection on a standard aEEG trace. Clearly, conventional EEG remains the gold standard for neonatal seizure detection, even if some seizures can be identified with aEEG recording.

One of the additional challenges for true neonatal EEG monitoring (rather than EEG recording) is that most centers do not have sufficient personnel for constant evaluation of the tracing, particularly outside of standard business hours. Neubauer et al correctly highlight that the combination of digitally displayed aEEG at the patient's bedside with simultaneous full conventional EEG recording may be the best clinical practice; bedside caregivers can monitor the aEEG in real-time and can consult the clinical neurophysiologist when needed for confirmation of any abnormal findings. Such collaboration between the neonatology and neurology teams is likely to result in the best possible neuromonitoring available for our smallest, most vulnerable patients.

**R. A. Shellhaas, MD, MS**

*References*

1. Shellhaas RA, Chang T, Tsuchida T, et al. The American clinical neurophysiology society's guideline on continuous electroencephalography monitoring in neonates. *J Clin Neurophysiol.* 2011;28:611-617.
2. Whitelaw A, White RD. Training neonatal staff in recording and reporting continuous electroencephalography. *Clin Perinatol.* 2006;33:667-677.
3. Rennie JM, Chorley G, Boylan GB, Pressler R, Nguyen Y, Hooper R. Non-expert use of the cerebral function monitor for neonatal seizure detection. *Arch Dis Child Fetal Neonatal Ed.* 2004;89:F37-F40.
4. Shah DK, Mackay MT, Lavery S, et al. Accuracy of bedside electroencephalographic monitoring in comparison with simultaneous continuous conventional electroencephalography for seizure detection in term infants. *Pediatrics.* 2008; 121:1146-1154.
5. Shellhaas RA, Saoita AI, Clancy RR. Sensitivity of amplitude-integrated electroencephalography for neonatal seizure detection. *Pediatrics.* 2007;120:770-777.

## Impact of Amplitude-Integrated Electroencephalograms on Clinical Care for Neonates With Seizures

Shellhaas RA, Barks AK (Univ of Michigan, Ann Arbor)
*Pediatr Neurol* 46:32-35, 2012

Amplitude-integrated electroencephalography (aEEG) was recently introduced into neonatal intensive care in the United States. We evaluated whether aEEG has changed clinical care for neonates with seizures. This study included all 202 neonates treated for seizures at our hospital from 2002-2007. Neonates monitored with aEEG (n = 67) were compared with contemporary control neonates who were not monitored, despite the availability of aEEG (n = 57), and a historic control group of neonates treated for seizures before our neonatal intensive care unit initiated aEEG (n = 78). Eighty-two percent of those receiving phenobarbital (137/167) continued treatment after discharge, with no difference among groups. Adjusted for gestational age and length of stay, no difference among groups was evident in number of neuroimaging studies or number of antiepileptic drugs per patient. Fewer patients undergoing aEEG, compared with contemporary (16/67 vs 29/57, respectively, $P = 0.001$) or historic (n = 38/78, $P = 0.002$) controls, were diagnosed clinically with seizures without electrographic confirmation. We conclude that aEEG did not increase neuroimaging tests, and did not alter antiepileptic drug use. However, diagnostic precision regarding neonatal seizures improved with aEEG because fewer neonates were treated for seizures based solely on clinical findings, without electrographic confirmation.

▶ Amplitude-integrated electroencephalography (aEEG) was intended primarily as a device for trending electroencephalographic background activity; however, it is frequently used as a tool for the detection of neonatal seizures. Because aEEG monitoring utilizes only 1 or 2 electrodes, it has limited sensitivity compared with conventional EEG, but its specificity appears to be more reliable with a very low false-positive rate.[1] In this retrospective study, the authors analyzed the impact of introducing aEEG into the clinical care of neonates with seizures. The only difference noted was that the percentage of infants who were treated for seizures based solely on clinical signs was significantly less in the cohort monitored with aEEG. The logical conclusion from this outcome would be that fewer neonates who were monitored with aEEG received antiepileptic therapy. However, overall the number of antiepileptic drugs prescribed per patient was the same regardless of whether monitoring was used. In the conclusion, the authors state that aEEG may prove important in decreasing the risk of neonates receiving unnecessary treatment. Based on their results, a different conclusion might be that aEEG monitoring did not affect resource utilization or short-term outcomes of neonates with seizures.

**L. A. Papile, MD**

*Reference*

1. Shah DK, Mackay MT, Lavery S, et al. Accuracy of bedside electroencephalographic monitoring in comparison with simultaneous continuous conventional electroencephalography for seizure detection in term infants. *Pediatrics.* 2008; 121:1146-1154.

## Neonatal Seizures: Treatment Practices Among Term and Preterm Infants

Glass HC, Kan J, Bonifacio SL, et al (Univ of California at San Francisco)
*Pediatr Neurol* 46:111-115, 2012

Neonatal seizures are common clinical conditions in both term and preterm neonates, yet no clinical management guidelines for direct care exist. We surveyed 193 international neurologists, neonatologists, and specialists in neonatal neurology or neonatal neurocritical care to assess management practices for seizures in preterm and term neonates. We found high reported rates of electroencephalogram and amplitude-integrated electroencephalogram (aEEG) monitoring to detect neonatal seizures, prevalent use of older anticonvulsant agents, and high rates of neuroimaging. Overall, responses were similar for term and preterm neonates. However, term neonates were likelier to be more heavily investigated, with higher use of magnetic resonance imaging and of electroencephalogram and aEEG monitoring of at-risk neonates. Continuous monitoring and cranial imaging of neonatal seizures now comprise the standard of care in many centers, although management practices vary widely. Early recognition and management of neonatal seizures and possible underlying injury may lead to increased opportunities for stopping seizures, protecting the brain, and improving developmental outcomes in at-risk neonates. The need for collaboration among neonatologists and neurologists is urgent, to address gaps in knowledge regarding management of neonatal seizures in term and preterm neonates.

▶ This report is a summary of the responses to a questionnaire addressing seizure management practices in preterm and term infants. Of the likely 400 to 500 individuals with access to the survey, 193 responded. Respondents were physicians from the United States, the United Kingdom, Canada, and Europe who had an interest in neonatal neurology.

Although the survey may not reflect the usual practices in seizure management in the United States, there are several interesting results contained in the survey answers. The first is that 19% of the respondents identified themselves as either a neonatal neurologist or a neonatal neurocritical care specialist. Thus, it would appear that a subspecialty focusing on acute neonatal neurologic conditions is rapidly evolving. Another noteworthy finding is the widespread use of either amplitude-integrated electroencephalography or electroencephalography monitoring of newborns considered to be at risk for seizures, including preterm infants of low gestational age or those with intraventricular hemorrhage as well as term infants with encephalopathy and those treated with extracorporeal membrane oxygenation. Only 10% of respondents relied on clinical observation alone to diagnose neonatal seizures. It may be that in the not-so-distant future brain monitoring will be considered as routine as blood pressure and heart rate monitoring for infants admitted to the neonatal intensive care unit.

L. A. Papile, MD

**Grade and laterality of intraventricular haemorrhage to predict 18–22 month neurodevelopmental outcomes in extremely low birthweight infants**
Merhar SL, Tabangin ME, Meinzen-Derr J, et al (Cincinnati Children's Hosp Med Ctr, OH)
*Acta Paediatr* 101:414-418, 2012

*Aim.*—To determine whether extremely low-birthweight (ELBW) infants with bilateral compared to unilateral intraventricular haemorrhage (IVH) have worse neurodevelopmental outcomes at 18–22 months.

*Methods.*—A total of 166 ELBW infants (<1000 g) admitted to a Cincinnati NICU from 1998 to 2005 with a head ultrasound showing Grade I–IV IVH and neurodevelopmental assessment at 18–22 months corrected age were included. Multivariable linear and logistic regression models were developed to determine the impact of laterality and grade of IVH and other clinical variables to predict scores on the Bayley Scales of Infant Development, Second Edition, Mental Development Index and Psychomotor Development Index and the combined outcome of neurodevelopmental impairment (NDI).

*Results.*—Infants with bilateral grade IV IVH had lower adjusted mean Bayley scores compared with infants with unilateral grade IV IVH. For grades I, II and III IVH, bilaterality of IVH was not associated with lower mean Bayley scores. Infants with grade IV IVH had the highest odds of NDI. The probability of NDI increased with sepsis and postnatal steroid use.

*Conclusion.*—ELBW infants with bilateral compared to those with unilateral grade IV IVH had worse neurodevelopmental outcomes. Infants with grades I–III IVH had similar outcomes whether they had unilateral or bilateral IVH.

▶ This study is a retrospective analysis of center-specific data collected as part of the National Institute of Child Health and Human Development's Neonatal Research Network's generic database for infants who weighed less than 1000 g at birth. Infants were included in the analysis if they had a head ultrasound at either 7 or 28 days of age that was read as demonstrating grades I to IV intraventricular hemorrhage (IVH) without evidence of white matter injury and a formal neurodevelopmental assessment at 18 to 22 months' corrected age. Of the 214 infants with grades I to IV IVH without evidence of white matter injury, 22% were not included in the analysis because they did not undergo a formal neurodevelopmental assessment. Among the 166 infants included in the analysis, the distribution of IVH was 67% grade I, 9% grade II, 11% grade

III, and 12% grade IV, a distribution similar to that reported by others. Interestingly, more that 50% of the lesions were bilateral. As expected, infants with bilateral grade IV IVH had lower Mental Developmental Index and Psychomotor Developmental Index scores on the Bayley Scales of Infant Development-II than those with unilateral grade IV IVH. However, the study lacks sufficient power to support the conclusion that the outcome of grades II to III IVH is similar for infants with unilateral or bilateral lesions.

**L. A. Papile, MD**

---

**Survival Without Disability to Age 5 Years After Neonatal Caffeine Therapy for Apnea of Prematurity**
Schmidt B, for the Caffeine for Apnea of Prematurity (CAP) Trial Investigators (McMaster Univ, Hamilton, Canada; et al)
*JAMA* 307:275-282, 2012

---

*Context.*—Very preterm infants are prone to apnea and have an increased risk of death or disability. Caffeine therapy for apnea of prematurity reduces the rates of cerebral palsy and cognitive delay at 18 months of age.

*Objective.*—To determine whether neonatal caffeine therapy has lasting benefits or newly apparent risks at early school age.

*Design, Setting, and Participants.*—Five-year follow-up from 2005 to 2011 in 31 of 35 academic hospitals in Canada, Australia, Europe, and Israel, where 1932 of 2006 participants (96.3%) had been enrolled in the randomized, placebo-controlled Caffeine for Apnea of Prematurity trial between 1999 and 2004. A total of 1640 children (84.9%) with birth weights of 500 to 1250 g had adequate data for the main outcome at 5 years.

*Main Outcome Measures.*—Combined outcome of death or survival to 5 years with 1 or more of motor impairment (defined as a Gross Motor Function Classification System level of 3 to 5), cognitive impairment (defined as a Full Scale IQ<70), behavior problems, poor general health, deafness, and blindness.

*Results.*—The combined outcome of death or disability was not significantly different for the 833 children assigned to caffeine from that for the 807 children assigned to placebo (21.1% vs 24.8%; odds ratio adjusted for center, 0.82; 95% CI, 0.65-1.03; *P* =.09). The rates of death, motor impairment, behavior problems, poor general health, deafness, and blindness did not differ significantly between the 2 groups. The incidence of cognitive impairment was lower at 5 years than at 18 months and similar in the 2 groups (4.9% vs 5.1%; odds ratio adjusted for center, 0.97; 95% CI, 0.61-1.55; *P* =.89).

*Conclusion.*—Neonatal caffeine therapy was no longer associated with a significantly improved rate of survival without disability in children with very low birth weights who were assessed at 5 years.

► The Caffeine for Apnea of Prematurity (CAP), a large-scale randomized clinical trial of 1640 infants born weighing between 500 and 1250 g at hospitals in

Canada, Australia, Europe, and Israel, showed a benefit of caffeine treatment on the primary study outcome (eg, composite of death before 18 months, cerebral palsy, cognitive delay, severe hearing loss, or bilateral blindness). The study also yielded some surprising initial results, including reduced rates of broncho-pulmonary dysplasia and retinopathy of prematurity, and improved neurodevel-opmental outcome at 18 to 21 months on the Bayley Scales of Infant Development-II (BSID-II).[1,2] Further analyses of CAP study data demonstrated that caffeine treatment is cost-effective.[3] Using a comprehensive battery of developmental tests for this study phase, these authors found an overall trend toward improved neurodevelopmental outcomes by age 5 unaccompanied by any detectable difference in disability-free survival between caffeine-treated infants and the control group. The poor ability of the BSID-II to predict school outcomes is a potential explanation of the study results. The impact of late envi-ronmental and health factors on outcome is an alternative explanation. A note-worthy finding is that subgroup analyses showed fewer caffeine-treated infants with any evidence of cerebral palsy, and caffeine treatment was also associated with better scores on the Gross Motor Classification Scale. As Maitre and Stark note in the accompanying editorial,[4] these findings might have longer-term implications for motor development. In summary, the CAP study provides powerful evidence for early benefits of caffeine treatment of infants born at or below 1250 g and that the current report, indicating overall null neurodevelop-mental findings at age 5 notwithstanding, leaves open the possibility of later health or neurodevelopmental benefits of neonatal caffeine therapy. I look forward to future reports of even later outcomes of CAP study subjects.

**L. J. Van Marter, MD, MPH**

*References*

1. Schmidt B, Roberts RS, Davis P, et al. Caffeine for apnea of prematurity. *N Engl J Med.* 2006;354:2112-2121.
2. Schmidt B, Roberts RS, Davis P, et al. Long term effects of caffeine therapy for apnea of prematurity. *N Engl J Med.* 2007;357:1893-1902.
3. Dukhovny D, Lorch SA, Schmidt B, et al. Economic evaluation of caffeine for apnea of prematurity. *Pediatrics.* 2011;127:e146-e155.
4. Maitre N, Stark A. Neuroprotection for premature infants?: another perspective on caffeine. *JAMA.* 2012;307:304-305.

---

## Neurologic Outcomes in Very Preterm Infants Undergoing Surgery

Filan PM, Hunt RW, Anderson PJ, et al (Royal Children's Hosp, Melbourne, Australia; Murdoch Children's Res Inst, Melbourne, Australia)
*J Pediatr* 160:409-414, 2012

---

*Objective.*—To investigate the relationship between surgery in very preterm infants and brain structure at term equivalent and 2-year neuro-developmental outcome.

*Study Design.*—A total of 227 infants born at <30 weeks gestation or at a birth weight of <1250 g were prospectively enrolled into a longitudinal observational cohort for magnetic resonance imaging and developmental follow-up. The infants were categorized retrospectively into either a nonsurgical group (n = 178) or a surgical group (n = 30). Nineteen infants were excluded because of incomplete or unsuitable data. The surgical and nonsurgical groups were compared in terms of clinical demographic data, white matter injury, and brain volume at term. Neurodevelopmental outcome was assessed at age 2 years.

*Results.*—Compared with the nonsurgical group, the infants in the surgical group were smaller and more growth-restricted at birth, received more respiratory support and oxygen therapy, and had longer hospital stays. They also had smaller brain volumes, particularly smaller deep nuclear gray matter volumes. Infants who underwent bowel surgery had greater white matter injury. Mental Developmental Index scores were lower in the surgical group, whereas Psychomotor Developmental Index scores did not differ between the groups. The Mental Developmental Index difference became nonsignificant after adjustment for confounding variables.

*Conclusion.*—Preterm infants exposed to surgery and anesthesia had greater white matter injury and smaller total brain volumes, particularly smaller deep nuclear gray matter volumes. Surgical exposure in the preterm infant should alert the clinician to an increased risk for adverse cognitive outcome.

▶ A systemic inflammatory response associated with surgery has been described in adults and children undergoing cardiac surgery. Concerns regarding a similar response occurring in preterm infants undergoing a surgical procedure have been raised because immature oligodendroglia in the preterm infant's brain appear to be particularly vulnerable to inflammation-mediated injury. In addition to inflammation, there are concerns about the potential for anesthesia-induced neuronal apoptosis in the developing brain. It is estimated that 10% to 20% of very preterm infants undergo a surgical procedure requiring general anesthesia before discharge from the neonatal unit.

The Victoria Infant Brain Study was a prospective study in which infants underwent magnetic resonance imaging (MRI) at term corrected age and a formal neurodevelopmental assessment at 2 years corrected age using the Bayley Scales of Infant Development II (BSID-II). In this report, the MRI findings and BSID-II scores were compared for the cohort of study infants who had undergone a surgical procedure requiring general anesthesia and those who did not. A secondary analysis related to the type of surgery procedure also was done.

The increased incidence of moderate to severe white matter injury and reduced brain volumes noted in the surgical cohort most likely is multifactorial in origin. The surgical cohort had a significantly lower birth weight z score than the nonsurgical cohort, indicating a greater degree of in utero growth restriction. However, the reduction in deep nuclear gray matter volume in the surgical cohort may be related, at least in part, to exposure to anesthesia and perhaps sedatives that are used in neonatal practice.

**L. A. Papile, MD**

## Neonatal Intensive Care Unit Stress Is Associated with Brain Development in Preterm Infants

Smith GC, Gutovich J, Smyser C, et al (Washington Univ School of Medicine, St Louis, MO; et al)
*Ann Neurol* 70:541-549, 2011

*Objective.*—Although many perinatal factors have been linked to adverse neurodevelopmental outcomes in very premature infants, much of the variation in outcome remains unexplained. The impact on brain development of 1 potential factor, exposure to stressors in the neonatal intensive care unit, has not yet been studied in a systematic, prospective manner.

*Methods.*—In this prospective cohort study of infants born at <30 weeks gestation, nurses were trained in recording procedures and cares. These recordings were used to derive Neonatal Infant Stressor Scale scores, which were employed to measure exposure to stressors. Magnetic resonance imaging (brain metrics, diffusion, and functional magnetic resonance imaging) and neurobehavioral examinations at term equivalent postmenstrual age were used to assess cerebral structure and function. Simple and partial correlations corrected for confounders, including immaturity and severity of illness, were used to explore these relations.

*Results.*—Exposure to stressors was highly variable, both between infants and throughout a single infant's hospital course. Exposure to a greater number of stressors was associated with decreased frontal and parietal brain width, altered diffusion measures and functional connectivity in the temporal lobes, and abnormalities in motor behavior on neurobehavioral examination.

*Interpretation.*—Exposure to stressors in the Neonatal Intensive Care Unit is associated with regional alterations in brain structure and function. Further research into interventions that may decrease or mitigate exposure to stressors in the neonatal intensive care unit is warranted.

▶ One of the focuses of developmentally supportive care for preterm infants is to minimize physiological stress by modifying the infant's environment. Whether one subscribes to the concept of developmentally supportive care, there is mounting evidence that repeated stress, especially during the early period of infant development, has long-lasting effects on the central nervous system.[1,2] The data regarding infant exposure to stressors in this article suggest that this exposure is unacceptably high and may have long-lasting consequences. During the first 28 days of life, the daily number of procedures, such as any attempts at vascular access or intubation and radiology or diagnostic studies, ranged from 3 to 20, indicating that some infants were exposed to an extremely stressful procedure every 72 minutes. Using MRI, the authors examined brain metrics, diffusion, and functional connectivity at term equivalent age in a cohort of extremely preterm infants. The findings that a high level of stress exposure is associated with differences in the brain on both an anatomic and a functional level suggest that the differences associated with stress are not only structural, but also alter the function of the brain and thus may potentially adversely affect neurodevelopment.

**L. A. Papile, MD**

*References*

1. Grunau R. Early pain in preterm infants. A model of long-term effects. *Clin Perinatol.* 2002;29:373-394.
2. Als H, Duffy FH, McAnulty GB, et al. Early experience alters brain function and structure. *Pediatrics.* 2004;113:846-857.

---

**Infant regulation of intake: the effect of free glutamate content in infant formulas**

Ventura AK, Beauchamp GK, Mennella JA (Monell Chemical Senses Ctr, Philadelphia, PA)
*Am J Clin Nutr* 95:875-881, 2012

---

*Background.*—We recently discovered that infants randomly assigned to a formula high in free amino acids (extensive protein hydrolysate formula; ePHF) during infancy consumed less formula to satiation and gained less weight than did infants fed an isocaloric formula low in free amino acids (cow milk formula; CMF).

*Objective.*—Because ePHF and CMF differ markedly in concentrations of free glutamate, we tested the hypothesis that the higher glutamate concentrations in ePHF promote satiation and satiety.

*Design.*—In this counterbalanced, within-subject study, infants <4 mo of age ($n = 30$) visited our laboratory for 3 sets of 2 consecutive infant-led formula meals over 3 test days. Infants were fed 1 of 3 isocaloric formulas during each first meal: CMF, ePHF, or CMF with added free glutamate to approximate concentrations in ePHF (CMF+glu). When infants signaled hunger again, they were fed a second meal of CMF. From these data, we calculated satiety ratios for each of the 3 formulas by dividing the intermeal interval by the amount of formula consumed during that particular first meal.

*Results.*—Infants consumed significantly less CMF+glu ($P < 0.02$) and ePHF ($P < 0.04$) than CMF during the first meals. They also showed greater levels of satiety after consuming CMF+glu or ePHF: satiety ratios for CMF+glu ($P < 0.03$) and ePHF ($P < 0.05$) were significantly higher than for CMF.

*Conclusion.*—These findings suggest a role of free glutamate in infant intake regulation and call into question the claim that formula feeding impairs infants' abilities to self regulate energy intake. This trial was registered at clinicaltrials.gov as NCT00957892.

▶ Concern about the obesity epidemic and its origins in early life is prompting a closer evaluation of what and how much babies eat. Breast-fed babies are thought to self-regulate more than bottle-fed babies, and this has been conjectured as one of the reasons for less obesity among breast-fed infants. Whether the composition of a feeding and the taste of formula may relate to satiety and less intake is the subject of this article, which presents an interesting concept: free glutamate concentrations in formula may lead to earlier satiety. In this study, 3 formulas were tested, which included a standard cow's milk formula, an extensive protein hydrolysate formula, and a cow's milk formula with added glutamate. All the formulas were isocaloric. Using a design whereby each baby received all 3 formulas, it was found that the babies appeared to be satiated earlier with the hydrolyzed formula and the cow's milk formula with the added glutamate. The authors aptly discuss several aspects of the reasons behind this. One potential factor is the taste. For those readers who have ever tasted some of the protein hydrolysate formulas, it is immediately clear: for many adults, they taste "awful." As mentioned by the authors, most babies less than 4 months of age do not seem to mind the taste, but previous studies of satiety are lacking. The parents' stopping the feedings earlier with the hydrolysate formulas may still be a factor, although the investigators tried to control for this. For some sensitive parents, there is no easy hiding of the taste or smell of these formulas. The fact that the added free glutamate to the cow's milk formula had an effect is of interest. Whether the "umami"[1] or meaty, savory taste that this amino acid may confer affected the infants or parents is questionable. As stated by the authors, a more likely reason relates to receptors that may be related to satiety centers, but these mechanisms in babies have not yet been fully investigated, and this remains conjecture. Nevertheless, the fact that glutamate addition to cow's milk formula appeared to result in greater satiety is of interest and may be an important finding with implications for controlling intake and subsequent obesity.

**J. Neu, MD**

*Reference*

1. Lindemann B. A taste for umami. *Nat Neurosci.* 2000;3:99-100.

---

**Effects of fetal antiepileptic drug exposure: Outcomes at age 4.5 years**
Meador KJ, For the NEAD Study Group (Emory Univ, Atlanta, GA; et al)
*Neurology* 78:1207-1214, 2012

---

*Objective.*—To examine outcomes at age 4.5 years and compare to earlier ages in children with fetal antiepileptic drug (AED) exposure.

*Methods.*—The NEAD Study is an ongoing prospective observational multicenter study, which enrolled pregnant women with epilepsy on AED monotherapy (1999—2004) to determine if differential long-term neurodevelopmental effects exist across 4 commonly used AEDs (carbamazepine, lamotrigine, phenytoin, or valproate). The primary outcome is IQ at 6 years of age. Planned analyses were conducted using Bayley Scales of Infant Development (BSID at age 2) and Differential Ability Scale (IQ at ages 3 and 4.5).

*Results.*—Multivariate intent-to-treat (n = 310) and completer (n = 209) analyses of age 4.5 IQ revealed significant effects for AED group. IQ for children exposed to valproate was lower than each other AED. Adjusted means (95% confidence intervals) were carbamazepine 106 (102−109), lamotrigine 106 (102−109), phenytoin 105 (102−109), valproate 96 (91−100). IQ was negatively associated with valproate dose, but not other AEDs. Maternal IQ correlated with child IQ for children exposed to the other AEDs, but not valproate. Age 4.5 IQ correlated with age 2 BSID and age 3 IQ. Frequency of marked intellectual impairment diminished with age except for valproate (10% with IQ <70 at 4.5 years). Verbal abilities were impaired for all 4 AED groups compared to nonverbal skills.

*Conclusions.*—Adverse cognitive effects of fetal valproate exposure persist to 4.5 years and are related to performances at earlier ages. Verbal abilities may be impaired by commonly used AEDs. Additional research is needed.

▶ Recently published studies by Molgaard-Nielsen and Haavid,[1] Holmes et al,[2] and Meador et al[3,4] evaluated the risks of congenital anomalies and neurodevelopmental outcomes following maternal antiepileptic drug (AED) exposure during pregnancy.

Between 1999 and 2004, the Neurodevelopmental Effects of Antiepileptic Drugs (NEAD) study prospectively enrolled pregnant women with epilepsy on monotherapy into what is now an ongoing comprehensive observational study of childhood neurodevelopmental outcomes. At age 4.5 years, children born to mothers who received valproate therapy during pregnancy were found to be at greatest risk of intellectual impairment, and the effects appeared to be dose dependent. This study validates the previously published NEAD study outcomes at 3 years of age[3] in which valproate therapy was associated with, on average, a 6-point to 9-point reduction in IQ; and in contrast to those treated with other antiepileptics, among infants born to valproate-treated mothers, the child's later IQ appeared to be independent of his or her mother's IQ. An important finding of this study is that cognitive impairments improved over time among infants exposed to most antiepileptic drugs (AEDs), but not for infants of valproate-treated mothers; in the valproate group, 10% of the infants had later evidence of marked intellectual impairment (ie, IQ less than 70).

Previously published reports have shown increased risk of major congenital anomalies,[4] including spina bifida, atrial septal defect, cleft palate, hypospadias, polydactyly, and craniosynostosis, associated with first-trimester fetal exposure to valproate.

Among a population-based Danish cohort of 837 795 infants born between 1996 and 2008, Molgaard-Nielsen and Hviid[1] found risk-adjusted analyses of maternal AED consumption during pregnancy revealed no increased risk of major congenital anomalies among infants born to mothers treated with newer-generation AEDs, including oxcarbazepine, topiramate, gabapentin, and levetiracetam.

Holmes et al[2] examined the fetal effects of antiepileptic polytherapies and found that the risk of malformations among infants exposed to lamotrigine and carbamazepine as polytherapy exceeded the risks of monotherapy only when the AED polytherapy included valproate.

These data argue strongly for avoiding, whenever possible, maternal use of valproate as AED therapy during pregnancy, a goal that is likely to be more attainable in the context of the availability of newer AEDs.

**L. J. Van Marter, MD, MPH**

*References*

1. Molgaard-Nielsen D, Hviid A. Newer-generation antiepileptic drugs and the risk of major birth defects. *JAMA.* 2011;305:1996-2002.
2. Holmes LB, Mittendorf R, Shen A, Smith CR, Hernandez-Diaz S. Fetal effects of anticonvulsant polytherapies. *Arch Neurol.* 2011;68:1275-1281.
3. Meador KJ, Baker GA, Browning N, et al. Cognitive function at 3 years of age after fetal exposure to antiepileptic drugs. *N Engl J Med.* 2009;360:1597-1605.
4. Meador KJ, Baker GA, Browning N, et al. Valproic acid monotherapy in pregnancy and major congenital malformations. *N Engl J Med.* 2010;362:2185-2193.

## Normal gut microbiota modulates brain development and behavior

Heijtz RD, Wang S, Anuar F, et al (Karolinska Institutet, Stockholm, Sweden; Genome Inst of Singapore; et al)

*Proc Natl Acad Sci U S A* 108:3047-3052, 2011

Microbial colonization of mammals is an evolution-driven process that modulates host physiology, many of which are associated with immunity and nutrient intake. Here, we report that colonization by gut microbiota impacts mammalian brain development and subsequent adult behavior. Using measures of motor activity and anxiety-like behavior, we demonstrate that germ free (GF) mice display increased motor activity and reduced anxiety, compared with specific pathogen free (SPF) mice with a normal gut microbiota. This behavioral phenotype is associated with altered expression of genes known to be involved in second messenger pathways and synaptic long-term potentiation in brain regions implicated in motor control and anxiety-like behavior. GF mice exposed to gut microbiota early in life display similar characteristics as SPF mice, including reduced expression of PSD-95 and synaptophysin in the striatum. Hence, our results suggest that the microbial colonization process initiates signaling mechanisms that affect neuronal circuits involved in motor control and anxiety behavior (Fig 4).

▶ The cliché "gut feeling" is one commonly used and implies an association between behavior and the brain. We have known that there is a strong relationship between intestinal physiology and the brain. In the last several years, an association has been established between intestinal microbes and local physiology affecting processes such as motility. But whether these commensal intestinal microbes actually play a role in brain development and behavior has only recently been provided attention. This study is one of the first to extensively evaluate the influence of intestinal bacteria on the chemistry and development of the

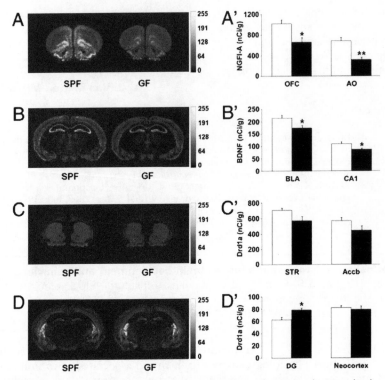

FIGURE 4.—GF mice show altered expression of anxiety and synaptic plasticity-related genes. (A) Representative autoradiograms showing NGFI-A mRNA expression at the level of the frontal cortex of SPF and GF mice (OFC, orbital frontal cortex; AO, anterior olfactory region). (A′) Bars show expression of NGFI-A mRNA (nCi/g) in the OFC and AO of SPF and GF mice. (B) Representative autoradiograms showing BDNF mRNA expression at the level of amygdala and dorsal hippocampus of SPF and GF mice (BLA, basolateral amygdala; CA1, CA1 region of the dorsal hippocampus). (B′) Bars show expression of BDNF mRNA (nCi/g) in the BLA and CA1 region of SPF and GF mice. (C) Representative autoradiograms showing dopamine D1 receptor (Drd1a) mRNA expression at the level of the striatum and nucleus accumbens of SPF and GF mice (STR, striatum; Accb, nucleus accumbens, shell region). (C′) Bars show expression of Drd1a mRNA (nCi/g) in the STR and Accb of SPF and GF mice. (D) Representative autoradiograms showing Drd1a mRNA expression at the level of the dorsal hippocampus of SPF and GF mice (DG, dentate gyrus; PtCx, parietal cortex, somatosensory area). (D′) Bars show expression of Drd1a mRNA (nCi/g) in the DG and PtCx of SPF and GF mice. All data (A′−D′) are expressed as means ± SEM, $n = 8$ per group. Filled bars represent GF mice. Open bars represent SPF mice. *$P < 0.05$, *$P < 0.001$ compared with SPF mice. (Reprinted from Heijtz RD, Wang S, Anuar F, et al. Normal gut microbiota modulates brain development and behavior. *Proc Natl Acad Sci U S A.* 2011;108:3047-3052. Copyright 2011 National Academy of Sciences, U.S.A.)

brain. In a comparison of germ-free with normally raised pathogen-free mice, the germ-free mice exhibited less anxiety and "bolder" activity. When the investigators colonized adult germ-free animals with normal gut bacteria, this had no effect on their behavior. If germ-free animals were colonized early in life, the behavioral effects could be reversed.

From a molecular regulation perspective, 2 genes associated with anxiety were found to be down-regulated in several regions in the brain of germ-free animals. Synaptic plasticity genes were also affected in various parts of the brain (Fig 4).

In a comprehensive gene analysis of 5 different brain regions, approximately 40 genes were affected by the presence of gut bacteria. Neurotransmitters as well as molecules involved in synaptogenesis were affected by the presence or absence of intestinal microbes.

Another article published recently[1] using antibiotics to disrupt intestinal microbiota similarly showed that the microbiota influences brain chemistry and behavior independent of the autonomic nervous system, gastrointestinal specific neurotransmitters, or inflammation. These are very important studies that beg the question of what are obstetricians, neonatologists, and pediatricians doing to the developing brain when the intestinal microbial ecology is altered with frequent and sometimes indiscriminant use of antibiotics. Could this be a link to neurobehavioral disorders such as autism, schizophrenia, and anxiety?

**J. Neu, MD**

*Reference*

1. Bercik P, Denou E, Collins J, et al. The intestinal microbiota affect central levels of brain-derived neurotropic factor and behavior in mice. *Gastroenterology*. 2011; 141:599-609.

---

**Current Role of Cryotherapy in Retinopathy of Prematurity: A Report by the American Academy of Ophthalmology**
Simpson JL, Melia M, Yang MB, et al (Univ of California, Irvine; Jaeb Ctr for Health Res, Tampa, FL; Univ of Cincinnati, OH; et al)
*Ophthalmology* 119:873-877, 2012

---

*Objective.*—To evaluate the role of cryotherapy in the current treatment of retinopathy of prematurity (ROP).

*Methods.*—Literature searches of PubMed and the Cochrane Library were conducted on December 2, 2009, for articles published after 1984. The searches included all languages and retrieved 187 relevant citations. Thirteen articles were deemed relevant to the assessment question and were rated according to the strength of evidence. Four articles reported results from 2 large multicenter randomized clinical trials, and the remaining 9 articles reported results of 3 small randomized trials that directly compared cryotherapy and laser.

*Results.*—Neither of the multicenter randomized clinical trials was a direct comparison of cryotherapy with laser. These studies were used to evaluate the comparative trials based on treatment criteria, study populations, and clinical results. Higher percentages of poor structural and functional outcomes generally were seen in eyes treated with cryotherapy compared with eyes undergoing laser treatment. Higher rates of systemic complications and myopia also were identified after treatment with cryotherapy.

*Conclusions.*—Despite a relative paucity of level I evidence directly comparing cryotherapy and laser treatment for threshold ROP, the literature suggests that neonatal facilities should gain access to laser technology and laser-trained ophthalmic staff to achieve better outcomes for treatment of the disease.

▶ According to the oft-quoted words of George Santayana, "Those who cannot remember the past are condemned to repeat it." The history of retinopathy of prematurity (ROP), originally described as retrolental-fibroplasia (RLF), a proliferative retinal vascular disease, and the leading preventable cause of blindness, is an encapsulated story of the history of neonatal-perinatal medicine. It also exemplifies the dangers of making decisions with incomplete data and understanding of a particular problem. Hence, after the recognition that there was an association between oxygen therapy and RLF, oxygen was restricted in the delivery room and for the care of preterm infants. The end result was a combination of increased mortality, notably on the first day of life, and an increase in cerebral palsy with minimal effect on blindness. Oxygen therapy was therefore liberalized but could be better monitored with continuous transcutaneous monitors and subsequently saturation monitors.

The landmark Cryotherapy for Retinopathy of Prematurity (CRYO-ROP) Study was stopped early because of an indisputable benefit of the cryotherapy. Favorable outcomes occurred in 75% of the cryotherapy-treated eyes, compared with 53% of control eyes.[1] The cohort was diligently followed and benefits for structure and function sustained through 15 years.[2,3]

The article by Simpson and colleagues represents an ophthalmic technology assessment, the goal of which is to evaluate the peer-reviewed, published scientific literature to help refine the important questions to be answered by future investigations and to define what is well established. The goals are accomplished in the report, which concludes that cryotherapy has outlived its usefulness and been replaced by laser photocoagulation delivered via an indirect ophthalmoscope.[4,5] Laser requires less general anesthesia and more easily accesses the posterior pole in addition to improving visual acuity and structural outcomes. Nonetheless, laser is still damaging to the developing retina, and a new blush of therapies is undergoing evaluation. Preliminary data from the use of intravitreal bevacizumab (an anti–vascular endothelial growth factor [VEGF] monoclonal) has been very encouraging in terms of the rapidity of action and the beautiful normal vascularization of the retina.[6,7] However, long-term visual outcomes are not yet available, few patients have been treated, and concerns about the effects of VEGF inhibition if the monoclonal enters the systemic circulation have not yet been answered. However, we may be on the cusp of a new era in therapy for ROP. Remember, the prime goal is to prevent ROP.

**A. A. Fanaroff, MBBCh, FRCPE**

*References*

1. Multicenter trial of cryotherapy for retinopathy of prematurity. Preliminary results. Cryotherapy for Retinopathy of Prematurity Cooperative Group. *Arch Ophthalmol.* 1988;106:471-479.
2. Multicenter trial of cryotherapy for retinopathy of prematurity. One-year outcome—structure and function. Cryotherapy for Retinopathy of Prematurity Cooperative Group. *Arch Ophthalmol.* 1990;108:1408-1416.

3. Palmer EA, Hardy RJ, Dobson V, et al; Cryotherapy for Retinopathy of Prematurity Cooperative Group. 15-year outcomes following threshold retinopathy of prematurity: final results from the multicenter trial of cryotherapy for retinopathy of prematurity. *Arch Ophthalmol.* 2005;123:311-318.
4. Shalev B, Farr AK, Repka MX. Randomized comparison of diode laser photocoagulation versus cryotherapy for threshold retinopathy of prematurity: seven-year outcome. *Am J Ophthalmol.* 2001;132:76-80.
5. Azad RV, Pasumala L, Kumar H, et al. Prospective randomized evaluation of diode-laser and cryotherapy in prethreshold retinopathy of prematurity. *Clin Experiment Ophthalmol.* 2004;32:251-254.
6. Mintz-Hittner HA, Kennedy KA, Chuang AZ; BEAT-ROP Cooperative Group. Efficacy of intravitreal bevacizumab for stage 3+ retinopathy of prematurity. *N Engl J Med.* 2011;364:603-615.
7. Moshfeghi DM, Berrocal AM. Retinopathy of prematurity in the time of bevacizumab: incorporating the BEAT-ROP results into clinical practice. *Ophthalmology.* 2011;118:1227-1228.

## Association of Antenatal Corticosteroids With Mortality and Neurodevelopmental Outcomes Among Infants Born at 22 to 25 Weeks' Gestation

Carlo WA, for the Eunice Kennedy Shriver National Institute of Child Health and Human Development Neonatal Research Network (Univ of Alabama, Birmingham; et al)
*JAMA* 306:2348-2358, 2011

*Context.*—Current guidelines, initially published in 1995, recommend antenatal corticosteroids for mothers with preterm labor from 24 to 34 weeks' gestational age, but not before 24 weeks due to lack of data. However, many infants born before 24 weeks' gestation are provided intensive care.

*Objective.*—To determine if use of antenatal corticosteroids is associated with improvement in major outcomes for infants born at 22 and 23 weeks' gestation.

*Design, Setting, and Participants.*—Cohort study of data collected prospectively on inborn infants with a birth weight between 401 g and 1000 g (N=10 541) born at 22 to 25 weeks' gestation between January 1, 1993, and December 31, 2009, at 23 academic perinatal centers in the United States. Certified examiners unaware of exposure to antenatal corticosteroids performed follow-up examinations on 4924 (86.5%) of the infants born between 1993 and 2008 who survived to 18 to 22 months. Logistic regression models generated adjusted odds ratios (AORs), controlling for maternal and neonatal variables.

*Main Outcome Measures.*—Mortality and neurodevelopmental impairment at 18 to 22 months' corrected age.

*Results.*—Death or neurodevelopmental impairment at 18 to 22 months was significantly lower for infants who had been exposed to antenatal corticosteroids and were born at 23 weeks' gestation (83.4% with exposure to antenatal corticosteroids vs 90.5% without exposure; AOR, 0.58 [95% CI,

0.42-0.80]), at 24 weeks' gestation (68.4% with exposure to antenatal corticosteroids vs 80.3% without exposure; AOR, 0.62 [95% CI, 0.49-0.78]), and at 25 weeks' gestation (52.7% with exposure to antenatal corticosteroids vs 67.9% without exposure; AOR, 0.61 [95% CI, 0.50-0.74]) but not in those infants born at 22 weeks' gestation (90.2% with exposure to antenatal corticosteroids vs 93.1% without exposure; AOR, 0.80 [95% CI, 0.29-2.21]). If the mothers had received antenatal corticosteroids, the following events occurred significantly less in infants born at 23, 24, and 25 weeks' gestation: death by 18 to 22 months; hospital death; death, intraventricular hemorrhage, or periventricular leukomalacia; and death or necrotizing enterocolitis. For infants born at 22 weeks' gestation, the only outcome that occurred significantly less was death or necrotizing enterocolitis (73.5% with exposure to antenatal corticosteroids vs 84.5% without exposure; AOR, 0.54 [95% CI, 0.30-0.97]).

*Conclusion.*—Among infants born at 23 to 25 weeks' gestation, antenatal exposure to corticosteroids compared with nonexposure was associated with a lower rate of death or neurodevelopmental impairment at 18 to 22 months.

▶ When Liggins and Howie[1] launched their 1972 trial of antenatal glucocorticoid treatment for the prevention of respiratory distress syndrome, the likely benefit of steroids to the fetus at 22 to 25 weeks' gestation could scarcely have been imagined. In fact, the assumption that the extremely preterm fetus was unlikely to derive benefit from maternal antenatal corticosteroid (ACS) treatment persisted for decades. This study, conducted in the context of the Eunice Kennedy Shriver National Institute of Child Health and Human Development's Neonatal Research Network, adds to a growing body of evidence that antenatal glucocorticoid treatment of women threatening preterm delivery benefits is advantageous to extremely, as well as moderately, preterm infants and confers multisystem benefits. This observational cohort study evaluated outcomes among 4294 survivors at 18 to 22 months (from 10 000 infants who were born at 22 to 25 weeks' gestation between 1993 and 2009). Infants born at 22 weeks' gestation did not appear to benefit from maternal ACS treatment, although 95% confidence limits for adjusted odds ratios were wide and small subgroup numbers limited analytic power. ACS-exposed infants born at 23, 24, or 25 weeks' gestation, however, clearly showed greater likelihood of survival free of neurodevelopmental impairment at 18 to 22 months of age. These authors have rigorously addressed an important question and, in the process, have scored another point for the ACS team.

**L. J. Van Marter, MD, MPH**

*Reference*

1. Liggins GC, Howie RN. A controlled trial of antepartum glucocorticoid treatment for prevention of the respiratory distress syndrome in premature infants. *Pediatrics.* 1972;50:515-525.

# 9  Behavior and Pain

**Analgesic Effect of Breast Milk Versus Sucrose for Analgesia During Heel Lance in Late Preterm Infants**
Simonse E, Mulder PGH, van Beek RHT (Amphia Hosp, Breda, Netherlands)
*Pediatrics* 129:657-663, 2012

*Objective.*—The purpose of this trial was to investigate whether breast milk (either breastfed or bottle-fed) has a better analgesic effect than sucrose in newborns born at a postmenstrual age between 32 and 37 weeks.

*Methods.*—We conducted a randomized controlled trial at a secondary care neonatal unit in the Netherlands on 71 preterm neonates (postmenstrual age at birth 32–37 weeks), undergoing heel lance with an automated piercing device. Newborns were randomly assigned to breast milk (either breastfed or bottle-fed) administered during heel lance or oral sucrose administered before heel lance. We assessed the Premature Infant Pain Profile (PIPP) score (range, 0–21) to investigate whether there was a difference in pain score between neonates receiving breast milk and those receiving sucrose solution.

*Results.*—There was no significant difference in mean PIPP score between neonates receiving breast milk (6.1) and those receiving sucrose (5.5), with a mean difference of 0.6 (95% confidence interval $-1.6$ to 2.8; $P = .58$).

*Conclusions.*—From this study, it cannot be concluded that breast milk has a better analgesic effect than sucrose in late preterm infants. From the results, it follows with 95% confidence that the analgesic effect of breast milk is not > 1.6 points better and not > 2.8 points worse on the PIPP scale (SD 3.7) than the analgesic effect of sucrose in late preterm infants.

▶ This article reports on a trial from the Netherlands on late preterm infants undergoing heel lance who were randomized to receive either a 25% oral sucrose solution or the same volume of breast milk before the procedure to determine a difference on Premature Infant Pain Profile (PIPP) scores. This study showed no difference between neonates receiving breast milk and those receiving sucrose. The authors stated in the discussion that from their study, it could not be concluded that breast milk has a better analgesic effect than sucrose in later preterm infants.

However, in the same issue of *Pediatrics*, the next article from Brazil[1] attempted to test a similar hypothesis using a slightly different statistical approach called a "non-inferiority randomized trial." Noninferiority trials are intended to show that the effect of a new treatment is not worse than that of an active control by more than a specified margin. Noninferiority trials may be necessary when a placebo group cannot be ethically included, but it should be recognized that the results of such trials are not as credible as those from a superiority trial. This trial found that by also using PIPP scores and crying time, the effects of expressed breast milk were inferior to those of 25% glucose. It is difficult to tell why the results of these 2 studies differed, but the statistical technique used in the second study could be considered.

In another study from England,[2] in addition to using a PIPP score, the primary outcome was pain-specific brain activity evoked by onetime locked heel lance recorded with electroencephalography and identified by principal component analysis. Although the PIPP score was lower in infants who received the sucrose, the electroencephalography indicators for pain were not different from those infants who received sucrose and those who did not receive sucrose. These data, according to the authors, suggest that oral sucrose does not significantly affect activity in neonatal brain or spinal cord nociceptive circuits and therefore might not be an effective analgesic drug. They also stated that the ability of sucrose to reduce clinical observational scores after noxious events in newborn infants should not be interpreted as pain relief.

These are somewhat contradictory studies. If the PIPP scores are not reflective of true pain as suggested in the study from England, then use of sucrose or breast milk for analgesia may provide a feeling of security that the pain is being addressed. However, if the nervous response to pain is still present after feeding, it is possible that this false sense of security may actually lead to pain-induced injury in the patient.

Simple pain relief obviously is controversial, but it is also an area of great importance. I am glad to see it is getting some attention, but clarity has not yet come from the studies, despite a pretty strong suggestion that sucrose may at least blunt some of the grimacing and crying activities seen in these babies.

**J. Neu, MD**

*References*

1. Bueno M, Stevens B, de Camargo PP, Toma E, Krebs VL, Kimura AF. Breast milk and glucose for pain relief in preterm infants: a noninferiority randomized controlled trial. *Pediatrics.* 2012;129:664-670.
2. Slater R, Cornelissen L, Fabrizi L, et al. Oral sucrose as an analgesic drug for procedural pain in newborn infants: a randomised controlled trial. *Lancet.* 2010;376: 1225-1232.

**Oral Sucrose and "Facilitated Tucking" for Repeated Pain Relief in Preterms: A Randomized Controlled Trial**
Cignacco EL, Sellam G, Stoffel L, et al (Univ of Basel, Switzerland; Univ Hosp Bern, Switzerland; et al)
*Pediatrics* 129:299-308, 2012

*Objectives.*—To test the comparative effectiveness of 2 nonpharmacologic pain-relieving interventions administered alone or in combination across time for repeated heel sticks in preterm infants.

*Methods.*—A multicenter randomized controlled trial in 3 NICUs in Switzerland compared the effectiveness of oral sucrose, facilitated tucking (FT), and a combination of both interventions in preterm infants between 24 and 32 weeks of gestation. Data were collected during the first 14 days of their NICU stay. Three phases (baseline, heel stick, recovery) of 5 heel stick procedures were videotaped for each infant. Four independent experienced nurses blinded to the heel stick phase rated 1055 video sequences presented in random order by using the Bernese Pain Scale for Neonates, a validated pain tool.

*Results.*—Seventy-one infants were included in the study. Interrater reliability was high for the total Bernese Pain Scale for Neonates score (Cronbach's $\alpha$: 0.90–0.95). FT alone was significantly less effective in relieving repeated procedural pain ($P < .002$) than sucrose (0.2 mL/kg). FT in combination with sucrose seemed to have added value in the recovery phase with lower pain scores ($P = .003$) compared with both the single-treatment groups. There were no significant differences in pain responses across gestational ages.

*Conclusions.*—Sucrose with and without FT had pain-relieving effects even in preterm infants of <32 weeks of gestation having repeated pain exposures. These interventions remained effective during repeated heel sticks across time. FT was not as effective and cannot be recommended as a nonpharmacologic pain relief intervention for repeated pain exposure.

▶ All would agree that continued painful procedures have deleterious effects on long-term outcome. We have come a long way since the primitive theories that babies don't perceive pain and the brutal surgical assaults on neonates without the benefit of anesthesia or analgesia. All providers should now acknowledge that neonates, even very preterm neonates, experience pain and should make every effort to minimize noxious stimuli. They must be aware of how to assess and relieve neonatal pain and stress. As noted in this abstract, sucrose has become a cornerstone of the relief of pain for minor procedures. The facilitated tucking supported the sucrose but alone was not effective. In support of this Swiss study, Kristoffersen et al[1] evaluated the use of sucrose for pain relief when inserting feeding tubes in preterm infants. Using the well-established Premature Infant Pain Profile as the assessment tool, they reported that pain relief was best achieved by combining a pacifier with 30% sucrose. Similarly, sucrose has been effective in evaluating retinopathy.[2,3]

Despite many such randomized trials documenting effectiveness, sucrose has not been universally accepted for relief of discomfort with minor procedures, such as heel sticks and placement of intravenous lines. In fact, there are some cogent arguments that sucrose appears to but does not in fact relieve pain.

The Slater study[4] strongly recommended stopping the practice of giving sucrose for the relief of multiple minor procedures. They challenged and criticized prior studies that relied on changes in facial expression as a measurement of relief of pain, noting that this was an unreliable and inaccurate measure of pain relief. Their technique was to directly measure noxious receptor activity in the brain recorded with electroencephalogram and spinal cord nociceptive reflex withdrawal in addition to the usual behavioral and physiologic pain scores. They noted ongoing brain and spinal cord activity, even after the administration of sucrose.

So the big question is to sweeten or not? Having witnessed enough apparent relief with "sweeties" and cognizant that sucrose will not do any harm, I am still prepared to use it until a better alternative becomes available. Most of the evidence supports such a position, but we must recognize that the measurement of pain using the behavioral characteristics is imperfect.

**A. A. Fanaroff, MBBCh, FRCPE**

*References*

1. Kristoffersen L, Skogvoll E, Hafström M. Pain reduction on insertion of a feeding tube in preterm infants: a randomized controlled trial. *Pediatrics*. 2011;127: e1449-e1454.
2. Kandasamy Y, Smith R, Wright IM, Hartley L. Pain relief for premature infants during ophthalmology assessment. *J AAPOS*. 2011;15:276-280.
3. O'Sullivan A, O'Connor M, Brosnahan D, McCreery K, Dempsey EM. Sweeten, soother and swaddle for retinopathy of prematurity screening: a randomized placebo controlled trial. *Arch Dis Child Fetal Neonatal Ed*. 2010;95:F419-F422.
4. Slater R, Cornelissen L, Fabrizi L, et al. Oral sucrose as an analgesic drug for procedural pain in newborn infants: a randomised controlled trial. *Lancet*. 2010;376: 1225-1232.

---

**Rapid Sequence Induction is Superior to Morphine for Intubation of Preterm Infants: A Randomized Controlled Trial**
Norman E, Wikström S, Hellström-Westas L, et al (Lund Univ and Lund Univ Hosp, Sweden; Uppsala Univ, Sweden; et al)
*J Pediatr* 159:893-899, 2011

---

*Objectives.*—To compare rapid sequence intubation (RSI) premedication with morphine for intubation of preterm infants.

*Study Design.*—Preterm infants needing semi-urgent intubation were enrolled to either RSI (glycopyrrolate, thiopental, suxamethonium, and remifentanil, n = 17) or atropine and morphine (n = 17) in a randomized trial. The main outcome was "good intubation conditions" (score ≤10 assessed with intubation scoring), and secondary outcomes were procedural duration, physiological and biochemical variables, amplitude-integrated electroencephalogram, and pain scores.

*Results.*—Infants receiving RSI had superior intubation conditions (16/17 versus 1/17, $P < .001$), the median (IQR) intubation score was 5 (5-6) compared with 12 (10.0-13.5, $P < .001$), and a shorter procedure duration of 45 seconds (35-154) compared with 97 seconds (49-365, $P = .031$). The morphine group had prolonged heart rate decrease (area under the curve, $P < .009$) and mean arterial blood pressure increase (area under the curve, $P < .005$ and %change: mean ± SD 21% ± 23% versus −2% ± 22%, $P < .007$) during the intubation, and a subsequent lower mean arterial blood pressure 3 hours after the intubation compared with baseline $(P=.033)$, concomitant with neurophysiologic depression $(P<.001)$ for 6 hours after. Plasma cortisol and stress/pain scores were similar.

*Conclusion.*—RSI with the drugs used can be implemented as medication for semi-urgent intubation in preterm infants. Because of circulatory changes and neurophysiological depression found during and after the intubation in infants given morphine, premedication with morphine should be avoided.

▶ In 2001, the International Evidence Based Group for Neonatal Pain published a consensus statement stating that "tracheal intubation without the use of analgesia or sedation should be performed only for resuscitation in the delivery room or for life-threatening situations associated with the unavailability of intravenous access."[1] Six years later, the American Academy of Pediatrics Committee on Fetus and Newborn issued the following consensus statement: "Every health care facility caring for neonates [should] implement an effective pain-prevention program and use pharmacologic and non-pharmacologic therapies for the prevention of pain associated with procedures."[2] Why then, nearly a decade after the initial statement, are we still discussing whether neonates should be premedicated prior to intubation? This is a procedure known to be not only painful but also associated with other adverse effects, including bradycardia, hypoxia, increased blood pressure and intracranial pressure, and potential neurologic complications such as intraventricular hemorrhage. Rapid sequence intubation (RSI) offers the potential benefits of eliminating pain and discomfort as well as reducing physiologic instability while allowing for a rapid and safe intubation. This study investigates the possibility of using a RSI premedication regimen when intubating preterm neonates as compared to many neonatologists' traditional "go-to" drug of choice, morphine. Although pain scores did not significantly differ between groups, the RSI group was found to have superior intubation conditions as well as a shorter procedure duration. The morphine group, on the contrary, had more severe and prolonged circulatory changes as well as a longer duration of neurophysiologic depression after intubation. Strict attention must be paid to the prescription, preparation, and administration of these RSI drugs, given the opportunity for medication errors with a multidrug regimen. With this in mind, it is not only possible but preferable to implement RSI as a premedication regimen for semiurgent intubations in preterm infants. It may be time to step out of our comfort zone and shelve morphine as our drug of choice.

**R. Chitkara, MD**

*References*

1. Anand KJ; International Evidence-Based Group for Neonatal Pain. Consensus statement for the prevention and management of pain in the newborn. *Arch Pediatr Adolesc Med.* 2001;155:173-180.
2. American Academy of Pediatrics Committee on Fetus and Newborn; American Academy of Pediatrics Section on Surgery; Canadian Paediatric Society Fetus and Newborn Committee. Prevention and management of pain in the neonate: an update. *Pediatrics.* 2006;118:2231-2241.

## Efficacy of tramadol versus fentanyl for postoperative analgesia in neonates

de Alencar AJC, Sanudo A, Sampaio VMR, et al (Federal Univ of Ceará, Fortaleza, Brazil; Federal Univ of São Paulo, Brazil; Albert Sabin Hosp, Fortaleza, Ceará, Brazil)
*Arch Dis Child Fetal Neonatal Ed* 97:F24-F29, 2012

*Objective.*—To assess, in newborn infants submitted to surgical procedures, the efficacy of two opioids—fentanyl and tramadol—regarding time to extubate, time to achieve 100 ml/kg of enteral feeding and pain in the first 72 h after surgery.

*Design.*—Controlled, blind, randomised clinical trial.

*Setting.*—Neonatal intensive care unit.

*Patients.*—160 newborn infants up to 28 days of life requiring major or minor surgeries.

*Interventions.*—Patients were randomised to receive analgesia with fentanyl (1–2 µg/kg/h intravenously) or tramadol (0.1–0.2 mg/kg/h intravenously) in the first 72 h of the postoperative period, stratified by surgical size and by patient's gender.

*Main Outcome Measures.*—Pain assessed by validated neonatal scales (Crying, Requires oxygen, Increased vital signs, Expression and Sleepless Scale and the Neonatal Facial Coding System), time until extubation and time to reach 100 ml/kg enteral feeding. Statistical analysis included repeated measures analysis of variance adjusted for confounding variables and Kaplan–Meier curve adjusted by a Cox model of proportional risks.

*Results.*—Neonatal characteristics were (mean ± SD) birth weight of 2924 ± 702 g, gestational age of 37.6 ± 2.2 weeks and age at surgery of 199 ± 63 h. The main indication of surgery was gastrointestinal malformation (85 newborns; 53%). Neonates who received fentanyl or tramadol were similar regarding time until extubation, time to reach 100 ml/kg of enteral feeding and pain scores in the first 72 h after surgery.

*Conclusion.*—Tramadol was as effective as fentanyl for postoperative pain relief in neonates but does not appear to offer advantages over fentanyl regarding the duration of mechanical ventilation and time to reach full enteral feeding.

*Trial Registration.*—NCT00713726.

▶ Among the most important challenges of newborn intensive care is the search for optimal approaches and therapies to evaluate and treat our tiny patients' pain. Although pain pathways are well established by 24 weeks' gestation, extremely preterm or very ill newborns are limited in the ways in which they can convey their discomfort. The analgesics most commonly used in treating newborn intensive care patients, morphine sulfate and fentanyl, have a significant number of undesirable side effects. This study evaluates the efficacy of tramadol, a relatively new opioid analgesic. As the investigators explain, "tramadol is a weak opioid that acts in the central nervous system and has a µ-receptor affinity 6000 times lower than morphine.[1] The drug releases serotonin from nerve terminals and increases synaptic reuptake of serotonin and norepinephrine, leading to the activation of cortex-spinal descendent tracts that modulate and inhibit pain afference to subcortical and cortical centres."[2] The authors also note that in the adult population, compared with other opioids, tramadol has been linked to a reduced risk of respiratory depression, gastrointestinal dysmotility, and dependence.[3,4] Although this study of 160 infants undergoing surgery in the first postnatal month found no benefit of tramadol over fentanyl in reducing the duration of ventilation and time to reach full enteral feeding, the lower side effect profile of tramadol is attractive and makes it a good candidate for study in the broader population of infants hospitalized in the newborn intensive care unit.

**L. J. Van Marter, MD, MPH**

*References*

1. Allegaert K, Simons SH, Vanhole C, Tibboel D. Developmental pharmacokinetics of opioids in neonates. *J Opioid Manag.* 2007;3:59-64.
2. Allegaert K, van den Anker JN, de Hoon JN, et al. Covariates of tramadol disposition in the first months of life. *Br J Anaesth.* 2008;100:525-532.
3. Lee CR, McTavish D, Sorkin EM. Tramadol. A preliminary review of its pharmacodynamic and pharmacokinetic properties, and therapeutic potential in acute and chronic pain states. *Drugs.* 1993;46:313-340.
4. Scott LJ, Perry CM. Tramadol: a review of its use in perioperative pain. *Drugs.* 2000;60:139-176.

# 10 Gastrointestinal Health and Nutrition

---

**Enteral feeding practices in very preterm infants: an international survey**
Klingenberg C, Embleton ND, Jacobs SE, et al (Univ Hosp of North Norway, Tromsø, Norway; Newcastle Hosps NHS Foundation Trust, Newcastle upon Tyne, UK; Royal Women's Hosp, Melbourne, Australia)
*Arch Dis Child Fetal Neonatal Ed* 97:F56-F61, 2012

---

*Objective.*—To evaluate enteral feeding practices in neonatal units in different countries and on different continents.

*Design.*—A web-based survey of 127 tertiary neonatal intensive care units in Australia, Canada, Denmark, Ireland, New Zealand, Norway, Sweden and the UK.

*Results.*—124 units (98%) responded. 59 units (48%) had a breast milk bank or access to donor human milk (Australia/New Zealand 2/27, Canada 6/29, Scandinavia 20/20 and UK/Ireland 31/48). The proportion of units initiating enteral feeding within the first 24 h of life was: 43/124 (35%) if gestational age (GA) <25 weeks, 53/124 (43%) if GA 25-27 weeks and 88/124 (71%) if GA 28-31 weeks. In general, Scandinavian units introduced enteral feeds the earliest, followed by UK/Ireland. Continuous feeding was routinely used for infants below 28 weeks' gestation in almost half of the Scandinavian units and in approximately one sixth of units in UK/Ireland, but rarely in Australia/New Zealand and Canada. Minimal enteral feeding for 4-5 days was common in Canada, but rare in Scandinavia. Target enteral feeding volume in a 'stable' preterm infant was 140-160 ml/kg/day in most Canadian units and 161-180 ml/kg/day or higher in units in the other regions. There were also marked regional differences in criteria for use and timing when human milk fortifier was added.

*Conclusions.*—This study highlights areas of uncertainty and demonstrates marked variability in feeding practices. It provides valuable data for planning collaborative feeding trials to optimise outcome in preterm infants.

▶ In their survey of tertiary neonatal units, Klingenberg and colleagues aimed to determine worldwide differences in feeding practices for premature infants. The provision of enteral nutrition for this population is fraught with complexity, both in the number of choices presented to clinicians (continuous vs bolus, trophic vs continuous, etc) and the lack of definitive evidence to guide these decisions. Additionally, the studies that are available often focus on single interventions, such as rate of advancement or route of administration, rather than comparisons of feeding practices as a whole. This survey of international clinical practice illustrates the end result of this complexity: variability to a startling degree.

With a robust response rate (98%) and an expansive survey base, this article clearly delineates practice differences both between countries and within them. Dramatic variations in the type of substrate, age of feeding commencement, route of administration, target feeding volume, and even discharge nutrition recommendations were demonstrated. Given the number of infants who demonstrate growth failure during their neonatal intensive care unit stay and the potential to improve outcomes by reducing variability, the authors convincingly call for multicenter trials to evaluate the optimal strategy to provide enteral nutrition. Additionally, the results highlight the opportunity for multicenter collaboration such as sharing of experiences about the use of donor human milk or discharge nutrition strategies. Importantly, as the authors disclose, this survey asked individuals for policy rather than actual nutrition received. Clearly, determining how policy translates into practice will need to be elucidated prior to any interventional trials. However, variations in growth outcomes[1] and morbidities such as necrotizing enterocolitis[2] have been associated with differences in feeding practices in other studies.

**R. J. Vartanian, MD**

*References*

1. Blackwell MT, Eichenwald EC, McAlmon K, et al. Interneonatal intensive care unit variation in growth rates and feeding practices in healthy moderately premature infants. *J Perinatol.* 2005;25:478-485.
2. Wiedmeier SE, Henry E, Baer VL, et al. Center differences in NEC within one health-care system may depend on feeding protocol. *Am J Perinatol.* 2008;25:5-11.

---

## The Effect of the Odor of Breast Milk on the Time Needed for Transition From Gavage to Total Oral Feeding in Preterm Infants

Yildiz A, Arikan D, Gözüm S, et al (AbantIzzetBaysal Univ, Bolu, Turkey; Atatürk Univ, Erzurum, Turkey; Akdeniz Univ School of Nursing, Antalya, Turkey)
*J Nurs Scholarsh* 43:265-273, 2011

---

*Purpose.*—The aim of this study was to investigate the effect of the application of the odor of breast milk in preterm infants during gavage feeding on the period of transition to total oral feeding.

*Design.*—This prospective experimental study was performed on a total of 80 preterm infants: 40 infants in the study group and 40 in the control group.

*Methods.*—This experimental study was performed in eastern Turkey at the Neonatal Intensive Care and Premature Unit of a university hospital between September 2007 and December 2008. The demographic data were collected via a questionnaire, and an intervention and follow-up table was prepared by the researcher based on relevant literature. The study was approved by the local institution, and written informed consent was obtained from all parents.

*Findings.*—The findings of the study indicated that the preterm infants who were stimulated by the odor of breast milk during gavage feeding transitioned to oral feeding 3 days earlier than control subjects. Moreover, the mean hospitalization time of these infants was 4 days shorter.

*Conclusions.*—The results show that stimulation with breast milk odor is an effective method for decreasing transition of preterm infants from gavage to oral feeding.

*Clinical Relevance.*—Nurses can train mothers to pump their breast milk, stimulate their infants with the odor of their breast milk, and feed it to their infants in the premature unit. This may lead to a quicker transition to oral feeding.

▶ Nonnutritive sucking is thought to be essential to the development of nutritive sucking and is also associated with weight gain.[1] Maternal odors are known to elicit rooting and nonnutritive sucking, and preterm infants can differentiate the odor of their mother's breast milk from that of another mother's breast milk.[2,3] In this study, the investigators evaluated the effect of stimulation with mother's own breast milk odor on the time for transition to total oral feeding.

Infants included in the study had a mean gestational age of 31 weeks, a mean birth weight of more than 1400 g, and were medically stable during the first 24 hours after birth. Infants in both the control and study cohort were gavage fed their mother's own breast milk. When the feeding process started in the study cohort, the stimulus of breast milk odor was initiated by placement of a sterile pad soaked in mother's own breast milk approximately 2 cm from the infant's nose. When the feeding was completed, the breast milk odor stimulus was removed. The intervention was carried out daily for 3 feedings until the infant graduated to oral feeding. All infants were transitioned from gavage feeding directly to breastfeeding.

Mean weight gained between hospitalization and discharge and the mean weights at the time of discharge were not significantly different between the study and control groups. However, the study group graduated to oral feedings at a mean of 9.4 days compared with 12.3 days for the control group. In addition, hospital stay was 20% shorter for the study group. This study confirms previous observations that stimulation with breast milk odors contributes to the development of sucking behavior in preterm infants, which in turn leads to relatively early tolerance of oral feeding and shortens hospital stays.[4]

**L. A. Papile, MD**

*References*

1. Lau C. Development of oral feeding skills in the preterm infant. *Arch Pediatr.* 2007;14:S35-S41.
2. Varendi H, Porter RH. Breast odour as the only maternal stimulus elicits crawling towards the odour source. *Acta Paediatr.* 2001;90:372-375.

3. Schleidt M, Genzel C. The significance of mother's perfume for infants in the first weeks of life. *Ethol Sociobiol*. 1990;11:145-154.
4. Pinelli J, Symington A. Non-nutritive sucking for promoting physiologic stability and nutrition in preterm infants. *Cochrane Database Syst Rev*. 2005;19:CD001071.

---

**Enteral feeding practices in very preterm infants: an international survey**
Klingenberg C, Embleton ND, Jacobs SE, et al (Univ Hosp of North Norway, Tromsø, Norway; Newcastle Hosps NHS Foundation Trust, Newcastle upon Tyne, UK; Royal Women's Hosp, Melbourne, Australia)
*Arch Dis Child Fetal Neonatal Ed* 97:F56-F61, 2012

---

*Objective.*—To evaluate enteral feeding practices in neonatal units in different countries and on different continents.

*Design.*—A web-based survey of 127 tertiary neonatal intensive care units in Australia, Canada, Denmark, Ireland, New Zealand, Norway, Sweden and the UK.

*Results.*—124 units (98%) responded. 59 units (48%) had a breast milk bank or access to donor human milk (Australia/New Zealand 2/27, Canada 6/29, Scandinavia 20/20 and UK/Ireland 31/48). The proportion of units initiating enteral feeding within the first 24 h of life was: 43/124 (35%) if gestational age (GA) <25 weeks, 53/124 (43%) if GA 25−27 weeks and 88/124 (71%) if GA 28−31 weeks. In general, Scandinavian units introduced enteral feeds the earliest, followed by UK/Ireland. Continuous feeding was routinely used for infants below 28 weeks' gestation in almost half of the Scandinavian units and in approximately one sixth of units in UK/Ireland, but rarely in Australia/New Zealand and Canada. Minimal enteral feeding for 4−5 days was common in Canada, but rare in Scandinavia. Target enteral feeding volume in a 'stable' preterm infant was 140−160 ml/kg/day in most Canadian units and 161−180 ml/kg/day or higher in units in the other regions. There were also marked regional differences in criteria for use and timing when human milk fortifier was added.

*Conclusions.*—This study highlights areas of uncertainty and demonstrates marked variability in feeding practices. It provides valuable data for planning collaborative feeding trials to optimise outcome in preterm infants.

▶ Enteral nutritional practices vary widely between neonatal intensive care units (NICUs) and even occasionally within individual NICUs. There is increased recognition of the importance of early nutrition in critically ill low birth weight babies, and the use of the enteral route has been a matter of considerable debate, despite the strong base of evidence that a lack of enteral feeding leads to intestinal atrophy and significant morbidity, including late-onset sepsis and necrotizing enterocolitis. An international Web-based survey was used to evaluate feeding practices in Australia/New Zealand, UK/Ireland, Canada, and Scandinavia. The study did not focus on parenteral practices. As expected, there was wide variability. But of interest was that the variability is partly explained by differences in access to donor human milk. Neonatologists would rather NOT introduce any feeding at all if a baby's own mother's milk or donor milk was not immediately available. So the question arises: why does the lack of immediate availability of donor milk preclude enteral feeding? Is there evidence from human studies that introduction of minimal feedings with formula rather than human milk for a few days while the mother's milk is coming in causes an increase in NEC or other morbidities? To my knowledge, such data are not available. However, data from animals show that intestinal atrophy occurs rapidly without enteral feedings and that lack of enteral feedings is associated with alterations in mesenteric artery blood flow and causes a higher risk for cholestasis. As mentioned by the authors, prolongation of intravenous nutrition (lack of enteral feeding) also is now known to be associated with late-onset sepsis and NEC. I agree with the authors that additional studies are needed, but in the meantime, finding ways to obtain the baby's own mother's milk early are needed. Furthermore, until studies show harm in the use of formula for minimal feedings to stimulate gut development and reduce gut atrophy for a couple of days as the babies' own mothers' milk becomes available, it appears prudent to provide some food rather than no food enterally. Furthermore, algorithms for feeding guidelines that are based on current evidence have been developed in many NICUs and should be used.

**J. Neu, MD**

---

**Impact of Early and High Amino Acid Supplementation on ELBW Infants at 2 Years**

Blanco CL, Gong AK, Schoolfield J, et al (Univ of Texas Health Science Ctr, San Antonio; et al)

*J Pediatr Gastroenterol Nutr* 54:601-607, 2012

---

*Objective.*—The aim of the present study was to examine the effects of early and high intravenous (IV) amino acid (AA) supplementation on growth, health, and neurodevelopment of extremely-low-birth-weight (ELBW) infants throughout their first 2 years of life.

*Methods.*—Infants were prospectively randomized in a double-masked fashion and treated for 7 days with either IV AA starting at 0.5 $g \cdot kg^{-1} \cdot day^{-1}$ and increased by 0.5 $g \cdot kg^{-1}$ every day to 3 $g \cdot kg^{-1} \cdot day^{-1}$ or starting at 2 $g \cdot kg^{-1} \cdot day^{-1}$ of IV AA and advanced by 1 $g \cdot kg^{-1}$ every day to 4 $g \cdot kg^{-1} \cdot day^{-1}$. Plasma AA concentrations were determined by reverse-phase high-performance liquid chromatography. Survivors were longitudinally assessed with Bayley II Scales of Infant Development and physical, social, and global health.

*Results.*—Forty-three of 51 survivors were studied. Mental Developmental Index (MDI) and Psychomotor Developmental Index were similar between groups; however, the early and high AA group had a lower MDI at 18 months. This difference disappeared at 2 years of age. The early and high AA group $z$ score means for weight, length, and head circumferences were significantly lower than the standard AA group at most visits.

Cumulative and single plasma AA concentrations correlated negatively with MDI and postnatal growth.

*Conclusions.*—ELBW infants who received early and high IV AA during the first week of life were associated with poor overall growth at 2 years.

▶ This is a study with results that are apparently contrary to the vast majority of evidence that has accumulated over the past several years that relates benefits and safety of early amino acid intake in very low birth weight infants.[1] These include better growth,[2] increased head circumference,[3] better nitrogen balance,[1] lower short-term morbidity,[4] and data that support an approximate 8-point increase in the Mental Developmental Index for every 1 g/kg increment in amino acid intake in the first week of life.[5] In this study, as mentioned by the authors, the sample size was not powered to test the hypothesis of either growth or neurodevelopmental outcome, there was large attrition of patients in the early amino acid group, and there were no differences in growth at the time of discharge, suggesting that any differences in growth that occurred in the early amino acid group after discharge to 18 months or 2 years was likely due to circumstances after discharge. It has taken neonatology over 2 decades to feel more comfortable with early aggressive nutrition, where the term "aggressive" is probably a misnomer because for the most part it represents a continuation of what these babies would be receiving at comparable gestational ages if they were still in utero. Lower amino acid intakes have clearly been shown to be catabolic, especially if also accompanied with low energy intake. Although we still have a lot to learn about the quality of amino acids we are providing both intravenously and enterally to very low birth weight infants to provide them with optimum intakes, it is clear that a large enough quantity needs to be provided and that this is between 3 to 4 g/kg/day for most very low birth weight infants starting as soon as possible after birth. Studies such as this should keep us aware that we need to do more good research in this area. They should not cause us to revert back to the days when we starved preterm babies by using techniques based on dogma rather than evidence.

**J. Neu, MD**

*References*

1. Hay WW, Thureen P. Protein for preterm infants: how much is needed? How much is enough? How much is too much? *Pediatr Neonatol.* 2010;51:198-207.
2. Valentine CJ, Fernandez S, Rogers LK, et al. Early amino-acid administration improves preterm infant weight. *J Perinatol.* 2009;29:428-432.
3. Poindexter BB, Langer JC, Dusick AM, Ehrenkranz RA; National Institute of Child Health and Human Development Neonatal Research Network. Early provision of parenteral amino acids in extremely low birth weight infants: relation to growth and neurodevelopmental outcome. *J Perinatol.* 2006;148:300-305.
4. Ehrenkranz RA, Das A, Wrage LA, et al; Eunice Kennedy Shriver National Institute of Child Health and Human Development Neonatal Research Network. Early nutrition mediates the influence of severity of illness on extremely LBW infants. *Pediatr Res.* 2011;69:522-529.
5. Stephens BE, Walden RV, Gargus RA, et al. First-week protein and energy intakes are associated with 18-month developmental outcomes in extremely low birth weight infants. *Pediatrics.* 2009;123:1337-1343.

## Impact of Early and High Amino Acid Supplementation on ELBW Infants at 2 Years

Blanco CL, Gong AK, Schoolfield J, et al (Univ of Texas Health Science Ctr, San Antonio; et al)

*J Pediatr Gastroenterol Nutr* 54:601-607, 2012

*Objective.*—The aim of the present study was to examine the effects of early and high intravenous (IV) amino acid (AA) supplementation on growth, health, and neurodevelopment of extremely-low-birth-weight (ELBW) infants throughout their first 2 years of life.

*Methods.*—Infants were prospectively randomized in a double-masked fashion and treated for 7 days with either IV AA starting at $0.5 \text{ g·kg}^{-1} \text{·day}^{-1}$ and increased by $0.5 \text{ g·kg}^{-1}$ every day to $3 \text{ g·kg}^{-1} \text{·day}^{-1}$ or starting at $2 \text{ g·kg}^{-1} \text{·day}^{-1}$ of IV AA and advanced by $1 \text{ g·kg}^{-1}$ every day to $4 \text{ g·kg}^{-1} \text{·day}^{-1}$. Plasma AA concentrations were determined by reverse-phase high-performance liquid chromatography. Survivors were longitudinally assessed with Bayley II Scales of Infant Development and physical, social, and global health.

*Results.*—Forty-three of 51 survivors were studied. Mental Developmental Index (MDI) and Psychomotor Developmental Index were similar between groups; however, the early and high AA group had a lower MDI at 18 months. This difference disappeared at 2 years of age. The early and high AA group $z$ score means for weight, length, and head circumferences were significantly lower than the standard AA group at most visits. Cumulative and single plasma AA concentrations correlated negatively with MDI and postnatal growth.

*Conclusions.*—ELBW infants who received early and high IV AA during the first week of life were associated with poor overall growth at 2 years (Fig 2).

▶ Once again, it appears to be possible to get too much of a good thing. Evidence that early protein supplementation for extremely low-birth-weight (ELBW) infants is associated with better glucose tolerance, faster weight gain, and improved head growth has led to widespread adoption of strategies for early and aggressive initiation of parenteral and enteral nutrition. Some experts have advocated administration of 2 g/kg/day of amino acids or more beginning immediately after birth, followed by rapid advancement to 3.5 to 4 g/kg/day. This is now a common practice in many nurseries. This report of long-term follow-up of subjects enrolled in a trial comparing early initiation of high amino acid intake to more gradual introduction of amino acids suggests that the early benefits of this approach may not be sustained. The strength of the conclusions from this study are limited by a small sample size (61 infants enrolled), subject attrition (32 subjects followed up at 18–24 months), and post hoc examination of neurodevelopmental and growth outcomes, which were not included in the original study design. External validity is limited by exclusion of infants greater than 24 weeks' gestation (after observation of a high mortality rate among infants < 24 weeks assigned to the early high amino acid group soon after initiation of

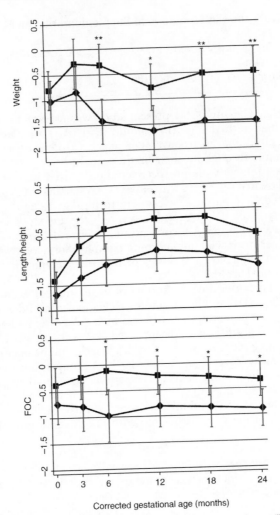

Corrected gestational age (months)

**FIGURE 2.**—z Scores for weight, length/height, and frontooccipital circumference (FOC) up to 2 years of age are shown. Diamonds represent early and high AA group, squares represent the standard AA group. *P < 0.05, **P < 0.01. (Reprinted from Blanco CL, Gong AK, Schoolfield J, et al. Impact of early and high amino acid supplementation on ELBW infants at 2 years. *J Pediatr Gastroenterol Nutr.* 2012;54:601-607, with permission from European Society for Pediatric Gastroenterology, Hepatology, and Nutrition and North American Society for Pediatric Gastroenterology, Hepatology, and Nutrition.)

the trial) and by the predominantly Hispanic study sample. Nonetheless, the unexpected finding of compromised growth in the group who received early high amino acid infusions is worrisome. As shown in Fig 2, z scores for weight, length, and head circumference were lower in the early high amino acid group ages 6, 12, 18, and 24 months. Because of the strong association between head size and neurodevelopmental status, the latter is particularly alarming. These data suggest that early initiation of high amino acid infusions may actually

be harmful to ELBW infants. There is clearly an urgent need for adequately powered randomized controlled trials, including long-term follow up, to determine the
optimal approach to early nutrition of these babies. Until better information is
available, a circumspect approach may be advisable.

**W. E. Benitz, MD**

---

**Impact of Personalized Feeding Program in 100 NICU Infants: Pathophysiology-based Approach for Better Outcomes**
Jadcherla SR, Peng J, Moore R, et al (Ohio State Univ College of Medicine, Columbus; Res Inst at Nationwide Children's Hosp, Columbus, OH; et al)
*J Pediatr Gastroenterol Nutr* 54:62-70, 2012

---

*Objectives.*—In neonatal intensive care unit infants referred for home-tube feeding methods, we evaluated the effect of an innovative diagnostic and management approach on feeding outcomes at discharge and 1 year, by comparing data from historical controls; we hypothesized that clinical and aerodigestive motility characteristics at evaluation were predictive of feeding outcomes at discharge; we assessed the economic impact of feeding outcomes.

*Patients and Methods.*—Patients (N = 100) who were referred for development of long-term feeding management strategy at 46.4 ± 13.1 weeks' postmenstrual age were compared with 50 historical controls that received routine care. The focused approach included swallow-integrated pharyng-oesophageal manometry, individualized feeding strategy, and prospective follow-up. Feeding success was defined as ability to achieve oral feedings at discharge and 1 year. Motility characteristics were evaluated in relation to feeding success or failure at discharge.

*Results.*—Higher feeding success was achieved in the innovative feeding program (vs historical controls) at discharge (51% vs 10%, $P < 0.0001$) and at 1 year (84.3% vs 42.9%, $P < 0.0001$), at a reduced economic burden ($P < 0.05$). Contributing factors to the innovative program's feeding success (vs feeding failure) were earlier evaluation and discharge (both $P < 0.05$), greater peristaltic reflex-frequency to provocation ($P < 0.05$), normal pharyngeal manometry ($P < 0.05$), oral feeding challenge success ($P < 0.05$), and suck-swallow-breath-esophageal swallow sequence ($P < 0.05$). Probability of feeding success demonstrated a prediction rate of 79.6%.

*Conclusions.*—Short-term and long-term feeding outcomes in complex neonates can be significantly improved with innovative feeding strategies at a reduced cost. Clinical and aerodigestive motility characteristics were predictive of outcomes.

▶ This study is a comparison of infants referred to a specialty center for feeding difficulties, who were treated with innovative methods compared with infants treated historically with the center's conventional approach. The innovative approach used diagnostic studies (including pharyngoesophageal manometry) combined with multidisciplinary input to tailor an individual, pathophysiology-based feeding strategy for each patient. The conventional approach also included other disciplines, but the feeding plans were determined by the attending physician of record. The use of esophageal manometry was exclusive to the innovative methods. The results are impressive in that for every 2.4 infants in the innovative program, 1 more infant achieved feeding success by discharge. Feeding success at the first birthday was 84.3% compared with 42.9% in the historical controls ($P < .0001$).

The innovative arm was then subdivided into infants who were not feeding orally at discharge compared with those who were. Infants with feeding success were of younger gestational age and were evaluated earlier than those with feeding failure. A logistic regression analysis identified associations between bronchopulmonary dysplasia and neuropathology and subsequent poor feeding outcomes (this is also relevant for interpreting the innovative vs conventional comparison, where more infants had BPD in the innovative group). Statistically significant differences in pharyngoesophageal manometry characteristics were identified between the success and failure groups. The authors' expertise with this technique allowed for incorporation of test results into the feeding plan development. However, lack of knowledge and familiarity with this technology limits extrapolation elsewhere.

The authors demonstrated that the innovative feeding program results in cost savings by avoiding gastrostomy tube placement. A more complex analysis of the direct costs of the implementation and maintenance of the innovative versus conventional programs would be interesting but difficult to do, especially since the social impact of feeding success would be difficult to factor. The results from this program are certainly impressive, but it is conjectural to believe that these improvements are replicable elsewhere using the same strategy. It would also be interesting to study whether these innovative approaches might be useful at the initiation of oral feeding as a preventative strategy for oral aversion in high-risk infants.

**R. Vartanian, MD**

---

**Impact of Personalized Feeding Program in 100 NICU Infants: Pathophysiology-based Approach for Better Outcomes**
Jadcherla SR, Peng J, Moore R, et al (Res Inst at Nationwide Children's Hosp, Columbus, OH; et al)
*J Pediatr Gastroenterol Nutr* 54:62-70, 2012

---

*Objectives.*—In neonatal intensive care unit infants referred for home-tube feeding methods, we evaluated the effect of an innovative diagnostic and management approach on feeding outcomes at discharge and 1 year, by comparing data from historical controls; we hypothesized that clinical and aerodigestive motility characteristics at evaluation were predictive of feeding outcomes at discharge; we assessed the economic impact of feeding outcomes.

*Patients and Methods.*—Patients (N = 100) who were referred for development of long-term feeding management strategy at 46.4 ± 13.1 weeks' postmenstrual age were compared with 50 historical controls that received routine care. The focused approach included swallow-integrated pharyngoesophageal manometry, individualized feeding strategy, and prospective follow-up. Feeding success was defined as ability to achieve oral feedings at discharge and 1 year. Motility characteristics were evaluated in relation to feeding success or failure at discharge.

*Results.*—Higher feeding success was achieved in the innovative feeding program (vs historical controls) at discharge (51% vs 10%, $P < 0.0001$) and at 1 year (84.3% vs 42.9%, $P < 0.0001$), at a reduced economic burden ($P < 0.05$). Contributing factors to the innovative program's feeding success (vs feeding failure) were earlier evaluation and discharge (both $P < 0.05$), greater peristaltic reflex-frequency to provocation ($P < 0.05$), normal pharyngeal manometry ($P < 0.05$), oral feeding challenge success ($P < 0.05$), and suck-swallow-breath-esophageal swallow sequence ($P < 0.05$). Probability of feeding success demonstrated a prediction rate of 79.6%.

*Conclusions.*—Short-term and long-term feeding outcomes in complex neonates can be significantly improved with innovative feeding strategies at a reduced cost. Clinical and aerodigestive motility characteristics were predictive of outcomes (Fig 1).

▶ Some of our most critically ill babies have severe levels of feeding intolerance, which prompts serious discussion of home gavage feedings or the placement of a gastrostomy tube. Objective criteria for when the decision is made to

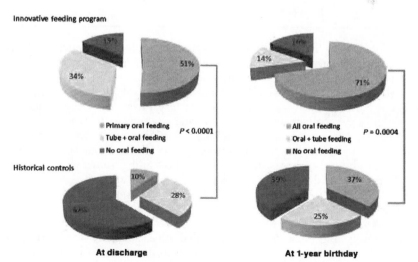

FIGURE 1.—Feeding success rate comparisons between innovative feeding program and historical controls. (Reprinted from Jadcherla SR, Peng J, Moore R, et al. Impact of personalized feeding program in 100 NICU infants: pathophysiology-based approach for better outcomes. *J Pediatr Gastroenterol Nutr.* 2012;54:62-70, with permission from European Society for Pediatric Gastroenterology, Hepatology, and Nutrition and North American Society for Pediatric Gastroenterology, Hepatology, and Nutrition.)

place a gastrostomy tube are not well described in the literature, and often there is great anxiety on the part of the parents and the physicians in these decisions.

This article describes a personalized feeding method, described locally at Ohio State as Dr Jadcherla's study, which involves the use of manometry to help decide which babies are reasonable candidates to try a staged feeding approach that often involves progression from continuous tube feedings to intermittent feedings with initial long feeding infusions progressing to shorter feeding infusions where babies begin to show hunger cues. Overall, the method appears to be personalized depending on the baby, but it still uses technologies developed and described by Jadcherla.

In this study, the individualized approach was compared to historical control babies. The results were striking, as shown in the Fig 1, with the personalized approach resulting in much greater success rates than the historical controls.

At this time, as mentioned by the authors, a more stringent study should be done in a more prospective manner. If validated, these techniques should provide a much clearer approach as to which infants should have gastrostomy tubes placed because of a high likelihood of failure and which infants should be placed on the personalized Jadcherla approach to feeding because they have a reasonable chance to succeed without gastrostomy.

**J. Neu, MD**

---

**Pediatricians', Obstetricians', Gynecologists', and Family Medicine Physicians' Experiences with and Attitudes about Breast-Feeding**
Anchondo I, Berkeley L, Mulla ZD, et al (Texas Tech Univ Health Sciences Ctr, El Paso)
*South Med J* 105:243-248, 2012

---

*Objectives.*—Investigate physicians' breast-feeding experiences and attitudes using a survey based on two behavioral theories: theory of reasoned action (TRA) and the health belief model (HBM).

*Methods.*—There were 73 participants included in the investigation. These participants were resident and faculty physicians from pediatrics, obstetrics/gynecology, and family medicine at a university campus, located on the US-Mexico border. The sample was reduced to 53 and 56 records for the attitude and confidence variables, respectively. Physicians answered a survey about their breast-feeding experiences and attitudes to learn about intention and ability applying constructs from TRA and HBM. An attitude scale, confidence variable (from self-efficacy items), and a lactation training index were created for the analysis.

*Results.*—Analysis of the association between physicians' breast-feeding experiences and their attitudes revealed physicians are knowledgeable about breast-feeding and have positive attitudes towards breast-feeding. They did not seem to remember how long they breast-fed their children or whether they enjoyed breast-feeding, but they wanted to continue breast-feeding. Physicians cite work as a main reason for not continuing to breast-feed.

*Conclusions.*—Physicians' attitudes toward breast-feeding are positive. They are expected to practice health-promotion behavior including breast-feeding; however, physicians' breast-feeding rates are low and although they are knowledgeable about breast-feeding their training lacks on didactic depth and hands-on experience. If physicians learn more about breast-feeding and breast-feed exclusively and successfully, the rates in the United States would increase naturally.

▶ Knowledge gained by physicians' breastfeeding their own babies may play a role in how they relate to their patients. Often the intensity of training programs, the lack of facilities, and attitudes of the physicians leads to suboptimal breast-feeding of their own babies. The authors point to the fact that even though initiation of breastfeeding is high among physicians, once they return to work, they cease breastfeeding. In fact, they refer to research that showed that in resident physicians, the rates of breastfeeding between female residents and male resident partners differed significantly. Although breast feeding initiation rates were similar between the 2 groups (83% vs 100%), the length of time that female residents breastfed was significantly shorter than that of partners/spouses (8% vs 50% by the child's first birthday).

This study involved a questionnaire focused on female residents and faculty physicians in pediatrics, obstetrics and gynecology, and family medicine in El Paso, Texas. The purpose of the study was to better understand the associations and implications in physicians' experiences in breastfeeding their children, their exposure to breast feeding training, and their attitudes toward breastfeeding.

This study found that physicians' breast feeding education and training are minimal. Most physicians attended only 2 breastfeeding lectures in medical school. Thus, physicians tend to have poor knowledge of breastfeeding. The attitudes of physicians about breastfeeding may also play an important role in the decisions of patients whether to breastfeed. However, this study shows that most physicians are not clear about their own breastfeeding attitudes. Although the physicians in this study believed that breastfeeding was important and demonstrated positive attitudes toward breastfeeding, there was a gap in the physicians' attitudes about exclusivity of breastfeeding: some considered it unrealistic to continue for more than 6 months after birth.

This study also found that work demands, including short maternity leave, volume of work, a lack of privacy, and other issues, were significant deterrents of physicians to continue breastfeeding.

It is clear that physicians in these specialties can have a huge effect on their patients. Their knowledge, experience, and attitudes about breastfeeding will clearly be transferred to their patients. Improved training, better understanding by peers and supervisors, as well as facilities for these mothers in the hospitals to care for their babies, to pump their milk, and other factors that would support them are in order.

**J. Neu, MD**

## 224 / Neonatal and Perinatal Medicine

**Should the use of probiotics in the preterm be routine?**
Millar M, Wilks M, Fleming P, et al (Dept of Infection, London, UK; Barts and
The London NHS Trust, London, UK; et al)
*Arch Dis Child Fetal Neonatal Ed* 97:F70-F74, 2012

Does the clinical trials' evidence of benefit justify the routine use of probiotics in the preterm infant? There are many uncertainties surrounding the use of probiotics in the preterm, including the mechanism(s) of action of probiotics, knowledge of who benefits and who might not, whether it is placement of large numbers of bacteria into the small intestine or colonisation that determines efficacy, the forms of microbial adaptation(s) and ecological consequences. There is also a current lack of defined products with associated evidence of safety in the preterm infant. It is argued that one cannot assume safety because of a lack of evidence of harm and that one should take a precautionary approach to the introduction of probiotics into routine neonatal practice. One should also consider how best one might monitor microbiological and ecological consequences and longer-term health outcomes before the introduction of this novel intervention into routine practice.

▶ This excellent review article is a must-read for all who care for infants in the neonatal intensive care unit (NICU). The authors acknowledge clinical trials' evidence of potential benefits of probiotic therapy and discuss some of the practical aspects important to consider, including the heterogeneity of preparations used in clinical trials (making aggregating in a meta-analysis difficult) as well as important current gaps in our knowledge, including the most beneficial strains, the ecological implications, the potential for cross-colonization, and potential adaptations of probiotic organisms. The authors share the cautionary tale of the disastrous effort, 50 years ago, to control outbreaks of *Staphylococcus aureus* by introducing *S aureus* 502A—an effort that resulted in the infection of many and the death of at least one infant.[1] In a vulnerable host, probiotics are capable of progressing to invasive infection, as documented by a recent report of *Bifidobacterium septicemia* in an extremely low birth weight infant.[2] Undoubtedly, the safest current means of introducing "friendly bacteria" to babies is via maternal milk.[3] I advocate for redoubling our efforts to make mother's milk the source of enteral nutrition for all of our NICU babies and to continue to study the benefits and risks of probiotic therapy in newborns.

**L. J. Van Marter, MD, MPH**

*References*

1. Houck PW, Nelson JD, Kay JL. Fatal septicemia due to Staphylococcus aureus 502A. Report of a case and review of the infectious complications of bacterial interference programs. *Am J Dis Child.* 1972;123:45-48.
2. Jenke A, Ruf EM, Hoppe T, Heldmann M, Wirth S. Bifidobacterium septicaemia in an extremely low-birthweight infant under probiotic therapy. *Arch Dis Child Fetal Neonatal Ed.* 2012;97:F217-F218.
3. Beattie LM, Weaver LT. Mothers, babies and friendly bacteria. *Arch Dis Child Fetal Neonatal Ed.* 2011;96:F160-F163.

## Should the use of probiotics in the preterm be routine?
Millar M, Wilks M, Fleming P, et al (Dept of Infection, London, UK; Barts and The London NHS Trust, UK; et al)
*Arch Dis Child Fetal Neonatal Ed* 97:F70-F74, 2012

Does the clinical trials' evidence of benefit justify the routine use of probiotics in the preterm infant? There are many uncertainties surrounding the use of probiotics in the preterm, including the mechanism(s) of action of probiotics, knowledge of who benefits and who might not, whether it is placement of large numbers of bacteria into the small intestine or colonisation that determines efficacy, the forms of microbial adaptation(s) and ecological consequences. There is also a current lack of defined products with associated evidence of safety in the preterm infant. It is argued that one cannot assume safety because of a lack of evidence of harm and that one should take a precautionary approach to the introduction of probiotics into routine neonatal practice. One should also consider how best one might monitor microbiological and ecological consequences and longer-term health outcomes before the introduction of this novel intervention into routine practice.

▶ The exuberance raised over the possible use of probiotics in preterm babies to prevent necrotizing enterocolitis (NEC) and even decrease mortality could present the possibility of another misadventure in neonatal care. This review and others[1,2] provide reasons to temper this enthusiasm and to proceed with caution. Some of the caveats raised include uncertainties about the pathogenesis of NEC, the unknown impact of probiotics on early development, ecologic consequences of widespread use of probiotics, microbial adaptations consequent on use of probiotics, and impact of unintended cross-colonization on outcome(s). We don't know which probiotic to use, and one probiotic dose is not equivalent to another. We don't know much about the mechanisms or long-term consequences; most of the studies to date are underpowered. We are still awaiting the results of larger controlled trials.[3] It is of concern to me that these agents are unregulated and well-studied preparations that show safety in a preterm infant population are not available. Nevertheless, neonatologists in various parts of the world, including the United States, are beginning to use whatever preparations may be available to them. Who will bear the burden if and when these unregulated agents begin showing unanticipated adverse consequences?

**J. Neu, MD**

*References*

1. Neu J. Routine probiotics for premature infants: let's be careful! *J Pediatr.* 2011; 158:672-674.
2. Caplan M. Are probiotics ready for prime time? *JPEN J Parenter Enteral Nutr.* 2012;36:6S.
3. Garland SM, Tobin JM, Pirotta M, et al; ProPrems Study Group. The ProPrems trial: investigating the effects of probiotics on late onset sepsis in very preterm infants. *BMC Infect Dis.* 2011;11:210.

## Bifidobacterium septicaemia in an extremely low-birthweight infant under probiotic therapy

Jenke A, Ruf E-M, Hoppe T, et al (Witten/Herdecke Univ, Wuppertal, Germany; Laboratoriumsmedizin Köln, Dres. Wisplinghoff, Cologne, Germany)
*Arch Dis Child Fetal Neonatal Ed* 97:F217-F218, 2012

*Background.*—Although probiotics have been shown to be effective in preventing necrotizing enterocolitis, limitations in all the relevant studies suggest that the risks and benefits of such therapy should be carefully considered.

*Case Report.*—At 7 weeks gestational age (GA) a monochorial-diamnial monozygotic twin pregnancy was identified. Intrauterine laser ablation therapy was done at 16 weeks GA to treat fetofetal transfusion syndrome. Premature rupture of membranes and uncontrolled labor at 27/5 weeks prompted a cesarean section. The index patient was the second twin and weighed 600 g at birth. She was given a dose of surfactant and successfully extubated 18 hours later. Enteral feeding of her mother's unpasteurized fortified breast milk was begun on day 1. The infant's hemodynamically significant patent arterial duct was closed successfully on day 5 using indomethacin 0.7 mg/kg. The probiotic Infloran was given beginning on day 9. On the infant's 18th day, gastric remnants and abdominal distention developed, and her C-reactive protein level was 1.7 mg/dl, with a white blood cell count of 78/nl. Cultures were obtained of the peripheral aerobic and anaerobic blood, urine, and throat. The infant was given cefotaxime and vancomycin empirically and enteral feedings were halted. After 6 hours, she was intubated because of apnea; her circulatory status remained stable. No intramural gas was noted, but her abdomen was distended and tender and her C-reactive protein level had increased to 8.5 mg/dl. Metronidazole was added. On day 21 the blood cultures grew *Bifidobacterium* spp, and further typing using mass spectrometry and strain-specific polymerase chain reaction (PCR) revealed there were two different strains: *Bifidobacterium longum* and the probiotic *infantis* strain. No direct complications developed thereafter, but the infant had postinflammatory stenosis of the left colonic flexure that required colostomy 6 weeks later.

*Conclusions.*—The clinical significance of *Bifidobacterium* spp as the cause of this infant's problems appears clear, based on the close correlation between her clinical symptoms, blood culture results, and heightened inflammatory markers. The incidence of sepsis related to *Bifidobacterium* spp may be underestimated, so clinicians should be alert to the possibility and implement appropriate culture conditions as needed.

▶ Despite being only a case report of 1 patient, this represents a very important finding. There has been significant controversy over the use of probiotics in neonates, and both the European Society of Pediatric Gastroenterology and Nutrition and American Academy of Pediatrics Committee on Nutrition have not recommended their use despite very strong claims based on meta-analyses where up to 10 different probiotics were evaluated. All of the studies so far have claimed safety. This case report raises an important point—some of the probiotics that are being provided to preterms cannot be cultured using standard techniques. In this case report, polymerase chain reaction was used and detected *Bifidobacterium longum* and the probiotic infantis strain. The fact that this occurred in the presence of clinical symptoms and increase in C-reactive protein supports the likelihood of translocation of this probiotic from the gastrointestinal tract into the bloodstream and also suggests that this was the cause of the baby's symptoms. In the United States, probiotics are being used routinely in some neonatal intensive care units. This is not considered a drug by the US Food and Drug Administration, and quality standards of many of the products on the market are not monitored. One probiotic is not the same as another. Thus, caution is warranted, and the time for use of these agents in preterm infants awaits additional safety and efficacy data.

**J. Neu, MD**

---

**The Human Microbiome and Its Potential Importance to Pediatrics**
Johnson CL, Versalovic J (Baylor College of Medicine, Houston, TX; Texas Children's Hosp, Houston)
*Pediatrics* 129:950-960, 2012

The human body is home to more than 1 trillion microbes, with the gastrointestinal tract alone harboring a diverse array of commensal microbes that are believed to contribute to host nutrition, developmental regulation of intestinal angiogenesis, protection from pathogens, and development of the immune response. Recent advances in genome sequencing technologies and metagenomic analysis are providing a broader understanding of these resident microbes and highlighting differences between healthy and disease states. The aim of this review is to provide a detailed summary of current pediatric microbiome studies in the literature, in addition to highlighting recent findings and advancements in studies of the adult microbiome. This review also seeks to elucidate the development of, and factors that could lead to changes in, the composition and function of the human microbiome (Fig 3).

▶ Johnson and Versalovic provide a very nice clinician-oriented review of new developments related to the microbiome as it relates to pediatrics. Over the last few years, this has become an area of intensive investigation partially based on newly developed sequencing technologies that now make it possible to identify microorganisms that either cannot or are extremely difficult to isolate using culture-based techniques. We are also developing a much greater appreciation of how the myriad of microbial cells and genes that are our commensals and symbionts interact with our somatic cells to form a superorganism. Some of the

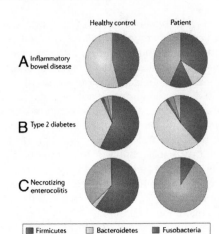

**FIGURE 3.**—Disease states reveal phylum-level differences compared with healthy controls. Comparisons of the relative abundances of predominant bacterial phyla in IBD, type 2 diabetes, and NEC compared with healthy controls. Fecal samples from infants with NEC and patients with type 2 diabetes were compared with healthy controls revealing a predominance of Proteobacteria in patients with NEC. Cecal samples from patients with IBD were compared with healthy controls, and relative abundances were assessed. (Reproduced with permission from Spor A, Koren O, Ley R. Unravelling the effects of the environment and host genotype on the gut microbiome. *Nat Rev Microbiol.* 2011;9[4]:281.) Secondary perm to Nat Rev Microbiol. (Reproduced with permission from Pediatrics, Johnson CL, Versalovic J. The human microbiome and its potential importance to pediatrics. *Pediatrics.* 2012;129:950-960. Copyright © 2012 by the American Academy of Pediatrics.)

aspects of this review that deserve additional emphasis include the points that are made about cesarean section versus vaginal delivery. The data on this suggest that colonization patterns differ according to mode of delivery. Whether this may have an effect on subsequent health remains speculative, but epidemiologic data suggest that babies born by cesarean section have higher odds of development of certain diseases when compared with vaginally delivered infants.[1] Another interesting point that the authors make is that antibiotics may reduce the microbial diversity of the intestinal community, and complete recovery of initial bacterial community composition is rarely achieved. They illustrate differences in microbial composition at the phylum level in inflammatory bowel disease, type 2 diabetes, and necrotizing enterocolitis, suggesting that these may play important roles in the pathophysiology of these diseases (Fig 3). One caveat to what is mentioned in their article is the statement that "probiotic formulations are generally believed to be safe and the American Academy of Pediatrics (AAP) has supported the administration of probiotics for the treatment of acute gastroenteritis and the prevention of antibiotic–associated diarrhea." This needs to be qualified. When one carefully examines the AAP article on the use of probiotics,[2] concerns are raised for immunocompromised individuals and other special situations. In neonatology, probiotic use is becoming much more common, but it needs to be remembered that not all probiotics are alike, and recent studies of probiotics in preterm infants need to be mentioned here. The AAP report states: "Another point that makes the data problematic is that the combinations of probiotics used in the Lin et al studies[3]—are not available in the United States. Not all probiotics have been studied; therefore all probiotics cannot be generally recommended."[2]

So overall, this is an excellent review that should be read by pediatric clinicians.

**J. Neu, MD**

*References*

1. Neu J, Rushing J. Cesarean versus vaginal delivery: long-term infant outcomes and the hygiene hypothesis. *Clin Perinatol.* 2011;38:321-331.
2. Thomas DW, Greer FR; American Academy of Pediatrics Committee on Nutrition, American Academy of Pediatrics Section on Gastroenterology, Hepatology, and Nutrition. Probiotics and prebiotics in pediatrics. *Pediatrics.* 2010;126:1217-1231.
3. Lin HC, Hsu CH, Chen HL, et al. Oral probiotics prevent necrotizing enterocolitis in very low birth weight preterm infants: a multicenter, randomized, controlled trial. *Pediatrics.* 2008;122:693-700.

## Incidence and Timing of Presentation of Necrotizing Enterocolitis in Preterm Infants

Yee WH, the Canadian Neonatal Network (Univ of Calgary, Alberta, Canada; et al)
*Pediatrics* 129:e298-e304, 2012

*Objectives.*—To examine the variation in the incidence and to identify the timing of the presentation of necrotizing enterocolitis (NEC) in a cohort of preterm infants within the Canadian Neonatal Network (CNN).

*Methods.*—This was a population-based cohort of 16 669 infants with gestational age (GA) <33 weeks, admitted to 25 NICUs participating in the CNN between January 1, 2003, and December 31, 2008. Variations in NEC incidence among the participating NICUs for the study period were examined. We categorized early-onset NEC as occurring at <14 days of age and late-onset NEC occurring at ≥14 days. Multivariate logistic regression analysis was performed to identify risk factors for early-onset NEC.

*Results.*—The overall incidence of NEC was 5.1%, with significant variation in the risk adjusted incidence among the participating NICUs in the CNN. Early-onset NEC occurred at a mean of 7 days compared with 32 days for late-onset NEC. Early-onset NEC infants had lower incidence of respiratory distress syndrome, patent ductus treated with indomethacin, less use of postnatal steroids, and shorter duration of ventilation days. Multivariate logistic regression analysis identified that greater GA and vaginal delivery were associated with increased risk of early-onset NEC.

*Conclusions.*—Among infants <33 weeks' gestation, NEC appears to present at mean age of 7 days in more mature infants, whereas onset of NEC is delayed to 32 days of age in smaller, lower GA infants. Further studies are required to understand the etiology of this disease process.

▶ This study, using a large cohort of 16 669 infants reiterates much of what is known about the timing of necrotizing enterocolitis (NEC): if a baby is born late preterm, the disease occurs earlier after birth than if the baby is very preterm. NEC is also associated with many other variables that are related to very preterm birth, again not a surprise. One caveat provided by the authors is that this study could not delineate between stage 3 surgical NEC and spontaneous intestinal perforation. There are other caveats not mentioned by the authors, and a very important one is our ability to diagnose NEC. Although most neonatologists state they can readily diagnose this disease, it is not always that easy. Does an absence of pneumatosis or portal venous gas on a radiograph preclude the diagnosis of NEC? Should a distended abdomen with bloody stools and a paucity of bowel gas and high levels of inflammatory markers be called *NEC*? Unfortunately, there are no highly specific and sensitive and predictive biomarkers available for use by neonatologists. Questions about the mechanistic pathophysiology of the disease are also raised by this phenomenon. Is early-onset NEC in later preterms associated with a greater confidence in feeding these infants? In the less mature infants, is the late onset secondary to acquisition of a certain set of microbiota that adversely interact with the developing intestine? This remains a mysterious disease. Nevertheless, this is the largest cohort to date that further validates the findings of Stoll et al from 1980.[1]

**J. Neu, MD**

*Reference*

1. Stoll BJ, Kanto WP Jr, Glass RI, Nahmias AJ, Brann AW Jr. Epidemiology of necrotizing enterocolitis: a case control study. *J Pediatr.* 1980;96:447-451.

---

**Investigation of the early intestinal microflora in premature infants with/ without necrotizing enterocolitis using two different methods**
Smith B, Bodé S, Skov TH, et al (Statens Serum Institut, Copenhagen, Denmark; Rigshospitalet, Copenhagen, Denmark; Univ of Copenhagen, Frederiksberg, Denmark)
*Pediatr Res* 71:115-120, 2012

---

*Introduction.*—The pathophysiology of necrotizing enterocolitis (NEC) is multifactorial, and gastrointestinal bacteria are thought to play an important role. In this study, the role of microflora in the gastrointestinal tract of neonates with NEC was assessed by comparing cases with controls.

*Results.*—Of the 163 neonates, 21 developed NEC. The risk of NEC decreased by 8% with each additional day of gestational age.

*Discussion.*—Typically, very few bacterial species could be cultured from the fecal specimens obtained. Gram-positive ($G^+$) bacteria dominated the samples in the NEC group, whereas in the control group mixed flora of $G^+$ and Gram-negative ($G^-$) bacteria were isolated. Surprisingly, molecular analysis using PCR-DGGE profiles did not confirm these differences. Our data suggest that $G^+$ bacteria in the intestine may play a role in the development of NEC in premature infants.

*Methods.*—One hundred and sixty three neonates born at <30 weeks of gestation were enrolled. Fecal samples taken during the first month of life were subjected to culture and PCR-denaturing gradient gel electrophoresis (PCR-DGGE). A total of 482 fecal samples were examined.

▶ In this study, fecal samples were collected longitudinally from 163 infants, 21 of whom had necrotizing enterocolitis (NEC) (21 of 163 [13%]). These were evaluated by standard culture-based techniques and a molecular technique that involved denaturing gel electrophoresis (DGGE) and methods that attempt to identify the subsequent bands. The authors state that there are differences between the NEC infants and the controls using the culture-based techniques, with more gram-positive microorganisms, especially *Staphylococcus* species identified in the babies with NEC. There are several caveats in this study. One is that the control infants are not described. Who are they? Were they simply all babies who did not develop NEC, or was there any attempt at matching the NEC babies with controls born at a similar gestational age, time, or other parameters? Severe bias could be introduced simply based on the fact that infants with NEC had a lower gestational age and therefore had a different length of time to develop a microflora. The non—culture-based technique was not very well described, and some of the newer sequencing technologies available were not used. The fact that more *Staphylococcus* species were cultured from the NEC babies is of interest, but the DGGE results showing no differences in number of bands, richness, or diversity is difficult to interpret because of the lack of case-control matching. I don't see much new that can be derived from this work.

**J. Neu, MD**

---

**Risk of Intussusception Following Administration of a Pentavalent Rotavirus Vaccine in US Infants**

Shui IM, Baggs J, Patel M, et al (Harvard Med School and Harvard Pilgrim Health Care Inst, Boston, MA; Ctrs for Disease Control and Prevention, Atlanta, GA; et al)
*JAMA* 307:598-604, 2012

---

*Context.*—Current rotavirus vaccines were not associated with intussusception in large prelicensure trials. However, recent postlicensure data from international settings suggest the possibility of a low-level elevated risk, primarily in the first week after the first vaccine dose.

*Objective.*—To examine the risk of intussusception following pentavalent rotavirus vaccine (RV5) in US infants.

*Design, Setting, and Patients.*—This cohort study included infants 4 to 34 weeks of age, enrolled in the Vaccine Safety Datalink (VSD) who received RV5 from May 2006-February 2010. We calculated standardized incidence ratios (SIRs), relative risks (RRs), and 95% confidence intervals for the association between intussusception and RV5 by comparing the rates of intussusception in infants who had received RV5 with the rates of intussusception in infants who received other recommended vaccines without concomitant RV5 during the concurrent period and with the expected number of intussusception visits based on background rates assessed prior to US licensure of the RV5 (2001-2005).

*Main Outcome Measure.*—Intussusception occurring in the 1- to 7-day and 1- to 30-day risk windows following RV5 vaccination.

*Results.*—During the study period, 786 725 total RV5 doses, which included 309 844 first doses, were administered. We did not observe a statistically significant increased risk of intussusception with RV5 for either comparison group following any dose in either the 1- to 7-day or 1- to 30-day risk window. For the 1- to 30-day window following all RV5 doses, we observed 21 cases of intussusception compared with 20.9 expected cases (SIR, 1.01; 95% CI, 0.62-1.54); following dose 1, we observed 7 cases compared with 5.7 expected cases (SIR, 1.23; 95% CI, 0.5-2.54). For the 1- to 7-day window following all RV5 doses, we observed 4 cases compared with 4.3 expected cases (SIR, 0.92; 95% CI, 0.25-2.36); for dose 1, we observed 1 case compared with 0.8 expected case (SIR, 1.21; 95% CI, 0.03-6.75). The upper 95% CI limit of the SIR (6.75) from the historical comparison translates to an upper limit for the attributable risk of 1 intussusception case per 65 287 RV5 dose-1 recipients.

*Conclusion.*—Among US infants aged 4 to 34 weeks who received RV5, the risk of intussusception was not increased compared with infants who did not receive the rotavirus vaccine.

▶ A recent study by Patel et al[1] sheds additional light on the previously reported association between rotavirus immunization and intussusception. In a cohort study of more than 300 000 infants aged 4 to 34 weeks who were enrolled in the Vaccine Safety Datalink (VSD) database, the authors of this study found no evidence of risk-adjusted occurrence of intussusception among infants who received the rotavirus (RV5) vaccine. This study differs from another surveillance study conducted in Australia that suggested an increased risk of intussusception 1 to 7 days following the first dose of RV5 (relative risk 5.3; 95% confidence interval, 1.1−15.4).[2] Furthermore, the case series by Patel et al[1] and the case-control study of intussusception and rotavirus vaccine (RV1) was conducted in Mexico and Brazil. In Mexico, both approaches suggested a 5-fold to 6-fold increase in intussusception risk within 7 days following the first dose of rotavirus vaccine. In Brazil, no increased risk was seen after the first dose, but a modest increase in risk was noted within a week following the second dose of rotavirus vaccine. The rate of rotavirus-associated intussusception was approximately 1 per 51 000 infants in Mexico and 1 per 68 000 in Brazil; however, the vaccine was estimated to have prevented a far greater number of hospitalizations (80 000) and deaths (1300). These studies provide evidence of a risk−benefit ratio favoring rotavirus immunization.

**L. J. Van Marter, MD, MPH**

*References*

1. Patel MM, López-Collada VR, Bulhões MM, et al. Intussusception risk and health benefits of rotavirus vaccination in Mexico and Brazil. *N Engl J Med.* 2011;364: 2283-2292.

2. Buttery JP, Danchin MH, Lee KJ, et al. Intussusception following rotavirus vaccine administration: post-marketing surveillance in the National Immunization Program in Australia. *Vaccine.* 2011;29:3061-3066.

## The early programming of metabolic health: is epigenetic setting the missing link?

Sebert S, Sharkey D, Budge H, et al (Univ Hosp Nottingham, UK)
*Am J Clin Nutr* 94:1953S-1958S, 2011

Adult health is dependent, in part, on maternal nutrition and growth during early life, which may independently affect insulin sensitivity, body composition, and overall energy homeostasis. Since the publication of the "thrifty phenotype hypothesis" by Hales and Barker (Diabetologia 1992;35: 595—601), animal experiments have focused on establishing the mechanisms involved, which include changes in fetal cortisol, insulin, and leptin secretion or sensitivity. Intrauterine growth retardation can be induced by either prolonged modest changes in maternal diet or by more severe changes in uterine blood supply near to term. These contrasting challenges result in different amounts of cellular stress in the offspring. In addition, shifts in the transcriptional activity of DNA may produce sustained metabolic adaptations. Within tissues and organs that control metabolic homeostasis (eg, hypothalamus, adipose tissue, stomach, skeletal muscle, and heart), a range of phenotypes can be induced by sustained changes in maternal diet via modulation of genes that control DNA methylation and by histone acetylation, which suggests epigenetic programming. We now need to understand how changes in maternal diet affect DNA and how they are conserved on exposure to oxidative stress. A main challenge will be to establish how the dietary environment interacts with the programmed phenotype to trigger the development of metabolic disease. This may aid in the establishment of nutrigenomic strategies to prevent the metabolic syndrome (Fig 1).

▶ The relationship of diet to DNA methylation, histone acetylation, and gene silencing due to microRNA has been well established. The fact that the fetal time period offers a major opportunity for these events to occur and thus programs the fetus for later health also is well known. However, there are concepts in this review that are new to me. The concept that fetal energy status as determined by mitochondrial function may determine DNA remodeling and set constitutive gene expression (Fig 1) is fascinating. Thus, epigenetic events may depend on mitochondrial division that depends on the PPAR receptor coactivator system and sirtuin. Mitochondrial functions such as the production of reactive oxygen species (ROS), the regulation of fat mass and obesity-associated gene (FTO), and mitochondrial regulation of other proteins are involved in DNA methylation and histone acetylation. This, in turn, can control transcriptional events that have epigenetic implications controlling subsequent health and disease including the metabolic phenotype. This is an intriguing concept that obviously needs further research.

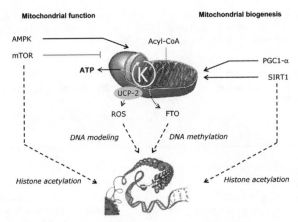

FIGURE 1.—Potential mechanisms by which changes in mitochondrial function contribute to metabolic and oxidative programming of epigenomic plasticity. AMPK, 5'-AMP activated kinase; PGC1-α, peroxisome proliferator−activated receptor co-activator 1-α; SIRT1, sirtuin 1; ROS, reactive oxygen species; mTOR, mammalian target of rapamycin; Acyl-CoA, acetyl-CoA carboxylase; UCP-2, uncoupling protein-2; FTO, fat mass and obesity associated gene. (Am J Clin Nutr. Sebert S, Sharkey D, Budge H, et al. The early programming of metabolic health: is epigenetic setting the missing link? *Am J Clin Nutr.* 2011;94:1953S-1958S, American Society for Nutrition.)

One issue not discussed in this review that remains one of the mysteries of nutritional epigenetics is the transgenerational transmission of epigenetic information. Hopefully more tenable concepts of why and how the diet of one's grand parent may affect one's epigenome will arise and be tested in future studies.

**J. Neu, MD**

## Why Feed Breast Milk From a Bottle?
Whitaker RC, Wright JA (Temple Univ, Philadelphia, PA; Univ of Washington School of Medicine, Seattle)
*Arch Pediatr Adolesc Med* 166:483-484, 2012

*Background.*—Pediatricians encourage breastfeeding of infants based on the clear evidence that infant weight and weight gain are linked to later obesity, and breastfed infants generally do not overeat. However, a study has found that among infants who were exclusively or predominantly fed breast milk, the monthly weight gain was higher among those who received a higher proportion of their breast milk feedings from the bottle. This suggests that infants fed breast milk from the bottle consume more breast milk than they would if they were fed from the breast. Ways to deliver infant feedings were explored.

*Reasons for Feeding Breast Milk by Bottle.*—Often mothers work outside the home and must return to their employment soon after delivery of their infant. This is a common situation for single mothers, who can be under great economic pressure, but also for married mothers. Those who want to provide breast milk for their infants can either breastfeed the child at work or pump and store milk to feed the infant later. Often workplaces are not supportive of the time required for mothers to pump breast milk, and the pumped milk must be stored appropriately and transported before it can be delivered to the infant by bottle. Thus pumped breast milk is costly, and parents may feel they need to encourage the infant to not leave any in the bottle. Mothers also often face the demands of caring for other children, maintaining the house, and performing other routines. Caregiving can be difficult to maintain while breastfeeding. Using a bottle helps mothers meet multiple work demands and allows others to help care for the infant.

Fathers and grandparents also enjoy feeding infants and bottles allow them to do so. This provides a break for the mother while encouraging bonding with the father and/or grandparent. It is important to balance the benefits of breastfeeding with the benefits of allowing fathers to be more involved in infant care by bottle-feeding.

Parents feel their child is well and they are doing a good job when the infant finishes off a meal. It is impossible to know how much an infant is receiving from breastfeeding, which can cause anxiety. Parents naturally want to know that their child is receiving sufficient food, and using a bottle can provide that reassurance.

*Conclusions.*—Other reasons may also lead a mother to choose to use bottle-feeding techniques to deliver breast milk. In addition, faced with the difficulties of providing breast milk and weighing its importance against family issues, mothers may choose to feed their infants formula. Therefore pediatricians should deliver their expert advice nonjudgmentally, being mindful of parents who have to choose to do what is possible rather than what is ideal.

▶ In a study done by authors from the Centers for Disease Control and Prevention,[1] an assessment was made to better understand the mechanisms behind breastfeeding and childhood obesity. Infants were followed up from birth to age 1 year and analyses were conducted to estimate infant weight gain by type of milk and feeding mode. Weights were reported on 3-month, 5-month, 7-month, and 12-month surveys. Compared with infants fed at the breast, infants fed nonhuman or breast milk by bottle gained more weight than those fed by breast alone. It was concluded that infant weight gain might be associated not only with the type of milk consumed but also by the fact that they were fed using a bottle. It was conjectured that a reason for the increased weight gain was because the parents want to see the bottle emptied and the babies would hence be overfed when a bottle was used compared to feeding directly from the breast.

In this article, the authors mention 3 reasons for not feeding mother's milk by breast, which include time constraints such with working mothers, mothers with other unpaid work (other children and family-related duties) who may be constrained by time factors, and fathers who want to feed their infants. Additional reasons not mentioned by the authors may include maternal aversion to feeding directly from the breast or the occasional mother with anatomical challenges.

Whether the increased weight gain by the babies who are feeding by breast milk has any direct causality for adult obesity is not addressed by these studies and remains speculative. This study may have implications for manufacturers considering lowering the energy content of their formulas to mimic that of human milk in order to prevent obesity. Doing this may not matter if the baby simply just eats more or is given more than what he or she would receive from the breast.

**J. Neu, MD**

*Reference*

1. Li R, Magadia J, Fein SB, Grummer-Strawn LM. Risk of bottle-feeding for rapid weight gain during the first year of life. *Arch Pediatr Adolesc Med.* 2012;166: 431-436.

---

**Functional Impairments at School Age of Children With Necrotizing Enterocolitis or Spontaneous Intestinal Perforation**
Roze E, Ta BDP, Van Der Ree MH, et al (Univ of Groningen, The Netherlands)
*Pediatr Res* 70:619-625, 2011

---

We aimed to determine motor, cognitive, and behavioral outcome at school age of children who had either necrotizing enterocolitis (NEC) or spontaneous intestinal perforation (SIP). This case-control study included infants with NEC Bell's stage IIA onward, infants with SIP, and matched controls (1996–2002). At school age, we assessed motor skills, intelligence, visual perception, visuomotor integration, verbal memory, attention, behavior, and executive functions. Of 93 infants with NEC or SIP, 28 (30%) died. We included 52 of 65 survivors for follow-up. At mean age of 9 y, we found that 68% of the children had borderline or abnormal scores on the Movement Assessment Battery for Children (*versus* 45% of controls). Their mean total intelligence quotient (IQ) was 86 ± 14 compared with 97 ± 9 in the controls. In addition, attention and visual perception were affected ($p < 0.01$ and $p = 0.02$). In comparison to controls, surgically treated children were at highest risk for adverse outcome. In conclusion, at school age, the motor functions and intelligence of many children with NEC or SIP were borderline or abnormal and, specifically, attention and visual perception were impaired. Children with NEC or SIP form a specific risk group for functional impairments at school age even though the majority does not have overt brain pathology.

▶ There are several important and novel aspects of this study. One is the fact that this is a 9-year neurodevelopmental follow-up of children who had either medical or surgical necrotizing enterocolits (NEC) or babies with spontaneous intestinal perforations (SIPs). The comparisons of NEC with SIP are also of major interest. Here they find that the neurodevelopmental outcomes of both surgical NEC and SIP are both poor and comparable. Despite medical NEC not showing a statistically significant difference from other matched preterm babies, the trend is certainly in that direction, and with a greater number of subjects in this study, this probably would have been statistically significant. A very important point made by the authors is that the neurodevelopmental outcome of surgical NEC is as serious as severe brain lesions such as periventricular leukomalacia. The authors very aptly call for magnetic resonance imaging (MRI) studies in neonates to help clarify mechanisms. I strongly agree but think that other studies related to biomarkers of brain injury that correlate to MRI findings need to be done to better address the mechanisms.

**J. Neu, MD**

---

**Comparison of the efficacy of serum amyloid A, C-reactive protein, and procalcitonin in the diagnosis and follow-up of necrotizing enterocolitis in premature infants**
Çetinkaya M, Özkan H, Köksal N, et al (Uludag Univ, Bursa, Turkey)
*J Pediatr Surg* 46:1482-1489, 2011

---

*Purpose.*—The aim of this study was to compare the efficacy of serum amyloid A (SAA) with that of C-reactive protein (CRP), and procalcitonin (PCT) in diagnosis and follow-up of necrotizing enterocolitis (NEC) in preterm infants.

*Methods.*—A total of 152 infants were enrolled into this observational study. The infants were classified into 3 groups: group 1 (58 infants with NEC and sepsis), group 2 (54 infants with only sepsis), and group 3 (40 infants with neither sepsis nor NEC, or control group). The data including whole blood count, CRP, PCT, SAA, and cultures that were obtained at diagnosis (0 hour), at 24 and 48 hours, and at 7 and 10 days were evaluated.

*Results.*—A total of 58 infants had a diagnosis of NEC. Mean CRP (7.4 ± 5.2 mg/dL) and SAA (46.2 ± 41.3 mg/dL) values of infants in group 1 at 0 hour were significantly higher than those in groups 2 and 3. Although the area under the curve of CRP was higher at 0 hour in infants with NEC, there were no significant differences between groups with respect to the areas under the curve of SAA, CRP, and PCT at all measurement times. Levels of SAA decreased earlier than CRP and PCT in the follow-up of NEC (mean SAA levels were 45.8 ± 45.2, 21.9 ± 16.6, 10.1 ± 8.3, and 7.9 ± 5.1 mg/dL at evaluation times, respectively). Levels of CRP and SAA of infants with NEC stages II and III were significantly higher than those with only sepsis and/or NEC stage I.

*Conclusions.*—Serum amyloid A, CRP, and PCT all are accurate and reliable markers in diagnosis of NEC, in addition to clinical and radiographic findings. Higher CRP and SAA levels might indicate advanced stage of NEC. Serial measurements of SAA, CRP, and PCT, either alone or in combination, can be used safely in the diagnosis and follow-up of NEC.

▶ Biomarkers that accurately predict the full expression of necrotizing enterocolitis (NEC) are badly needed.[1] This article adds another test (serum amyloid

A) that we might be able to use to evaluate those babies we suspect as having NEC but do not have the classic clear signs of "stage 2 or 3" NEC. Nevertheless, it baffles me to know that the authors were able to determine a "time 0" when they first diagnosed a condition as being sepsis or NEC and to know that this actually reflected the time of onset of the disease. Diagnostic biomarkers have been evaluated by others recently, and surprisingly the authors do not refer to one of the most important of these studies that evaluated urinary intestinal fatty acid binding protein (IFABP), claudin 3 and fecal calprotectin,[2] 2 of which actually showed results comparable to, if not better than, the results shown by these authors using relatively noninvasive tests. A couple of concerning issues are first, that they use the term "NEC Stage 1." Although highly prevalent in the literature, this is a nonspecific term that could apply to such a large number of babies and should be totally removed from our diagnostic vernacular. The fact that the sensitivity of the mentioned tests is high is encouraging in terms of a screening test, but the specificities tend to be lower than IFABP or calprotectin[2] is of interest. It is pleasing to know that researchers are pursuing better diagnostic biomarkers for NEC, but we are still not there.

**J. Neu, MD**

*References*

1. Neu J, Walker WA. Necrotizing enterocolitis. *N Engl J Med.* 2011;364:255-264.
2. Thuijls G, Derikx JP, van Wijck K, et al. Non-invasive markers for early diagnosis and determination of the severity of necrotizing enterocolitis. *Ann Surg.* 2010;251: 1174-1180.

---

**Changes in immunomodulatory constituents of human milk in response to active infection in the nursing infant**
Riskin A, Almog M, Peri R, et al (Bnai Zion Med Ctr, Haifa, Isreal)
*Pediatr Res* 71:220-225, 2012

---

*Introduction.*—To investigate whether immunologic factors in breast milk change in response to nursing infants infection.

*Results.*—Total CD45 leukocyte count dropped from 5,655 (median and interquartile range: 1,911; 16,871) in the acute phase to 2,122 (672; 6,819) cells/ml milk after recovery with macrophage count decreasing from 1,220 (236; 3,973) to 300 (122; 945) cells/ml. Tumor necrosis factor-α (TNFα) levels decreased from 3.66 ± 1.68 to 2.91 ± 1.51 pg/ml. The decrease in lactoferrin levels was of borderline statistical significance. Such differences were not recorded in samples of the controls. Interleukin-10 levels decreased in the sick infants' breast milk after recovery, but also in the healthy controls, requiring further investigation. Secretory immunoglobulin A levels did not change significantly in the study or control group.

*Discussion.*—During active infection in nursing infants, the total number of white blood cells, specifically the number of macrophages, and TNFα levels increase in their mothers' breast milk. These results may support the dynamic nature of the immune defense provided by breastfeeding sick infants.

*Methods.*—Breast milk from mothers of 31 infants, up to 3 months of age, who were hospitalized with fever, was sampled during active illness and recovery. Milk from mothers of 20 healthy infants served as controls.

▶ The interplay between the infant's health status and the response in the mother's milk in this study is highly reminiscent of the concept that Kleinman and Walker[1] introduced more than 30 years ago, termed the *enteromammary system*, wherein antigen presented from the infant to the maternal gut via contact between the mother and the baby is brought into proximity to the mother's lymphoid follicles. This, in turn, commits lymphoblasts to specific immunoglobulin A (IgA) production, which then migrate to the breast and secrete SIgA, which is ingested by the infant. Furthermore, in this concept, T cells, B cells, and macrophages also are thought extruded into the breast milk and are immunologically active. At the time the enteromammary system was conceptualized, the basis was primarily from studies done in animals. This study nicely supports this concept by showing responses in human infants' mothers' milk (consisting of increased white blood cells, primarily macrophages, tumor necrosis factor alpha [TNF-α], and, to a lesser extent, lactoferrin and IgA) to infectious illness thought to originate from the infant.

The authors of this study aptly raise the possibility that some of the findings in the first milk samples from the mothers of the sick infants (eg, more CD45 cells and higher TNF-α levels, especially in comparison with those found in the controls) actually reflect a nonspecific stress response of the mothers whose infants were hospitalized. Although this is unlikely given the nature of the response, it cannot be ruled out.

This study provides support to the dynamic nature of human milk and how the mother's immune system adjusts to her infant's infectious status.

**J. Neu, MD**

*Reference*

1. Kleinman RE, Walker WA. The enteromammary immune system: an important new concept in breast milk host defense. *Dig Dis Sci.* 1979;24:876-882.

---

**Antibiotic Exposure in the Newborn Intensive Care Unit and the Risk of Necrotizing Enterocolitis**

Alexander VN, Northrup V, Bizzarro MJ (Yale Univ School of Medicine, New Haven, CT; Yale Ctr for Analytical Sciences, New Haven, CT)
*J Pediatr* 159:392-397, 2011

---

*Objective.*—To determine whether duration of antibiotic exposure is an independent risk factor for necrotizing enterocolitis (NEC).

*Study Design.*—A retrospective, 2:1 control-case analysis was conducted comparing neonates with NEC to those without from 2000 through 2008.

Control subjects were matched on gestational age, birth weight, and birth year. In each matched triad, demographic and risk factor data were collected from birth until the diagnosis of NEC in the case subject. Bivariate and multivariate analyses were used to assess associations between risk factors and NEC.

*Results.*—One hundred twenty-four cases of NEC were matched with 248 control subjects. Cases were less likely to have respiratory distress syndrome ($P = .018$) and more likely to reach full enteral feeding ($P = .028$) than control subjects. Cases were more likely to have culture-proven sepsis ($P = .0001$). Given the association between sepsis and antibiotic use, we tested for and found a significant interaction between the two variables ($P = .001$). When neonates with sepsis were removed from the cohort, the risk of NEC increased significantly with duration of antibiotic exposure. Exposure for >10 days resulted in a nearly threefold increase in the risk of developing NEC.

*Conclusions.*—Duration of antibiotic exposure is associated with an increased risk of NEC among neonates without prior sepsis (Fig).

▶ I am fascinated by this article and the previous work by Cotten et al[1] that also showed a relationship between the use of antibiotics and the development of necrotizing enterocolitis (NEC). Fig 1 very nicely shows this relationship. Another study by Wang et al[2] also looked at the microbial diversity with NEC and found that there was a decrease in microbial diversity at the time of NEC and that this was also associated with a greater previous use of antibiotics. Another study of NEC and the evaluation of the fecal microbiota prior to the development of NEC[3] showed alteration in the Firmicute to Proteobacteria phyla prior to the development of NEC, along with some interesting differences noted on more in-depth sequencing analysis of the microbiome. Unfortunately, the study by Mai et al[3] did not have enough patients to do a full analysis of

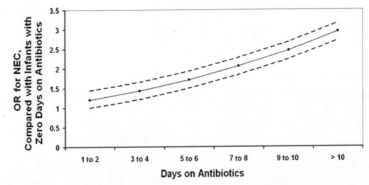

FIGURE.—OR of developing necrotizing enterocolitis (Y-axis) as the cumulative duration of antibiotic exposure increases (X-axis) in neonates without a prior diagnosis of culture-proven sepsis. The comparison group is neonates with zero days of antibiotic exposure. The *dotted lines* represent 95% CIs. A statistically significant increase is observed. (Reprinted from Journal of Pediatrics, Alexander VN, Northrup V, Bizzarro MJ. Antibiotic exposure in the newborn intensive care unit and the risk of necrotizing enterocolitis. *J Pediatr.* 2011;159:392-397. Copyright 2011, with permission from Elsevier.)

antibiotic usage prior to the development of the disease, but a quick look at the differences in antibiotic usage in the controls and cases suggests more antibiotics were also used in the NEC cases. This article is important from several perspectives. First, it shows the relationship between antibiotic usage and the development of NEC. This should raise interesting research questions about what this does to the microbial ecology of the gastrointestinal tract and how this eventually becomes destructive to the intestine. It also raises a warning about the overuse of antibiotics in this very vulnerable population.

**J. Neu, MD**

*References*

1. Cotten CM, Taylor S, Stoll B, et al; NICHD Neonatal Research Network. Prolonged duration of initial empirical antibiotic treatment is associated with increased rates of necrotizing enterocolitis and death for extremely low birth weight infants. *Pediatrics.* 2009;123:58-66.
2. Wang Y, Hoenig JD, Malin KJ, et al. 16S rRNA gene-based analysis of fecal microbiota from preterm infants with and without necrotizing enterocolitis. *ISME J.* 2009;3:944-954.
3. Mai V, Young CM, Ukhanova M, et al. Fecal microbiota in premature infants prior to necrotizing enterocolitis. *PLoS One.* 2011;6:e20647.

---

**Absence of gastrointestinal pathogens in ileum tissue resected for necrotizing enterocolitis**

Ullrich T, Tang Y-W, Correa H, et al (Vanderbilt Univ, Nashville, TN; et al)
*Pediatr Infect Dis J* 31:413-414, 2012

---

Necrotizing enterocolitis (NEC) is one of the most common gastrointestinal emergencies in premature infants and has been linked with viral antigens in as much as 40% of cases in single-center cohorts. We examined 28 tissue sections from surgically resected ileum from 27 preterm infants with NEC from 2 separate institutions for 15 common bacterial, viral, and parasitic gastrointestinal pathogens using multiplex reverse transcriptase polymerase chain reaction amplification and suspension array detection methods. We did not detect infectious enteritis pathogens in any of the NEC tissues and conclude that gastrointestinal pathogens are a rare cause of NEC.

▶ The search for a specific pathogen that causes necrotizing enterocolitis (NEC) is not a new one. Over the 40 or so years since this disease has become highly prevalent, there have been numerous attempts to relate the cause of NEC to various bacteria and viruses. None have been found to be consistently present. This article evaluates 28 tissue sections resected from patients with NEC. A polymerase chain reaction (PCR)-based pathogen screen is used in an attempt to identify known gastrointestinal pathogens. It is not a surprise that this screen did not identify known pathogens in these NEC patients. Why? There are several reasons, including the ones provided by the authors (eg, lack of sensitivity of the assay). Another reason is that there may not be a microbial pathogen that causes NEC, but rather the host response to an overgrowth of symbionts or commensals that may readily become pathogenic under the right conditions (eg, development of a quorum that incites an exaggerated response via toll receptors). Another simple reason is that only probes to known microbes were used. With the advent of the Human Microbiome Project, it is known that most of the microbial taxa in the human gastrointestinal tract have not yet been identified. So, the experiment by these investigators was analogous to trying to identify a criminal by looking at only a small percentage of the entire population, without having any ideas about the identities of the other percentage of the population and whether criminals may exist in that segment. Of interest in this regard is a recent article by Mai et al[1] using 16S pyrosequencing that showed thus far unidentified microbial taxa present in feces from babies with NEC that were not found in closely matched controls. The quest for finding pathogens in NEC is far from over.

**J. Neu, MD**

*Reference*

1. Mai V, Young CM, Ukhanova M, et al. Fecal microbiota in premature infants prior to necrotizing enterocolitis. *PLoS One*. 2011;6:e20647.

# 11 Hematology and Bilirubin

---

**Late-type vitamin K deficiency bleeding: experience from 120 patients**
Ozdemir MA, Karakukcu M, Per H, et al (Erciyes Univ, Talas, Kayseri, Turkey)
*Childs Nerv Syst* 28:247-251, 2012

---

*Background.*—Deficiency of vitamin K predisposes to early, classic, or late vitamin K deficiency bleeding (VKDB), of which late VKDB may be associated with serious and life-threatening intracranial bleeding. Late VKDB is characterized with intracranial bleeding in infants aged 2–24 weeks due to severe vitamin K deficiency, occurring primarily in exclusively breast-fed infants. Late VKDB is still an important cause of mortality and morbidity in developing countries.

*Materials and Methods.*—We presented 120 cases of late VKDB, which were evaluated at Erciyes University Medical Faculty Hospital between June 1990 and June 2006.

*Results.*—Signs and symptoms of the patients were bulging fontanels (70%); irritabilities (50%); convulsions (49%); bleeding and ecchymosis (47%); feeding intolerance, poor sucking, and vomiting (46%); diarrhea (34%); jaundice (11%); and pallor (9%), and among these infants, 21% received medication before the diagnosis (10%, antibiotics; 3%, simethicone; 4%, paracetamol; and 4%, phenobarbital). Intracranial hemorrhage in 88 (73%) patients has been observed. The hemorrhage was subdural in 34 (28%) cases, intracerebral in 28 (23%), subarachnoid in 17 (14%), intraventricular in 9 (8%), intracerebral and subdural in 12 (10%), subdural and subarachnoid in 6 (5%), and combination of intracerebral, subdural, and intraventricular in 14 (12%), and the mortality rate was 31%.

*Conclusion.*—Although late VKDB leads to significant morbidity and mortality, it can be avoided by providing vitamin K prophylaxis to all newborns. Administration of vitamin K (1 mg) at birth can prevent intracranial bleeding and other hemorrhagic manifestations.

▶ Hemorrhagic disease of the newborn has been recognized for over a century and prophylactic therapy available for over half a century, yet the disorder persists. According to McNinch,[1] "At the start of the 20th century the mechanisms of haemostasis were virtually unknown. Townsend had coined the term 'Haemorrhagic disease of the newborn' in 1894 but it was not until the discovery of vitamin K ('Koagulation vitamin') by Dam and others in the 1930s that the condition became understood, allowing treatment and prophylaxis." Hemorrhagic disease of the newborn has been replaced by the term *vitamin K−dependent bleeding* (VKDB), as the etiologic basis is solely vitamin K deficiency. VKDB, especially the late-onset form, is a potent cause of neonatal intracranial hemorrhage and one of the leading acquired disorders of hemostasis. Although the incidence of VKDB in neonates has dramatically decreased in the developed world since the adoption of routine vitamin K prophylaxis, in developing countries the incidence is still high. Ozdemir in Turkey has accumulated a series of 120 patients over 16 years, but almost 75% have intracranial bleeding, and the mortality rate was 31% with no data presented on the long-term morbidity. From the literature, even with early recognition and surgical evacuation of intracranial bleeding, these cases are associated with high mortality rate and neurological disabilities.[2]

In New Zealand, Darlow et al[3] surveyed the prevalence of VKDB from 1998 to 2008. There were 8 confirmed classic cases with an overall incidence of 1.24 per 100 000 births; none had received vitamin K prophylaxis, 7 were fully breastfed, and all fully recovered. There were 9 confirmed late-onset cases with an overall incidence of 1.40 per 100 000 births; 8 had received no vitamin K, 8 were fully breastfed, 6 had liver disease, and 4 suffered an intracranial hemorrhage. They reaffirmed that VKDB is virtually confined to fully breastfed infants not given vitamin K at birth. Late-onset cases were frequently associated with liver disease.

The universal message is to ensure that all babies receive vitamin K at birth. Coagulation studies need to be monitored in babies with liver disease, and repeat dosing may be necessary for these infants. This will reduce VKDB to its bare minimum.

**A. A. Fanaroff, MBBCh, FRCPE**

*References*

1. McNinch A. Vitamin K deficiency bleeding: early history and recent trends in the United Kingdom. *Early Hum Dev.* 2010;86:63-65.
2. Zidan AS, Abdel-Hady H. Surgical evacuation of neonatal intracranial hemorrhage due to vitamin K deficiency bleeding. *J Neurosurg Pediatr.* 2011;7:295-299.
3. Darlow BA, Phillips AA, Dickson NP. New Zealand surveillance of neonatal vitamin K deficiency bleeding (VKDB): 1998-2008. *J Paediatr Child Health.* 2011;47:460-464.

---

**Economic evaluation alongside the Premature Infants in Need of Transfusion randomised controlled trial**

Kamholz KL, the Premature Infants in Need of Transfusion Study Group (Boston Med Ctr, MA; et al)

*Arch Dis Child Fetal Neonatal Ed* 97:F93-F98, 2012

---

*Background.*—The Premature Infants in Need of Transfusion (PINT) Outcome Study showed no significant difference in the primary outcome of death or neurodevelopmental impairment (NDI) in extremely low birthweight (ELBW) infants. However, a post-hoc analysis expanding the definition of NDI to include borderline intellectual functioning (Mental

Development Index (MDI) < 85) found an improvement in outcomes in the group maintained at higher haemoglobin levels.

*Objective.*—To determine the cost effectiveness of more frequent red blood cell transfusions (high-Hb threshold) compared with less frequent transfusions (low-Hb threshold) in ELBW infants.

*Design/Methods.*—The authors performed an economic evaluation using patient-level data collected during the PINT randomised trial. The authors measured comprehensive costs from a third-party payer's perspective over a time horizon from birth through 18–21 months corrected age.

*Results.*—The average total cost in the high-Hb threshold group was CAN$149 767 compared with CAN$150 227 in the low-Hb threshold group (difference of CAN$460, $p = 0.96$). Cost-effectiveness analysis estimated savings of CAN$6879 for every additional infant surviving without severe NDI. There was a 48% chance that the high-Hb threshold reduced costs while improving outcome and a 90% chance that it would be cost effective at a willingness-to-pay threshold of CAN$250 000 per additional survivor without severe NDI. Post-hoc analysis defining cognitive delay as MDI score < 85, instead of < 70, revealed savings in the high-Hb threshold group of CAN$4457 per additional survivor without NDI. Results were robust to deterministic sensitivity analyses.

*Conclusion.*—A high-Hb threshold for transfusion, as measured in ELBW PINT study infants through 18 months corrected gestational age, may be an economically appealing intervention. The estimates were associated with moderate statistical uncertainty that should be targeted in larger, future studies.

► The Premature Infants in Need of Transfusion (PINT) study[1] evaluated the impact of a more versus less aggressive approach to transfusion of infants whose birth weight was below 1000 g. Using a consensus-based algorithm that accounted for postnatal age and degree of respiratory support, as expected, investigators found that infants randomized to the restrictive transfusion group indeed received fewer transfusions than those assigned to the liberal transfusion group. The PINT study investigators found no difference in the composite primary outcome that incorporated death before neonatal intensive care unit discharge, severe retinopathy of prematurity, bronchopulmonary dysplasia, and severe brain injury on cranial ultrasound. Follow-up at 18 to 24 months of age,[2] likewise, revealed no difference between groups in the composite death or severe impairment (Mental Development Index [MDI] < 70); however, a post hoc analysis evaluating MDI less than 85 showed a benefit among infants randomized to the liberal transfusion group. Investigators leading these economic analyses found a 46% chance that a liberal transfusion approach would be a cost-savings, at an estimate of CAN$6879 for each additional infant surviving without cerebral palsy or severe cognitive (MDI < 70), visual, or hearing impairment; savings fell to CAN$4457 if MDI less than 85 was applied. In analyzing not only hospital days, but also nurse-to-patient ratio, this study added a level of sophistication not commonly applied in economic analyses of newborn care. As with other approaches, economic evaluations have their limitations and can arrive at incorrect conclusions via flawed assumptions or methods. Still, I find this study's findings very illuminating: Through meticulously detailed analyses, the investigators provide an example that validates the importance of considering economic analyses, as well as primary clinical endpoints, of randomized trials in the evidence used to evaluate the potential benefits of a particular clinical intervention.

L. J. Van Marter, MD, MPH

References

1. Kirpalani H, Whyte RK, Andersen C, et al. The Premature Infants in Need of Transfusion (PINT) study: a randomized, controlled trial of a restrictive (low) versus liberal (high) transfusion threshold for extremely low birth weight infants. *J Pediatr.* 2006;149:301-307.
2. Whyte RK, Kirpalani H, Asztalos EV, et al. Neurodevelopmental outcome of extremely low birth weight infants randomly assigned to restrictive or liberal hemoglobin thresholds for blood transfusion. *Pediatrics.* 2009;123:207-213.

## Acute physiological effects of packed red blood cell transfusion in preterm infants with different degrees of anaemia

Fredrickson LK, Bell EF, Cress GA, et al (Univ of Iowa, Iowa City; et al)
*Arch Dis Child Fetal Neonatal Ed* 96:F249-F253, 2011

*Objective.*—The safe lower limit of haematocrit or haemoglobin that should trigger a red blood cell (RBC) transfusion has not been defined. The objective of this study was to examine the physiological effects of anaemia and compare the acute responses to transfusion in preterm infants who were transfused at higher or lower haematocrit thresholds.

*Methods.*—The authors studied 41 preterm infants with birth weights 500–1300 g, who were enrolled in a clinical trial comparing high ('liberal') and low ('restrictive') haematocrit thresholds for transfusion. Measurements were performed before and after a packed RBC transfusion of 15 ml/kg, which was administered because the infant's haematocrit had fallen below the threshold defined by study protocol. Haemoglobin, haematocrit, RBC count, reticulocyte count, lactic acid and erythropoietin were measured before and after transfusion using standard methods. Cardiac output was measured by echocardiography. Oxygen consumption was determined using indirect calorimetry. Systemic oxygen transport and fractional oxygen extraction were calculated.

*Results.*—Systemic oxygen transport rose in both groups following transfusion. Lactic acid was lower after transfusion in both groups. Oxygen consumption did not change significantly in either group. Cardiac output and fractional oxygen extraction fell after transfusion in the low haematocrit group only.

*Conclusions.*—These study's results demonstrate no acute physiological benefit of transfusion in the high haematocrit group. The fall in cardiac output with transfusion in the low haematocrit group shows that these infants had increased their cardiac output to maintain adequate tissue oxygen delivery in response to anaemia and, therefore, may have benefitted from transfusion.

▶ When it comes to neonatal intensive care unit patients, the question of when and if to administer blood transfusion continues to be vexing. When caring for babies whose circulating blood volumes can be as low as 40 mL (not quite 2.5 tablespoons) who have hematopoietic potential unable to keep up with phlebotomy losses, it is clear that some babies will require and others will benefit from transfusion. The question is, which babies should be transfused and what products should be administered? This study reports the acute physiologic effects of packed red blood cell (PRBC) transfusion among preterm infants born between 500 and 1300 g and enrolled in the Iowa Transfusion Trial[1] who reached thresholds at greater or lesser levels of anemia; mechanically ventilated group hematocrit thresholds were 34% and 46%, and nonventilated group thresholds were 22% and 30% for restrictive and liberal approaches to transfusion, respectively. The investigators found evidence of reduced cardiac output and fractional oxygen extraction with PRBC transfusion of infants in the low hematocrit group. Both groups experienced increased systemic oxygen transport and reduced lactate levels following transfusion. This is an impressive effort that adds to our understanding of the effects of PRBC transfusion. It also raises additional questions. For example, in an era in which we are increasingly cognizant of the potential adverse effects of oxygen, should we view the increase in systemic oxygen transport a benefit or risk of transfusion?

**L. J. Van Marter, MD, MPH**

*Reference*

1. Bell EF, Strauss RG, Widness JA, et al. Randomized trial of restrictive versus liberal guidelines for red blood cell transfusion in preterm infants. *Pediatrics.* 2005;115:1685-1691.

---

**Furosemide for Packed Red Cell Transfusion in Preterm Infants: A Randomized Controlled Trial**
Balegar VKK, Kluckow M (Royal North Shore Hosp, Sydney, Australia)
*J Pediatr* 159:913-918, 2011

---

*Objective.*—To assess the effect of furosemide administered with packed red blood cell transfusion on cardiopulmonary variables of hemodynamically stable, electively transfused preterm infants beyond the first week of life.

*Study Design.*—A randomized, stratified, double-blind, placebo-controlled trial of intravenous furosemide (1 mg/kg) versus placebo (normal saline) just before "top-up" packed red blood cell transfusion (20 mL/kg over 4 hours) in a tertiary neonatal intensive care unit.

*Results.*—The primary outcome was a change in fraction of inspired oxygen ($FiO_2$) during the 24 hours posttransfusion compared with the

6-hour pretransfusion period. Secondary outcomes were functional echocardiographic and clinical/biochemical variables. Of 51 consecutive preterm infants with mean ( ± SD) birth weights of 900 g ( ± 28); enrollment weights of 1342 g ( ± 432); birth gestation of 27 weeks ( ± 1); and postmenstrual age of 32 weeks ( ± 4), 40 completed the study. Pretransfusion variables were comparable between the furosemide (n = 21) and placebo (n = 19) groups. There was a small but significant increase ($P < .05$) in posttransfusion $FiO_2$ in placebo (relative increase of 7%, equivalent to an absolute increase from 0.27 to 0.29) compared with the furosemide group. Other variables were similar. No infant received open-label furosemide.

*Conclusions.*—Routine furosemide in electively transfused preterm infants confers minimal clinical benefits. Prevention of a clinically insignificant $FiO_2$ rise needs to be balanced against potential adverse effects.

▶ Another common practice withers in the light of empirical evidence. Previous observations of the effects of giving furosemide along with packed red blood cell transfusions to extremely low birth weight infants in the first 2 weeks after birth found no clear benefit from that common practice.[1] This randomized controlled trial extends those conclusions to older preterm infants as well. While both of these trials could be criticized for the small sample sizes (20 and 40 in the prior and current studies, respectively) and the consequent lack of statistical power to detect modest differences between the furosemide- and placebo-treated groups, neither study suggested any difference in respiratory or hemodynamic measures that might become statistically and clinically significant with continued enrollment. In this study, furosemide did blunt a very modest increase in oxygen requirement 24 hours after transfusion, from 27% to 29% in the placebo group, but this effect was evident only at a postmenstrual age of 32 weeks or more. Neither study examined effects on outcomes more than 24 hours after transfusion, so it remains possible that later benefits escaped notice. Nonetheless, extrapolation of demonstrated benefits of furosemide in anemic adults receiving transfusions has proven misleading. Transfusion of red blood cells to preterm infants in volumes of 15 to 20 mL/kg body weight, over a period of 3 to 4 hours (5 mL/kg/h), can be achieved safely without necessity for concurrent diuretic therapy.

**W. E. Benitz, MD**

*Reference*

1. Sarkar S, Dechert R, Becker MA, Attar MA, Schumacher RE, Donn SM. Double-masked, randomized, placebo-controlled trial of furosemide after packed red blood cell transfusion in preterm infants. *J Neonatal Perinatal Med.* 2008;1:13-19.

## Understanding and managing breast milk jaundice

Preer GL, Philipp BL (Boston Univ School of Medicine, MA)
*Arch Dis Child Fetal Neonatal Ed* 96:F461-F466, 2011

The breastfed infant with prolonged unconjugated hyperbilirubinaemia can present a vexing clinical dilemma. Although it is a frequently observed and usually benign finding, prolonged jaundice in the breastfed newborn requires a thoughtful evaluation that excludes possible pathological aetiologies. While recommendations for the treatment of unconjugated hyperbilirubinaemia in the first 7 days of life are straightforward, the approach to the breastfeeding infant with jaundice that persists beyond the immediate neonatal period is less clearly delineated. A sound understanding of bilirubin physiology and familiarity with current literature must guide the management of the otherwise well breastfeeding infant with prolonged unconjugated hyperbilirubinaemia.

▶ This is a very worthwhile review of a subject everyone working in the neonatal intensive care unit thinks he or she understands, but about which few actually possess an in-depth knowledge: breast milk jaundice. We often are challenged with the diagnostic and management dilemma of the breast-fed term infant who achieves bilirubin levels or duration of jaundice that exceeds expectations, pushing the limits of guidelines and the comfort zones of caregivers. This highly informative review provides not only a systematic approach to differentiating pathogenic causes of prolonged unconjugated hyperbilirubinemia from breastfeeding associated with jaundice, but also helps to delineate breast milk jaundice from "not enough breastfeeding" jaundice.

**L. J. Van Marter, MD, MPH**

# 12 Renal, Metabolism, and Endocrine Disorders

**Tight Glycemic Control With Insulin in Hyperglycemic Preterm Babies: A Randomized Controlled Trial**
Alsweiler JM, Harding JE, Bloomfield FH (Univ of Auckland, New Zealand)
*Pediatrics* 129:639-647, 2012

*Objective.*—The optimal treatment of neonatal hyperglycemia is unclear. The aim of this trial was to determine whether tight glycemic control with insulin improves growth in hyperglycemic preterm infants, without increasing the incidence of hypoglycemia.

*Methods.*—Randomized, controlled, nonblinded trial of 88 infants born at <30 weeks' gestation or <1500 g who developed hyperglycemia (2 consecutive blood glucose concentrations (BGC) >8.5 mmol/L, 4 hours apart) and were randomly assigned to tight glycemic control with insulin (target BGC 4—6 mmol/L, "tight" group) or standard practice (restrictive guidelines for starting insulin, target BGC 8—10 mmol/L, "control" group). The primary outcome was linear growth rate to 36 weeks' postmenstrual age.

*Results.*—Eighty-eight infants were randomly assigned (tight group $n = 43$; control group $n = 45$). Infants in the tight group had a lesser lower leg growth rate ($P < .05$), but greater head circumference growth ($P < .0005$) and greater weight gain ($P < .001$) to 36 weeks' postmenstrual age than control infants. Tight group infants had lower daily BGC (median [interquartile range] 5.7 [4.8—6.7] vs 6.5 [5.1—8.2] mmol/L, $P < .001$) and greater incidence of hypoglycemia (BGC <2.6 mmol/L) (25/43 vs 12/45, $P < .01$) than controls. There were no significant differences in nutritional intake, or in the incidences of mortality or morbidity.

*Conclusions.*—Tight glycemic control with insulin in hyperglycemic preterm infants increases weight gain and head growth, but at the expense of reduced linear growth and increased risk of hypoglycemia. The balance of risks and benefits of insulin treatment in hyperglycemic preterm neonates remains uncertain.

▶ There is no consensus with regard to the definition of hyperglycemia, but this report adds fuel to the fire that insulin therapy should be used only when all other

251

methods fail when dealing with hyperglycemia, regardless of definition, in the preterm neonate. Alsweiler et al found that tight glycemic control with insulin in hyperglycemic preterm infants was associated with increased weight gain and head growth but at the expense of reduced linear growth and increased risk of hypoglycemia. The randomized trial of Beardsall et al[1] with continuous monitoring of blood glucose was discontinued by the data and safety monitoring board before complete enrollment because of an increased incidence of hypoglycemia and an excess of dilation of the cerebral ventricles and parenchymal lesions seen on cranial ultrasound images in addition to a trend toward more deaths in the early-insulin group. There was a higher mortality rate in the early-insulin group at 28 days of age in the intention-to-treat analysis (11.9% vs 5.7%, $P < .02$). The cerebral lesions cannot directly be attributed to the hypoglycemia and may be due to the hyperglycemia or the underlying cause of the hypoglycemia. Long-term follow-up may yield answers, but as reduction in hypoglycemia was not accompanied by significant effects on major morbidities, overall the potential harm of tight glucose control with insulin greatly exceeds any perceived benefits. Other methods should, therefore, be tried to prevent and treat hyperglycemia. For example, using sequential cohorts, Mahaveer et al[2] demonstrated that increasing early protein intake is associated with a reduction in insulin-treated hyperglycemia (from 53% to 26%) in infants less than 29 weeks' gestation.

There is, however, an urgent need for further well-conducted randomized trials. Two Cochrane reviews address the prevention and treatment of hyperglycemia.[3,4] In the first, Sinclair et al concluded "There is insufficient evidence from trials comparing lower with higher glucose infusion rates to inform clinical practice. Large randomized trials are needed, powered on clinical outcomes including death, major morbidities and adverse neurodevelopment." With regard to insulin infusion they noted "The evidence reviewed does not support the routine use of insulin infusions to prevent hyperglycemia in VLBW neonates. Further randomized trials of insulin infusion may be justified. They should enroll extremely low birth weight neonates at very high risk for hyperglycemia and neonatal death. They might use real time glucose monitors if these are validated for clinical use. Refinement of algorithms to guide insulin infusion is needed to enable tight control of glucose concentrations within the target range."[3] Bottino et al, reviewing the literature on interventions for hyperglycemia, concluded "evidence from randomized trials in hyperglycemic VLBW neonates is insufficient to determine the effects of treatment on death or major morbidities. It remains uncertain whether the hyperglycemia per se is a cause of adverse clinical outcomes or how the hyperglycemia should be treated." They offered similar comments to those by Sinclair et al regarding the need for randomized trials. All the above frustrates the clinician who wants to know when and how.

**A. A. Fanaroff, MBBCh, FRCPE**

*References*

1. Beardsall K, Vanhaesebrouck S, Ogilvy-Stuart AL, et al. Early insulin therapy in very-low-birth-weight infants. *N Engl J Med.* 1873;2008:359.
2. Mahaveer A, Grime C, Morgan C. Increasing early protein intake is associated with a reduction in insulin-treated hyperglycemia in very preterm infants. *Nutr Clin Pract.* 2012;27:399-405.

3. Sinclair JC, Bottino M, Cowett RM. Interventions for prevention of neonatal hyperglycemia in very low birth weight infants. *Cochrane Database Syst Rev.* 2011;(10):CD007615.
4. Bottino M, Cowett RM, Sinclair JC. Interventions for treatment of neonatal hyperglycemia in very low birth weight infants. *Cochrane Database Syst Rev.* 2011;(10): CD007453.

## Tight Glycemic Control With Insulin in Hyperglycemic Preterm Babies: A Randomized Controlled Trial

Alsweiler JM, Harding JE, Bloomfield FH (Univ of Auckland, New Zealand)
*Pediatrics* 129:639-647, 2012

*Objective.*—The optimal treatment of neonatal hyperglycemia is unclear. The aim of this trial was to determine whether tight glycemic control with insulin improves growth in hyperglycemic preterm infants, without increasing the incidence of hypoglycemia.

*Methods.*—Randomized, controlled, nonblinded trial of 88 infants born at <30 weeks' gestation or <1500 g who developed hyperglycemia (2 consecutive blood glucose concentrations (BGC) >8.5 mmol/L, 4 hours apart) and were randomly assigned to tight glycemic control with insulin (target BGC 4—6 mmol/L, "tight" group) or standard practice (restrictive guidelines for starting insulin, target BGC 8—10 mmol/L, "control" group). The primary outcome was linear growth rate to 36 weeks' postmenstrual age.

*Results.*—Eighty-eight infants were randomly assigned (tight group $n =$ 43; control group $n = 45$). Infants in the tight group had a lesser lower leg growth rate ($P < .05$), but greater head circumference growth ($P < .0005$) and greater weight gain ($P < .001$) to 36 weeks' postmenstrual age than control infants. Tight group infants had lower daily BGC (median [interquartile range] 5.7 [4.8—6.7] vs 6.5 [5.1—8.2] mmol/L, $P < .001$) and greater incidence of hypoglycemia (BGC <2.6 mmol/L) (25/43 vs 12/45, $P < .01$) than controls. There were no significant differences in nutritional intake, or in the incidences of mortality or morbidity.

*Conclusions.*—Tight glycemic control with insulin in hyperglycemic preterm infants increases weight gain and head growth, but at the expense of reduced linear growth and increased risk of hypoglycemia. The balance of risks and benefits of insulin treatment in hyperglycemic preterm neonates remains uncertain.

▶ As mentioned by the authors of this article, insulin usage has become widespread in neonatal nurseries with very few data to support its use. Many early low birth weight infants experience hyperglycemia shortly after birth, with the etiology related to endogenous immature mechanisms for glucose metabolism, the high stresses associated with intensive care, and the use of glucocorticoids and other drugs that increase blood glucose levels. Potential benefits of providing insulin to these infants include control of the hyperglycemia, the growth enhancement benefits of insulin, and control of the oftentimes associated hyperkalemia. In adult intensive care, where since 2001 several randomized controlled trials have examined the effect of tight glucose control in ICU patients,[1] only 1 study showed an overall survival benefit. Tight glucose control is labor intensive and increases the incidence of hypoglycemia, which could have profound effects, especially if cerebral perfusion is poor. Another large, open-label randomized trial of neonates in the United Kingdom[2] was discontinued by the data and safety monitoring board before complete enrollment (389 infants were enrolled; the investigators aimed to recruit 500 patients) because of safety concerns (eg, an excess of dilation of the cerebral ventricles and parenchymal lesions seen on cranial ultrasound images and a trend toward more deaths in the early-insulin group). In an accompanying commentary it was stated: "On the basis of the results of higher mortality at 28 days of age and the increased incidence of hypoglycemia in the early-insulin group, the routine early use of insulin to achieve tighter control of glucose levels cannot be recommended."[3]

This article provides additional fodder for discouraging the use of routine insulin. Despite the better weight gain and occipitofrontal head circumference growth in the insulin group, for the babies who received insulin routinely, the growth advantage appeared to be largely due to increase in fat rather than lean body mass. This treatment also increased the incidence of potentially harmful hypoglycemia and was associated with many more blood draws for glucose monitoring. Thus, routine insulin infusions should not be considered as safe or effective treatment in hyperglycemic preterm neonates. With select neonates who have severe hyperglycemia, guidelines should be developed that use limitations in glucose infusions, discourage the use of glucocorticoids when not needed, and use noninvasive means to limit blood glucose increasing stress in these infants.

**J. Neu, MD**

*References*

1. Elia M, De Silva A. Tight glucose control in intensive care units: an update with an emphasis on nutritional issues. *Curr Opin Clin Nutr Metab Care.* 2008;11:465-470.
2. Beardsall K, Vanhaesebrouck S, Ogilvy-Stuart AL, et al. Early insulin therapy in very-low-birth-weight infants. *N Engl J Med.* 2008;359:1873-1884.
3. Kashyap S, Polin RA. Insulin infusions in very-low-birth-weight infants. *N Engl J Med.* 2008;359:1951-1953.

---

**Tight Glycemic Control With Insulin in Hyperglycemic Preterm Babies: A Randomized Controlled Trial**
Alsweiler JM, Harding JE, Bloomfield FH (Univ of Auckland, New Zealand)
*Pediatrics* 129:639-647, 2012

---

*Objective.*—The optimal treatment of neonatal hyperglycemia is unclear. The aim of this trial was to determine whether tight glycemic control with insulin improves growth in hyperglycemic preterm infants, without increasing the incidence of hypoglycemia.

*Methods.*—Randomized, controlled, nonblinded trial of 88 infants born at <30 weeks' gestation or <1500 g who developed hyperglycemia (2 consecutive blood glucose concentrations (BGC) >8.5 mmol/L, 4 hours apart) and were randomly assigned to tight glycemic control with insulin (target BGC 4–6 mmol/L, "tight" group) or standard practice (restrictive guidelines for starting insulin, target BGC 8–10 mmol/L, "control" group). The primary outcome was linear growth rate to 36 weeks' postmenstrual age.

*Results.*—Eighty-eight infants were randomly assigned (tight group $n =$ 43; control group $n = 45$). Infants in the tight group had a lesser lower leg growth rate ($P < .05$), but greater head circumference growth ($P < .0005$) and greater weight gain ($P < .001$) to 36 weeks' postmenstrual age than control infants. Tight group infants had lower daily BGC (median [interquartile range] 5.7 [4.8–6.7] vs 6.5 [5.1–8.2] mmol/L, $P < .001$) and greater incidence of hypoglycemia (BGC <2.6 mmol/L) (25/43 vs 12/45, $P < .01$) than controls. There were no significant differences in nutritional intake, or in the incidences of mortality or morbidity.

*Conclusions.*—Tight glycemic control with insulin in hyperglycemic preterm infants increases weight gain and head growth, but at the expense of reduced linear growth and increased risk of hypoglycemia. The balance of risks and benefits of insulin treatment in hyperglycemic preterm neonates remains uncertain.

▶ Infusion of insulin has been widely used to prevent or manage hyperglycemia in very low birth weight (VLBW) infants for many years. There is little doubt that this treatment is effective in allowing (or compelling) VLBW infants to tolerate higher glucose infusion rates and to correspondingly increase caloric intake. It has not been clear whether the babies benefit from this effect. We now have 2 randomized clinical trials that provide evidence on the matter. The first of these randomly assigned VLBW infants to routine insulin or no insulin, with adjustment of glucose infusion rates to target equivalent ranges of serum glucose concentrations.[1] In that trial, infants in the insulin infusion group were less likely to be hyperglycemic and received more carbohydrates, but rates of significant hypoglycemia and mortality in the first 28 days were higher. In this report, use of insulin in a more targeted fashion for infants with documented hyperglycemia was also associated with less hyperglycemia but more hypoglycemia. Infants in the insulin infusion group had greater weight gain and head growth but reduced linear growth, suggesting increased accretion of fat rather than lean mass. Although statistically significant in linear regression modeling, the regression coefficients associated with insulin infusion for these outcomes were not reported, so the magnitude of their contribution is indeterminate. In any case, the clinical significance of the small differences shown in the figure in original article is questionable. Insulin infusion did not lead to fewer complications, fewer days to full feedings, fewer hospital days, or better weights, lengths, or head circumferences at 36 weeks' postmenstrual age. The theoretical, and as yet undemonstrated, benefits of insulin infusion would not appear to outweigh the hazards posed by a higher incidence of hypoglycemia.

**W. E. Benitz, MD**

*Reference*

1. Beardsall K, Vanhaesebrouck S, Ogilvy-Stuart AL, et al. Early insulin therapy in very-low-birth-weight infants. *N Engl J Med*. 2008;359:1873-1884.

# 13 Miscellaneous

Association Between Hospital Recognition for Nursing Excellence and Outcomes of Very Low-Birth-Weight Infants
Lake ET, Staiger D, Horbar J, et al (Univ of Pennsylvania, PA; Dartmouth College, Hanover, NH; Univ of Vermont, Burlington; et al)
*JAMA* 307:1709-1716, 2012

*Context.*—Infants born at very low birth weight (VLBW) require high levels of nursing intensity. The role of nursing in outcomes for these infants in the United States is not known.

*Objective.*—To examine the relationships between hospital recognition for nursing excellence (RNE) and VLBW infant outcomes.

*Design, Setting, and Patients.*—Cohort study of 72 235 inborn VLBW infants weighing 501 to 1500 g born in 558 Vermont Oxford Network hospital neonatal intensive care units between January 1, 2007, and December 31, 2008. Hospital RNE was determined from the American Nurses Credentialing Center. The RNE designation is awarded when nursing care achieves exemplary practice or leadership in 5 areas.

*Main Outcome Measures.*—Seven-day, 28-day, and hospital stay mortality; nosocomial infection, defined as an infection in blood or cerebrospinal fluid culture occurring more than 3 days after birth; and severe (grade 3 or 4) intraventricular hemorrhage.

*Results.*—Overall, the outcome rates were as follows: for 7-day mortality, 7.3% (5258/71 955); 28-day mortality, 10.4% (7450/71 953); hospital stay mortality, 12.9% (9278/71 936); severe intraventricular hemorrhage, 7.6% (4842/63 525); and infection, 17.9% (11 915/66 496). The 7-day mortality was 7.0% in RNE hospitals and 7.4% in non-RNE hospitals (adjusted odds ratio [OR], 0.87; 95% CI, 0.76-0.99; $P = .04$). The 28-day mortality was 10.0% in RNE hospitals and 10.5% in non-RNE hospitals (adjusted OR, 0.90; 95% CI, 0.80-1.01; $P = .08$). Hospital stay mortality was 12.4% in RNE hospitals and 13.1% in non-RNE hospitals (adjusted OR, 0.90; 95% CI, 0.81-1.01; $P = .06$). Severe intraventricular hemorrhage was 7.2% in RNE hospitals and 7.8% in non-RNE hospitals (adjusted OR, 0.88; 95% CI, 0.77-1.00; $P = .045$). Infection was 16.7% in RNE hospitals and 18.3% in non-RNE hospitals (adjusted OR, 0.86; 95% CI, 0.75-0.99; $P = .04$). Compared with RNE hospitals, the adjusted absolute decrease in risk of outcomes in RNE hospitals ranged from 0.9% to 2.1%. All 5 outcomes were jointly significant ($P < .001$). The mean effect across all 5 outcomes was OR, 0.88 (95% CI, 0.83-0.94; $P < .001$). In a subgroup of

68 253 infants with gestational age of 24 weeks or older, the ORs for RNE for all 3 mortality outcomes and infection were statistically significant.

*Conclusion.*—Among VLBW infants born in RNE hospitals compared with non-RNE hospitals, there was a significantly lower risk-adjusted rate of 7-day mortality, nosocomial infection, and severe intraventricular hemorrhage but not of 28-day mortality or hospital stay mortality.

▶ Ask any parents of a baby hospitalized in a newborn intensive care unit (NICU) who among the multidisciplinary team of NICU caregivers makes the greatest difference in the health and well-being of their baby and the answer, almost certainly, will be the nurses! This study lends support to the view that nursing expertise and excellence are critically important to the outcomes of our most vulnerable patient population. In this cohort study of more than 72 000 infants hospitalized in NICUs of the Vermont-Oxford Network, infants hospitalized in Recognition for Nursing Excellence (RNE)—certified NICUs had lower 7-day risk-adjusted mortality rates and lower rates of nosocomial infection and severe intraventricular hemorrhage; overall and 28-day mortality were not significantly different between RNE and non-RNE units. The important contributions of nurses to direct patient care as well as the teamwork so necessary for optimal patient outcomes are increasingly recognized. Nevertheless, current work suggests that NICU safety culture varies greatly.[1] I applaud the authors of this study and suspect that the RNE designation is as much about recognizing the creation of institutional cultures that foster professional development among nurses, highly value the unique expertise of NICU nurses, and embrace nurses as key members of the collaborative NICU team as it is about the specific measures of nursing excellence.

**L. J. Van Marter, MD, MPH**

*Reference*

1. Profit J, Etchegaray J, Petersen LA, et al. Neonatal intensive care unit safety culture varies widely. *Arch Dis Child Fetal Neonatal Ed.* 2012;97:F120-F126.

---

**Association Between Hospital Recognition for Nursing Excellence and Outcomes of Very Low-Birth-Weight Infants**
Lake ET, Staiger D, Horbar J, et al (Univ of Pennsylvania, Philadelphia; Dartmouth College, Hanover, NH; Univ of Vermont, Burlington; et al)
*JAMA* 307:1709-1716, 2012

*Context.*—Infants born at very low birth weight (VLBW) require high levels of nursing intensity. The role of nursing in outcomes for these infants in the United States is not known.

*Objective.*—To examine the relationships between hospital recognition for nursing excellence (RNE) and VLBW infant outcomes.

*Design, Setting, and Patients.*—Cohort study of 72 235 inborn VLBW infants weighing 501 to 1500 g born in 558 Vermont Oxford Network hospital neonatal intensive care units between January 1, 2007, and December 31, 2008. Hospital RNE was determined from the American Nurses Credentialing Center. The RNE designation is awarded when nursing care achieves exemplary practice or leadership in 5 areas.

*Main Outcome Measures.*—Seven-day, 28-day, and hospital stay mortality; nosocomial infection, defined as an infection in blood or cerebrospinal fluid culture occurring more than 3 days after birth; and severe (grade 3 or 4) intraventricular hemorrhage.

*Results.*—Overall, the outcome rates were as follows: for 7-day mortality, 7.3% (5258/71 955); 28-day mortality, 10.4% (7450/71 953); hospital stay mortality, 12.9% (9278/71 936); severe intraventricular hemorrhage, 7.6% (4842/63 525); and infection, 17.9% (11 915/66 496). The 7-day mortality was 7.0% in RNE hospitals and 7.4% in non-RNE hospitals (adjusted odds ratio [OR], 0.87; 95% CI, 0.76-0.99; $P = .04$). The 28-day mortality was 10.0% in RNE hospitals and 10.5% in non-RNE hospitals (adjusted OR, 0.90; 95% CI, 0.80-1.01; $P = .08$). Hospital stay mortality was 12.4% in RNE hospitals and 13.1% in non-RNE hospitals (adjusted OR, 0.90; 95% CI, 0.81-1.01; $P = .06$). Severe intraventricular hemorrhage was 7.2% in RNE hospitals and 7.8% in non-RNE hospitals (adjusted OR, 0.88; 95% CI, 0.77-1.00; $P = .045$). Infection was 16.7% in RNE hospitals and 18.3% in non-RNE hospitals (adjusted OR, 0.86; 95% CI, 0.75-0.99; $P = .04$). Compared with RNE hospitals, the adjusted absolute decrease in risk of outcomes in RNE hospitals ranged from 0.9% to 2.1%. All 5 outcomes were jointly significant ($P < .001$). The mean effect across all 5 outcomes was OR, 0.88 (95% CI, 0.83-0.94; $P < .001$). In a subgroup of 68 253 infants with gestational age of 24 weeks or older, the ORs for RNE for all 3 mortality outcomes and infection were statistically significant.

*Conclusion.*—Among VLBW infants born in RNE hospitals compared with non-RNE hospitals, there was a significantly lower risk-adjusted rate of 7-day mortality, nosocomial infection, and severe intraventricular hemorrhage but not of 28-day mortality or hospital stay mortality (Tables 3 and 4).

▶ Most neonatologists are highly aware of how critical the nurse's role is for quality of patient care. The time each neonatologist spends directly at the bedside with each individual patient is usually minuscule compared to the nurse, hence, the higher the quality of nursing, the better the care of the patient. Very few studies have evaluated this in a scientific manner. In this study, an outcomes comparison was made between Vermont Oxford Affiliated hospital neonatal intensive care units (NICUs) that had achieved recognition for nursing excellence (RNE) versus hospitals that did not have this designation. Several interesting differences in outcomes for the infants were found. These included a lower risk of 7-day mortality, nosocomial infections, and severe intraventricular hemorrhage. At 28 days and for full hospital stay, mortality did not differ (Tables 3 and 4). Nevertheless, there were interesting differences that are likely related to the differences in RNE designation. RNE status was more strongly associated with survival for infants in the gestational age range in which the highest levels of intensive care are usually applied (ie, the smallest and most immature infants).

TABLE 3.—Odds Ratios Estimating the Association of Hospital RNE Status and NICU and Hospital Variables With Very Low-Birth-Weight Infant Outcomes[a]

| | Odds Ratio (95% CI) | | | | | |
|---|---|---|---|---|---|---|
| Outcomes | Unadjusted | P Value | Adjusted for Patient Characteristics | P Value | Adjusted for Patient, NICU, and Hospital Characteristics | P Value |
| Mortality | | | | | | |
| Within 7 d | 0.96 (0.86-1.06) | .41 | 0.84 (0.74-0.96) | .01 | 0.87 (0.76-0.99) | .04 |
| Within 28 d | 0.96 (0.87-1.05) | .35 | 0.87 (0.77-0.98) | .02 | 0.90 (0.80-1.01) | .08 |
| Before discharge | 0.95 (0.87-1.03) | .21 | 0.87 (0.78-0.97) | .01 | 0.90 (0.81-1.01) | .06 |
| Morbidity | | | | | | |
| Nosocomial infection | 0.88 (0.78-1.01) | .06 | 0.88 (0.76-1.00) | .06 | 0.86 (0.75-0.99) | .04 |
| Severe intraventricular hemorrhage | 0.90 (0.80-1.00) | .05 | 0.84 (0.75-0.95) | .01 | 0.88 (0.78-1.00) | .045 |

*Abbreviations*: NICU, neonatal intensive care unit; RNE, recognition for nursing excellence.
[a]Odds ratios and 95% CIs were derived from random-effects logistic regression models. All models control for year of birth. Infant risk adjusters were gestational age, gestational age squared, 1-minute Apgar score, small for gestational age, multiple birth, congenital malformation, vaginal delivery, prenatal care, race/ethnicity, and sex. NICU characteristics were adjusted for the natural log of volume of very low-birth-weight infants and level of care. Hospital characteristics were adjusted for hospital ownership and membership in the Council of Teaching Hospitals.

TABLE 4.—Odds Ratios Estimating the Association of Hospital RNE Status and NICU and Hospital Variables With Very Low-Birth-Weight Infant Outcomes Among Infants With Gestational Age of 24 Weeks or More at Birth[a]

| | Odds Ratio (95% CI) | | | | | |
|---|---|---|---|---|---|---|
| Outcomes | Unadjusted | P Value | Adjusted for Patient Characteristics | P Value | Adjusted for Patient, NICU, and Hospital Characteristics | P Value |
| Mortality (n = 67 497-67 517) | | | | | | |
| Within 7 d | 0.91 (0.81-1.02) | .10 | 0.81 (0.70-0.93) | .004 | 0.83 (0.72-0.96) | .01 |
| Within 28 d | 0.92 (0.83-1.02) | .11 | 0.85 (0.75-0.95) | .01 | 0.87 (0.77-0.99) | .03 |
| Before discharge | 0.91 (0.83-1.00) | .06 | 0.85 (0.76-0.96) | .01 | 0.87 (0.78-0.98) | .02 |
| Morbidity | | | | | | |
| Nosocomial infection (n = 64 201) | 0.87 (0.77-1.0) | .04 | 0.87 (0.75-0.99) | .04 | 0.86 (0.74-0.99) | .03 |
| Severe intraventricular hemorrhage (n = 61 030) | 0.89 (0.80-1.00) | .06 | 0.84 (0.74-0.96) | .01 | 0.88 (0.77-1.00) | .05 |

*Abbreviations*: NICU, neonatal intensive care unit; RNE, recognition for nursing excellence.
[a]Odds ratios and 95% CIs were derived from random-effects logistic regression models. All models control for year of birth. Infant risk adjusters were gestational age, gestational age squared, 1-min Apgar score, small for gestational age, multiple birth, congenital malformation, vaginal delivery, prenatal care, race/ethnicity, and sex. NICU characteristics were adjusted for volume of very low-birth-weight infants and level of care. Hospital characteristics were adjusted for hospital ownership and membership in the Council of Teaching Hospitals.

Although, as stated by the authors, one cannot fully rule out that RNE hospitals are also likely to have associated factors that improve the quality of care, and that teasing these out statistically may be a challenge. Many of the RNE hospitals also were higher-level NICUs and academic centers with considerable experience in caring for the sickest very low birth weight infants. Nevertheless, as stated by the authors, RNE is a way to increase the number of infants who receive high-quality care. Excellence in nursing is likely to have an aura effect; it also makes the care doctors provide better. This provides benefit for the preterm infants, but may also be highly applicable to other hospitalized patients, especially those receiving high-level intensive care.

**J. Neu, MD**

## Challenges in Setting Up Pediatric and Neonatal Intensive Care Units in a Resource-Limited Country

Basnet S, Adhikari N, Koirala J (Southern Illinois Univ School of Medicine, Springfield; Patan Academy Health Sciences, Kathmandu, Nepal)
*Pediatrics* 128:e986-e992, 2011

In collaboration with a host country and international medical volunteers, a PICU and an NICU were conceptualized and realized in the developing country of Nepal. We present here the challenges that were encountered during and after the establishment of these units. The decision to develop an ICU with reasonable goals in a developing country has to be made with careful assessments of need of that patient population and ethical principles guiding appropriate use of limited resources. Considerations during unit design include space allocation, limited supply of electricity, oxygen source, and clean-water availability. Budgetary challenges might place overall sustainability at stake, which can also lead to attrition of trained manpower and affect the quality of care. Those working in the PICU in resource-poor nations perpetually face the challenges of lack of expert support (subspecialists), diagnostic facilities (laboratory and radiology), and appropriate medications and equipment. Increasing transfer of severely ill patients from other health facilities can lead to space constraints, and lack of appropriate transportation for these critically ill patients increases the severity of illness, which leads to increased mortality rates. The staff in these units must make difficult decisions on effective triage of admissions to the units on the basis of individual cases, futility of care, availability of resources, and financial ability of the family.

► Having spent a considerable period of time in evolving but resource-limited countries, I highly recommend this article, not only for its description of the development of pediatric and neonatal intensive care units in Kathmandu, Nepal, but also to serve as a reminder of how fortunate we are to practice intensive care medicine in the developed world. The authors describe difficulties produced by the infrastructure (unreliable electrical power, lack of a clean water source, limited space, budget, equipment, personnel, and expertise) and budgetary challenges surrounding both development and maintenance. In my experience, there are additional issues, including dealing with ministries of health that view intensive care as an expense rather than as an investment, high taxation on imported medical devices and pharmaceuticals, and a limited ability to care for survivors of intensive care following discharge. Nevertheless, I commend the authors for describing how they went about accomplishing their goals and how they dealt with the obstacles and challenges of doing so.

**S. M. Donn, MD**

---

## Combining Kangaroo Care and Live Harp Music Therapy in the Neonatal Intensive Care Unit Setting
Schlez A, Litmanovitz I, Bauer S, et al (Meir Med Ctr, Kfar Saba, Israel)
*Isr Med Assoc J* 13:354-358, 2011

---

*Background.*—Music therapy has been recommended as an adjuvant therapy for both preterm infants and mothers during their stay in the neonatal intensive care unit (NICU), and has been shown to have beneficial effects.

*Objectives.*—To study the usefulness of combining live harp music therapy and kangaroo care (KC) on short-term physiological and behavioral parameters of preterm infants and their mothers in the NICU setting.

*Methods.*—Included in this study were stable infants born between 32 and 37 weeks of gestation, with normal hearing. Mother-infant dyads were randomly assigned to KC and live harp music therapy or to KC alone. Using repeated measures, neonatal and maternal heart rate, oxygen saturation and respiratory rate were recorded along with neonatal behavioral state and maternal anxiety state. Maternal age, ethnicity, education, and love of music were documented.

*Results.*—Fifty-two mother-infant dyads were tested. Compared with KC alone, KC and live harp music therapy had a significantly beneficial effect on maternal anxiety score (46.8 ± 10 vs. 27.7 ± 7.1, respectively, $P < 0.01$). Infants' physiological responses and behavior did not differ significantly. No correlation was found between mothers' age, ethnicity, years of education and affinity for music, and anxiety scores ($P = 0.2$ to 0.5 for all four variables).

*Conclusions.*—KC combined with live harp music therapy is more beneficial in reducing maternal anxiety than KC alone. This combined therapy had no apparent effect on the tested infants' physiological responses or behavioral state.

▶ A variety of techniques have been used in an attempt to improve preterm infants' physiological and neurobehavioral outcomes, including skin-to-skin contact (kangaroo care), newborn individualized developmental care, and control of ambient noise and light. However, there are few studies focusing on interventions that might reduce the anxiety and stress experienced by mothers of preterm infants. In this study, the authors explored the possibility that exposing both mothers and infants to music during kangaroo care would have a more beneficial effect for both maternal and infant physiologic parameters and for neonatal behavioral state and maternal anxiety than kangaroo care alone.

Mother—infant dyads were enrolled in the study if the infants had been born between 32 weeks and 37 weeks of gestation and had passed a hearing screen, and the mothers did not have a history of postpartum depression. Interestingly, one of the exclusion criteria for infants was an observed hyperresponsiveness to live music. A within-subject crossover design was used, with mother–infant dyads acting as their own controls. Each session lasted 30 minutes. A single musician performed live harp music in the style of lullabies.

The only finding of note was that maternal anxiety, as measured by the state-trait anxiety inventory, was less when mothers listened to soothing harp music while participating in kangaroo care. Regrettably, the effect of the harp music alone on maternal anxiety was not measured. In this era of high-tech interventions, additional studies exploring low-tech interventions that potentially promote the well-being of mothers of neonatal intensive care unit patients would be a welcome addition.

**L. A. Papile, MD**

---

## Factors associated with rehospitalizations of very low birthweight infants: Impact of a transition home support and education program

Vohr BR, Yatchmink YE, Burke RT, et al (Women and Infants Hosp, Providence, RI; The Warren Alpert Med School of Brown Univ, Providence, RI)

*Early Hum Dev* 88:455-460, 2012

*Objective.*—To determine the effects of a transition-home education and support program, BPD, and health insurance type on VLBW infant rehospitalizations at 3 and 7 months corrected age. It was hypothesized that the transition-home program would be associated with decreased rehospitalizations between Phase 1 and 2, and public health insurance and BPD would be associated with increased rehospitalizations.

*Methods.*—274 infants with birth weight<1500 g were enrolled in two successive years of a transition-home program (Phase 1—start-up) and (Phase 2—full implementation) and followed to 7 months CA.

*Results.*—The Phase 2 rehospitalization rates were lower but not statistically significant at both 3 months (20% and 15%; $p = 0.246$), and 7 months (24% and 17%; $p = 0.171$). Infants with public insurance had twice as many rehospitalizations by 3 months (28% versus 11%; $p = 0.018$) in Phase 1. In regression analyses the intervention effects did not achieve significance for the cohort at 3 months (OR = 0.63; CI = 0.33 to 1.20) or 7 months (OR = 0.61; CI = 0.33 to 1.13). BPD and public insurance did not reach significance in the models whereas siblings were significantly associated with increased odds of rehospitalization. In subgroup analyses for infants on pubic health insurance the intervention significantly decreased the odds of rehospitalization between Phase 1 and 2 (OR = 0.43; CI = 0.19 to 0.96) at 3 months.

*Conclusions.*—Our findings suggest that a transition-home program may be beneficial to reduce the rehospitalization rate for VLBW infants, and infants on public insurance may derive greater benefit.

▶ The transition home support and education program described in this article included a phone call within 48 hours of discharge from the newborn intensive care unit, the provision of postdischarge home visits by neonatal nurse practitioners (NNPs), and the availability 24/7 of project physicians and NNPs for telephone consultation with the primary care provider. In addition, comprehensive assessments were done in the follow-up clinic at 3 to 4 weeks, 3 to 4 months' corrected age, and 7 to 8 months' corrected age. Hospitalizations were defined as an admission for at least an overnight stay in the hospital and considered potentially preventable. Comparisons were made between phase 1 (the first 12 months of the program) and phase 2 (the second year of the program).

Overall, there was not a statistical difference in the rates of rehospitalization between phase 1 and phase 2. Not surprisingly, the presence of siblings in the home was the only factor that was significantly associated with rehospitalization. Although not statistically significant, the percentage of reduction in rehospitalizations between phase 1 and phase 2 for infants with public insurance was notable: 43% at 3 months' corrected age and 40% at 7 months' corrected age. Whether the cost savings resulting from a reduction in rehospitalizations for infants with public insurance would offset the cost of a transition home support program similar to the one outlined in this study is unknown.

**L. A. Papile, MD**

---

**Malpractice Risk According to Physician Specialty**
Jena AB, Seabury S, Lakdawalla D, et al (Massachusetts General Hosp, Boston; RAND, Santa Monica, CA; Univ of Southern California, Los Angeles, CA; et al)
*N Engl J Med* 365:629-636, 2011

---

*Background.*—Data are lacking on the proportion of physicians who face malpractice claims in a year, the size of those claims, and the cumulative career malpractice risk according to specialty.

*Methods.*—We analyzed malpractice data from 1991 through 2005 for all physicians who were covered by a large professional liability insurer with a nationwide client base (40,916 physicians and 233,738 physician-years of coverage). For 25 specialties, we reported the proportion of physicians who had malpractice claims in a year, the proportion of claims leading to an indemnity payment (compensation paid to a plaintiff), and the size of indemnity payments. We estimated the cumulative risk of ever being sued among physicians in high- and low-risk specialties.

*Results.*—Each year during the study period, 7.4% of all physicians had a malpractice claim, with 1.6% having a claim leading to a payment (i.e., 78% of all claims did not result in payments to claimants). The proportion of physicians facing a claim each year ranged from 19.1% in neurosurgery, 18.9% in thoracic–cardiovascular surgery, and 15.3% in general surgery to 5.2% in family medicine, 3.1% in pediatrics, and 2.6% in psychiatry. The mean indemnity payment was $274,887, and the median was $111,749. Mean payments ranged from $117,832 for dermatology to $520,923 for pediatrics. It was estimated that by the age of 65 years, 75% of physicians in low-risk specialties had faced a malpractice claim, as compared with 99% of physicians in high-risk specialties.

*Conclusions.*—There is substantial variation in the likelihood of malpractice suits and the size of indemnity payments across specialties. The cumulative risk of facing a malpractice claim is high in all specialties, although most claims do not lead to payments to plaintiffs. (Funded by the RAND Institute for Civil Justice and the National Institute on Aging.)

▶ This article reported the results of medical malpractice claims from 1991 to 2005 for physicians insured by a large medical malpractice insurance carrier. During this time, 40 916 physicians were insured, representing 233 738 physician-years of coverage. The authors sought to report the number of malpractice claims per year, the proportion resulting in an indemnity payment, and the size of the payment. Over this 15-year period, the average yearly incidence of malpractice claims was 7.4%, but only 1.6% resulted in a payment (about 80% of claims were dropped or dismissed without a payment made).

The specialty of pediatrics represents the good, the bad, and the ugly of malpractice risk. The good: only 3.1% of pediatricians were sued (compared with 19.1% of neurosurgeons and 18.9% of thoracic-cardiovascular surgeons), ranking us 24th of the 25 specialties represented. The bad: pediatrics had the highest amount of malpractice payments of all specialties. The ugly: the average payment was $520 924, considerably higher than the next highest specialty, and nearly double the mean for all specialties ($274 887).

These data differ slightly from those of the Physicians Insurers Association of America (PIAA), a consortium of liability insurance companies that pools closed claims data. In 2010, PIAA published data from closed claims from 1985 to 2009 and found pediatrics to be only the fifth-highest specialty in terms of indemnity payments ($271 784), with neurosurgery the highest ($323 227) and the mean at $212 722.[1] These differences could be explained by differing proportions of specialists within the respective databases, the longer duration of the PIAA study, and a more robust data set from the PIAA study.

Despite the differences, there are some similar messages. As a specialty, pediatrics is among the least frequently sued specialties. However, indemnity payments made to pediatric plaintiffs are among the highest. Why are pediatric claims so expensive? Damages cover the lifetime of the child and include not only the cost of care but also items such as lost wages. In addition, juries tend to be very sympathetic to families and children. A related issue is the long statute of limitations, which leaves pediatricians vulnerable to lawsuits for a much longer period of time than their counterparts in adult medicine.

The American tort system is outcomes based. Even appropriate care can result in a malpractice claim if the outcome is poor. One pediatrician in 3 will be sued. Having adequate liability insurance is essential.

**S. M. Donn, MD**

*Reference*

1. Physicians Insurers Association of America. *A Risk Management Review of Malpractice Claims-Pediatrics.* Rockville, MD: Physicians Insurers Association of America; 2010.

## Mandibular Distraction Osteogenesis in Infants Younger Than 3 Months

Scott AR, Tibesar RJ, Lander TA, et al (Tufts Univ School of Medicine, Boston, MA; Children's Hosps and Clinics of Minnesota, Minneapolis)

Arch Facial Plast Surg 13:173-179, 2011

*Objectives.*—To examine the long-term outcomes and complications in infants with upper airway obstruction and feeding difficulty who underwent bilateral mandibular distraction osteogenesis (MDO) within the first 3 months of life and to identify any preoperative characteristics that may predict the long-term outcome following early MDO intervention for airway obstruction.

*Methods.*—An institutional, retrospective medical chart review was performed. Inclusion criteria were bilateral MDO performed at an age younger than 3 months, with a minimum follow-up of 3 years. A quantitative outcome measures scale was developed, and patients were scored based on long-term postoperative complications as well as airway and feeding goals. Factors such as need for an additional surgical procedure were also considered.

*Results.*—Nineteen children were identified as having undergone MDO before 3 months of age and having more than 3 years of follow-up data. The mean age at distraction was 4.8 weeks (range, 5 days-12 weeks); the mean length of follow-up was 5.6 years (range, 37-122 months). Of these 19 patients, 14 had isolated Pierre Robin sequence (PRS) and 5 had syndromic PRS. All patients with isolated PRS had a good or intermediate long-term result. Infants with comorbidities such as developmental delay, seizures, or arthrogryposis had the poorest outcomes.

*Conclusions.*—Bilateral MDO is a relatively safe and effective means of treating airway obstruction and feeding difficulty in infants with PRS. The effects of this procedure, which carries a relatively low morbidity, persist through early childhood in most patients.

▶ Not long ago, supraglottic airway obstruction caused by posterior displacement of the tongue base was often an intractable problem in neonates with Pierre Robin sequence. Some infants could be treated with simple measures, such as prone positioning or use of nasopharyngeal airways (sometimes with continuous positive airway pressure or bilevel positive airway pressure). A definitive airway could be established by tracheostomy, but that procedure was often avoided because of well-placed fears of complications, ranging from disruption of speech development to sudden death from loss of the airway due to accidental decannulation or mucous plugging. Those fears led to tolerance of recurrent episodes of obstructive apnea or to attempts to stabilize the airway using surgical methods of dubious efficacy (eg, glossopexy). In the late 1990s, increasing experience with mandibular distraction osteotomy in older children and development of hardware small enough to permit the procedure in neonates led to reports of this approach in neonates. The results were transformative, and many (including me) quickly lost equipoise regarding the role of this procedure in management of severe airway obstruction from severe micrognathia. This report provides valuable outcome data and clinical perspective. For patients with isolated Pierre Robin sequence, airway stabilization is consistently achieved and persists well into childhood, realizing the goal of rapid elimination of obstructive apnea without the risks associated with tracheostomy. The authors caution that outcomes may not be so uniformly favorable in infants with multiple anomalies or neurological disease and suggest that tracheostomy may be preferred in those babies. They strongly advocate tracheostomy and feeding gastrostomy for infants with arthrogryposis, whose airway and feeding problems typically have numerous causes beyond micrognathia and tongue base displacement, which may be minor aspects of their incapacities. Accrual and sharing of experience with this procedure will allow further refinement of selection criteria, timing, technique, and postsurgical management. These early returns provide support for the perception that mandibular distraction offers a very effective and low-risk option for the management of severe Pierre Robin sequence.

**W. E. Benitz, MD**

---

**Neonatal Abstinence Syndrome and Associated Health Care Expenditures: United States, 2000-2009**
Patrick SW, Schumacher RE, Benneyworth BD, et al (Univ of Michigan Health System, Ann Arbor; et al)
*JAMA* 307:1934-1940, 2012

*Context.*—Neonatal abstinence syndrome (NAS) is a postnatal drug withdrawal syndrome primarily caused by maternal opiate use. No national estimates are available for the incidence of maternal opiate use at the time of delivery or NAS.

*Objectives.*—To determine the national incidence of NAS and antepartum maternal opiate use and to characterize trends in national health care expenditures associated with NAS between 2000 and 2009.

*Design, Setting, and Patients.*—A retrospective, serial, cross-sectional analysis of a nationally representative sample of newborns with NAS. The Kids' Inpatient Database (KID) was used to identify newborns with NAS by *International Classification of Diseases, Ninth Revision, Clinical Modification (ICD-9-CM)* code. The Nationwide Inpatient Sample (NIS) was used to identify mothers using diagnosis related groups for vaginal and cesarean deliveries. Clinical conditions were identified using *ICD-9-CM* diagnosis codes. NAS and maternal opiate use were described as an annual frequency per 1000 hospital births. Missing hospital charges (<5% of cases) were estimated using multiple imputation. Trends in health care utilization outcomes over time were evaluated using variance-weighted regression. All hospital charges were adjusted for inflation to 2009 US dollars.

*Main Outcome Measures.*—Incidence of NAS and maternal opiate use, and related hospital charges.

*Results.*—The separate years (2000, 2003, 2006, and 2009) of national discharge data included 2920 to 9674 unweighted discharges with NAS and 987 to 4563 unweighted discharges for mothers diagnosed with antepartum opiate use, within data sets including 784 191 to 1.1 million discharges for children (KID) and 816 554 to 879 910 discharges for all ages of delivering mothers (NIS). Between 2000 and 2009, the incidence of NAS among newborns increased from 1.20 (95% CI, 1.04-1.37) to 3.39 (95% CI, 3.12-3.67) per 1000 hospital births per year (*P* for trend <.001). Antepartum maternal opiate use also increased from 1.19 (95% CI, 1.01-1.35) to 5.63 (95% CI, 4.40-6.71) per 1000 hospital births per year (*P* for trend <.001). In 2009, newborns with NAS were more likely than all other hospital births to have low birthweight (19.1%; SE, 0.5%; vs 7.0%; SE, 0.2%), have respiratory complications (30.9%; SE, 0.7%; vs 8.9%; SE, 0.1%), and be covered by Medicaid (78.1%; SE, 0.8%; vs 45.5%; SE, 0.7%; all *P*<.001). Mean hospital charges for discharges with NAS increased from $39 400 (95% CI, $33 400-$45 400) in 2000 to $53 400 (95% CI, $49 000-$57 700) in 2009 (*P* for trend <.001). By 2009, 77.6% of charges for NAS were attributed to state Medicaid programs.

*Conclusion.*—Between 2000 and 2009, a substantial increase in the incidence of NAS and maternal opiate use in the United States was observed, as well as hospital charges related to NAS.

▶ Although primary care pediatricians confront daily the interactions between sociodemographic determinants of health and the presenting complaints of their patients, the more physiologically oriented milieu of the neonatal intensive care unit (NICU) sometimes results in the leaving of public health issues at the NICU door. This excellent article details how one such social determinant has direct and measurable effects on our population of patients. Patrick and colleagues use 2 large databases to establish the first nationally representative estimates of the clinical and financial burden of neonatal abstinence syndrome (NAS) and the changes of these over a 10-year period. They report dramatic increases in maternal opiate use and diagnosis of NAS, with the latter now affecting 0.3% of births studied. Infants with NAS were more likely to have low birth weight and respiratory complications, and most of their costs were borne by Medicaid. Addressing such major problems will require a coordinated approach between neonatologists, public health practitioners, and politicians. Arguably, neonatology will need to move beyond the specifics of therapy after the fact to advocate for appropriate preconceptual and prenatal care and to ensure that it does in fact reduce the burden of illness in our patients.

**J. Zupancic, MD**

## Neonatal Abstinence Syndrome and Associated Health Care Expenditures: United States, 2000-2009

Patrick SW, Schumacher RE, Benneyworth BD, et al (Univ of Michigan Health System, Ann Arbor; et al)
*JAMA* 307:1934-1940, 2012

*Context.*—Neonatal abstinence syndrome (NAS) is a postnatal drug withdrawal syndrome primarily caused by maternal opiate use. No national estimates are available for the incidence of maternal opiate use at the time of delivery or NAS.

*Objectives.*—To determine the national incidence of NAS and antepartum maternal opiate use and to characterize trends in national health care expenditures associated with NAS between 2000 and 2009.

*Design, Setting, and Patients.*—A retrospective, serial, cross-sectional analysis of a nationally representative sample of newborns with NAS. The Kids' Inpatient Database (KID) was used to identify newborns with NAS by *International Classification of Diseases, Ninth Revision, Clinical Modification (ICD-9-CM)* code. The Nationwide Inpatient Sample (NIS) was used to identify mothers using diagnosis related groups for vaginal and cesarean deliveries. Clinical conditions were identified using *ICD-9-CM* diagnosis codes. NAS and maternal opiate use were described as an annual frequency per 1000 hospital births. Missing hospital charges (<5% of cases) were estimated using multiple imputation. Trends in health care utilization outcomes over time were evaluated using variance-weighted regression. All hospital charges were adjusted for inflation to 2009 US dollars.

*Main Outcome Measures.*—Incidence of NAS and maternal opiate use, and related hospital charges.

*Results.*—The separate years (2000, 2003, 2006, and 2009) of national discharge data included 2920 to 9674 unweighted discharges with NAS and 987 to 4563 unweighted discharges for mothers diagnosed with antepartum opiate use, within data sets including 784 191 to 1.1 million discharges for children (KID) and 816 554 to 879 910 discharges for all ages of delivering mothers (NIS). Between 2000 and 2009, the incidence of NAS among newborns increased from 1.20 (95% CI, 1.04-1.37) to 3.39 (95% CI, 3.12-3.67) per 1000 hospital births per year (*P* for trend <.001). Antepartum maternal opiate use also increased from 1.19 (95% CI, 1.01-1.35) to 5.63 (95% CI, 4.40-6.71) per 1000 hospital births per year (*P* for trend <.001). In 2009, newborns with NAS were more likely than all other hospital births to have low birthweight (19.1%; SE, 0.5%; vs 7.0%; SE, 0.2%), have respiratory complications (30.9%; SE, 0.7%; vs 8.9%; SE, 0.1%), and be covered by Medicaid (78.1%; SE, 0.8%; vs 45.5%; SE, 0.7%; all *P*<.001). Mean hospital charges for discharges with NAS increased from $39 400 (95% CI, $33 400-$45 400) in 2000 to $53 400 (95% CI, $49 000-$57 700) in 2009 (*P* for trend <.001). By 2009, 77.6% of charges for NAS were attributed to state Medicaid programs.

*Conclusion.*—Between 2000 and 2009, a substantial increase in the incidence of NAS and maternal opiate use in the United States was observed, as well as hospital charges related to NAS.

▶ After extreme prematurity, neonatal abstinence syndrome (NAS) is one of the most prominent causes of prolonged newborn hospitalization. This article demonstrates the rising prevalence of NAS in the United States between 2000 and 2009 accompanied by marked increases in associated health care costs. The study was based on a retrospective serial cross-sectional analysis of a nationally representative sample of newborns with NAS. Over the study years, the incidence of antenatal maternal opiate use increased almost 5-fold, and there was an approximately 3-fold increase in incidence of NAS. Furthermore, infants with NAS were more likely in 2009 than in 2000 to have additional complications, including low birth weight, feeding problems, seizures, and respiratory complications; unsurprisingly, hospital charges per NAS case also increased. The prevalence of maternal opioid use and NAS was greatest in urban settings and the lowest-income ZIP code areas. These authors offer suggestions for decreasing NAS-associated costs, such as treating mothers with buprenorphine, rather than methadone; combining neonatal morphine treatment with other approaches, such as concurrent use of phenobarbital, clonidine, or breastfeeding; and caring for infants with NAS outside the neonatal intensive care unit. Increased scrutiny of health care expenditures has led to other suggestions for reducing health care costs,[1] such as the use of electronic medical records (EMR), using EMR information for more intensive monitoring, and interactions to increase medical adherence to treatment protocols, reducing the use of specialists, and providing services not traditionally covered by fee-for-service reimbursement (eg, e-mail, wireless monitoring) to enhance compliance and minimize complications. Could some of these reduce the costs associated with NAS? Perhaps so; however, this study argues for a broader approach. Although drug dependence and abuse occur in communities of all socioeconomic levels, the prevalence is greatest in the urban lower socioeconomic environment. With 75% of costs associated with NAS paid by Medicaid, the US government is faced with a powerful incentive to address the problem. The current approach of attempting to reduce health care costs by pressuring physicians and hospitals to use some of the measures listed in the abstract is not without merit. I would suggest that an equally valid way to reduce health care costs—and, in the process, enhance quality of life for many—would be to increase investment in initiatives that will reverse the culture of poverty, despair, and intergenerational health risks so prevalent in our inner cities.

**L. J. Van Marter, MD, MPH**

*Reference*

1. Emanuel EJ. Where are the health care cost savings? *JAMA.* 2012;307:39-40.

---

**Neonatal intensive care unit safety culture varies widely**
Profit J, Etchegaray J, Petersen LA, et al (Texas Children's Hosp, Houston; Univ of Texas Med School, Houston; Baylor College of Medicine, Houston, TX; et al)
*Arch Dis Child Fetal Neonatal Ed* 97:F120-F126, 2012

*Background.*—Variation in healthcare delivery and outcomes in neonatal intensive care units (NICUs) may be partly explained by differences in safety culture.
*Objective.*—To describe NICU care giver assessments of safety culture, explore variability within and between NICUs on safety culture domains, and test for association with care giver characteristics.

*Methods.*—NICU care givers in 12 hospitals were surveyed using the Safety Attitudes Questionnaire (SAQ), which has six scales: teamwork climate, safety climate, job satisfaction, stress recognition, perception of management and working conditions. Scale means, SDs and percent positives (percent agreement) were calculated for each NICU.

*Results.*—There was substantial variation in safety culture domains among NICUs. Composite mean score across the six domains ranged from 56.3 to 77.8 on a 100-point scale and NICUs in the top four NICUs were significantly different from the bottom four ($p < 0.001$). Across the six domains, respondent assessments varied widely, but were least positive on perceptions of management (3%—80% positive; mean 33.3%) and stress recognition (18%—61% positive; mean 41.3%). Comparisons of SAQ scale scores between NICUs and a previously published adult ICU cohort generally revealed higher scores for NICUs. Composite scores for physicians were 8.2 ($p = 0.04$) and 9.5 ($p = 0.02$) points higher than for nurses and ancillary personnel.

*Conclusion.*—There is significant variation and scope for improvement in safety culture among these NICUs. The NICU variation was similar to variation in adult ICUs, but NICU scores were generally higher. Future studies should validate whether safety culture measured with the SAQ correlates with clinical and operational outcomes in NICUs.

▶ More than 10 years after the Institute of Medicine documented the impact of medical error on outcomes in its report "To Err Is Human," safety[1] in neonatal intensive care units (NICUs) remains a core issue in improving quality. As in other areas of quality improvement, a major step in the improvement process is measurement of underlying issues that might be amenable to change. To date, such measurement in our field has typically focused on the incidence of adverse processes or outcomes and the changes that result from specific interventions to alter them. More recently, however, attention has begun to focus on the culture that forms the background and context for such quality lapses. Profit et al[2] assess the validity and applicability in the neonatology environment of the Safety Attitudes Questionnaire, a tool previously shown in other populations to measure a construct of safety culture. They surveyed more than 500 clinicians across multiple disciplines and 12 NICUs, with a good response rate of 86%. The study documents several findings that we as neonatologists might have predicted: NICUs vary in safety culture, there are multiple opportunities for improvement, different disciplines with the NICU assess the same culture differently, and NICUs that are high performing in one domain of safety culture tend to also perform well in others. The results of this study create opportunity; measurement of culture allows us to target and assess interventions that have the potential to change care at a level that may result in improvements on multiple dimensions of quality. This proposed link between assessment of safety culture, interventions to address identified deficiencies, and the outcomes that result is an important new research agenda for our community.

**J. Zupancic, MD**

*References*

1. Institute of Medicine. To err is human: building a safer health system. http://www. iom.edu/~/media/Files/Report%20Files/1999/To-Err-is-Human/To%20Err%20is %20Human%201999%20%20report%20brief.pdf. Published November 1999. Accessed June 28, 2012.
2. Profit J, Etchegaray J, Petersen LA, et al. The Safety Attitudes Questionnaire as a tool for benchmarking safety culture in the NICU. *Arch Dis Child Fetal Neonatal Ed.* 2012;97:F127-F132.

## NICU Care in the Aftermath of Hurricane Katrina: 5 Years of Changes

Barkemeyer BM (Louisiana State Univ Health Sciences Ctr, New Orleans)
*Pediatrics* 128:S8-S11, 2011

*Background.*—Hurricane Katrina caused more than 1800 deaths and over $80 billion in damage along the Gulf Coast in August 2005. A neonatal physician at University Hospital in downtown New Orleans before, during, and after Hurricane Katrina hit that region recounts how neonatology care was accomplished under trying conditions and how it evolved thereafter. The hospital cared primarily for inner-city indigent families.

*The Neonates.*—All neonatal intensive care unit (NICU) patients at University Hospital survived both the storm and the evacuation process. Two premature infants with progressive chronic lung disease dependent on high-frequency ventilators were the sickest being cared for. The morning after the storm, the lack of reliable power and running water forced their transport through floodwaters by canoe and fire truck to Children's Hospital, then to a third hospital when Children's closed. One infant was eventually hospitalized in Fort Worth, Texas, before being lost to follow-up, whereas the other spent 3 months in Baton Rouge, Louisiana, before returning to New Orleans. This infant was briefly hospitalized for a viral respiratory infection in the spring of 2006. One child was born preterm 4 days after Katrina made landfall to a mother who had been hospitalized before the storm with threatened preterm labor. The equipment used to care for her was powered by a portable generator and no routine services (blood gas determinations, laboratory studies, and radiographs) were performed. After 8 hours, she was transported along with 30 other NICU and well infants to Baton Rouge. Reuniting infants with their families was challenging because of the evacuation from the city and the relocations in areas other than New Orleans proper.

*The Hospital.*—University Hospital and nearby Charity Hospital were closed because of flood damage, and temporary emergency medical care was provided at various sites. Full-service health care returned only after several months of repairs. The first newborn infant after Katrina was delivered at University Hospital in February 2007, and neonatal care was upgraded stepwise from level 2 to level 3 as patient volume increased. Over the next 3 years, delivery numbers plateaued at a quarter of the volume before Katrina. In July 2010 the hospital closed the obstetric and neonatal care services because of the lower than anticipated number of births that resulted from the failure of many indigent residents to return to New Orleans and because of the establishment of other area hospitals as preferred sites for the delivery of obstetric care when University Hospital was closed.

*Evolution of NICU Care.*—All 3 major tertiary care NICUs were able to reopen and reestablish their roles fairly quickly after Katrina. However, of the 9 hospital NICUs present before Katrina, 1 remains closed, 1 reopened without obstetric and neonatal services, 2 were purchased by another system, and 1 reopened but subsequently closed, reducing the network of care to 4 hospitals and reducing the neonatology division from 12 staff members to 8.

New patterns in NICU patients developed after the hurricane. Hispanic workers flooded into the area, resulting in a significant increase in Hispanic NICU patients. Communication problems arose from cultural and language barriers. In addition, more of the infants cared for were suffering symptoms of withdrawal from opiates, reflecting the reported increase in the illicit use of prescription narcotics after Katrina.

Resident house staff served as key personnel in the prompt and safe evaluation of patients and in triage centers outside of New Orleans. However, the sudden loss of both patient population and training sites reduced educational opportunities. Most residents continued their training through the creativity of residency program directors, the hospitality of medical education leaders across the South, and new patient care opportunities provided by the migration of Katrina evacuees. Training programs returned as New Orleans became repopulated. Graduating medical students often committed to urban residency training programs in a leap of faith. However, shifts in medical facilities made it difficult to match trainees with appropriate patient care sites. New outpatient opportunities have arisen with the establishment of decentralized outpatient clinics.

*Assessment.*—Efforts to improve flood-protection systems continue in southern Louisiana, recognizing that there will always be the threat of hurricanes and other natural disasters. Hospitals have put into place mechanisms that allow the safe care or transport of critically ill patients. Depending on the risk associated with each hospital's location and physical plant, some hospitals have chosen to prepare for patient evaluation and others have planned for shelter in place. Hospitals that have chosen to evacuate NICU patients plan to use local, regional, and potentially national resources. Those that chose to shelter in place have preferred flood-zone status and enhanced physical plant preparations. Several layers of safeguards have been developed should local utilities fail, including raised generators to provide extended periods of electric power fueled by underground tanks, on-site wells to provide needed nonpotable water to cool chillers and provide human waste disposal, and stockpiling of food, potable water, and hospital supplies. An elevated heliport allows for necessary transport when typical ground routes are unavailable.

These efforts were tested in August 2008 when Hurricane Gustav threatened the Gulf Coast. Three million people sought shelter, area hospitals activated their evacuation or shelter-in-place plans, and neonatal patients were cared for effectively. The hurricane preparation in New Orleans was fine-tuned through this experience. Currently the hurricane protection and preparedness in New Orleans are significantly improved over the status pre-Katrina. Preparation is a key element, along with resiliency and resourcefulness of communities and individuals to meet these challenges.

▶ Every pediatric and neonatal care provider who lived in New Orleans in 2005 has personal stories similar to the ones so eloquently expressed by Dr Barkemeyer and his colleagues in the extraordinary August 2011 supplement to *Pediatrics*. In the 5 years since Katrina, local institutions in the Gulf Coast portion of Hurricane Alley have made significant preparations for the next storm. However, the recent devastation of Hurricane Irene along the East Coast demonstrates that few areas in our country are immune to some type of natural disaster. The important lesson to learn from the natural and man-made disasters of Katrina and the post-Katrina response are that every institution needs to have a plan to respond to natural or other disasters. Each plan should recognize the most likely disaster to occur in that region and be developed accordingly. Preparation, communication, and leadership are the most important aspects of any plan. In certain situations, "care in place" is an option, but provisions must be made if this option is not viable. When transport is necessary, it must be done preemptively, not waiting until the situation is untenable (ie, power is cut off). Not only do the patients need to move but also the caretakers (physicians, nurses, etc) must follow to allow safe care in a distant facility. An emergency declaration in our state now allows any licensed provider to practice in any hospital so that the cumbersome credentialing process is curtailed, thus making simultaneous movement of patients and providers possible.

One important aspect of an urban disaster was overlooked by every account in the supplement. We learned from Katrina that the isolation of a city means that supplies are cut off, including illegal drugs to those who depend on them. Once the usual supplies are exhausted, the drug-dependent population will seek drugs in health care facilities, putting health care workers in harm's way. A small minority of our own local populace becomes the enemy. Therefore, security must be an important part of any disaster plan.

Since Katrina, many hospitals and regional and national committees have modeled disaster preparation planning on a natural disaster with the assumption that health care providers will be available. It is possible that some disasters (eg, pandemic flu, nuclear attack) may limit the number of health care providers, and this contingency should also be considered in planning models.

The official reports indicated that 154 adults died in hospitals and other health care facilities during Katrina. There were no pediatric or neonatal deaths. This was in large part because of the brave commitment of many health care providers in the city as well as the wonderful transport teams who came from regional neonatal intensive care units as well as from many distant states to take our patients and left behind food, ice, and water. We shall be eternally grateful, and the entire pediatric community can be justifiably proud.

**J. P. Goldsmith, MD**

**Parental psychological well-being and cognitive development of very low birth weight infants at 2 years**

Huhtala M, PIPARI Study Group (Turku Univ Hosp, Finland; et al)
*Acta Paediatr* 100:1555-1560, 2011

*Aim.*—To assess the associations between cognitive development of very low birth weight (VLBW) infants and measures of parental psychological well-being.

*Methods.*—In this prospective cohort study, 182 VLBW infants born 1/2001-12/2006 at the Turku University Hospital, Finland, were followed up. At 2 years corrected age, cognitive development of the child was assessed using the Mental Development Index of Bayley Scales, and both parents filled in validated questionnaires defining parental psychological well-being (Beck Depression Inventory, Parenting Stress Index and Sense of Coherence Scale).

*Results.*—The cognitive delay of the infant was associated with paternal symptoms of depression ($p = 0.007$) and parenting stress ($p = 0.03$). Mothers of the infants with cognitive delay reported increased parenting stress related to the difficulty to accept the child ($p = 0.001$). Weak sense of coherence predicted depressive symptoms in both parents ($p < 0.0001$).

*Conclusion.*—Even if the fathers of VLBW infants experienced depressive symptoms less often than the mothers, the ability of the fathers to cope was significantly associated with the cognitive development of the infant. In addition, the fathers reported more parenting stress if the infant had a cognitive delay. The mothers reported more parenting stress related to accepting the VLBW infant with cognitive delay.

▶ Preterm birth is associated with an increased risk for maternal symptoms of anxiety, depression, and parenting stress.[1] It has been observed that the high degree of maternal stress associated with preterm birth is transient and is no longer evident by 2 years of age.[2] However, parenting stress may remain high in mothers of very low-birth-weight (VLBW) infants with delayed cognitive development. There are sparse data on paternal adaptation to the birth and subsequent care of VLBW infants.

This study evaluated the associations between cognitive development of VLBW infants at 2 years of age and symptoms of depression, parenting stress, and mental well-being in both mothers and fathers. Not surprisingly, depression was more common in mothers than fathers. Compared with fathers of normally developing VLBW infants, fathers of VLBW infants with delayed cognitive development expressed more depressive symptoms and parenting stress. The source of paternal stress was related to infant characteristics, suggesting that fathers of VLBW infants with developmental problems had difficulty finding ways to interact with their infants. In contrast, depressive symptoms in mothers were not associated with the cognitive development of their VLBW infants, implying that mothers have better coping mechanisms than fathers. It would be interesting to see if the psychological well-being of fathers improves when children with cognitive delay are older and have a greater capacity for interpersonal interactions.

**L. A. Papile, MD**

*References*

1. Davis L, Edwards H, Mohay H, Wollin J. The impact of very premature birth on the psychological health of mothers. *Early Hum Dev.* 2003;73:61-70.
2. Singer LT, Salvator A, Guo S, Collin M, Lilien L, Bayley J. Maternal psychological distress and parenting stress after the birth of a very low-birth-weight infant. *JAMA.* 1999;281:799-805.

**Patient Safety in the Context of Neonatal Intensive Care: Research and Educational Opportunities**
Raju TNK, Suresh G, Higgins RD (Eunice Kennedy Shriver Natl Inst of Child Health and Human Development, Bethesda, MD; Dartmouth-Hitchcock Med Ctr, Lebanon, NH)
*Pediatr Res* 70:109-115, 2011

Case reports and observational studies continue to report adverse events from medical errors. However, despite considerable attention to patient safety in the popular media, this topic is not a regular component of medical education, and much research needs to be carried out to understand the causes, consequences, and prevention of healthcare-related adverse events during neonatal intensive care. To address the knowledge gaps and to formulate a research and educational agenda in neonatology, the *Eunice Kennedy Shriver* National Institute of Child Health and Human Development invited a panel of experts to a workshop in August 2010. Patient safety issues discussed were the reasons for errors, including systems design, working conditions, and worker fatigue; a need to develop a "culture" of patient safety; the role of electronic medical records, information technology, and simulators in reducing errors; error disclosure practices; medicolegal concerns; and educational needs. Specific neonatology-related topics discussed were errors during resuscitation, mechanical ventilation, and performance of invasive procedures; medication errors including those associated with milk feedings; diagnostic errors; and misidentification of patients. This article provides an executive summary of the workshop.

▶ This article summarized the proceedings of a National Institute of Child Health and Human Development Workshop (in which I was privileged to be included), which defined and explored research and educational opportunities to improve patient safety in the neonatal intensive care unit. Drs Raju, Suresh, and Higgins did a masterful job condensing the content of this 2-day event. They summarized the major topics of discussion, including domains of errors and potential sources of errors and the factors enhancing injury risk, and provided a comprehensive list of the gaps in knowledge in patient safety and recommendations for future research.

I urge all neonatologists and those involved in neonatal intensive care to read this article, which implores us to design studies to both comprehend and prevent adverse events in neonatal intensive care. There is much to do.

**S. M. Donn, MD**

---

**Preterm Birth and Psychiatric Disorders in Young Adult Life**
Nosarti C, Reichenberg A, Murray RM, et al (King's College London, UK; et al)
*Arch Gen Psychiatry* 610-617, 2012

---

*Context.*—Preterm birth, intrauterine growth restriction, and delivery-related hypoxia have been associated with schizophrenia. It is unclear whether these associations pertain to other adult-onset psychiatric disorders and whether these perinatal events are independent.

*Objective.*—To investigate the relationships among gestational age, nonoptimal fetal growth, Apgar score, and various psychiatric disorders in young adult life.

*Design.*—Historical population-based cohort study.

*Setting.*—Identification of adult-onset psychiatric admissions using data from the National Board of Health and Welfare, Stockholm, Sweden.

*Participants.*—All live-born individuals registered in the nationwide Swedish Medical Birth Register between 1973 and 1985 and living in Sweden at age 16 years by December 2002 (n=1 301 522).

*Main Outcome Measures.*—Psychiatric hospitalization with nonaffective psychosis, bipolar affective disorder, depressive disorder, eating disorder, drug dependency, or alcohol dependency, diagnosed according to the *International Classification of Diseases* codes for 8 through 10. Cox proportional hazards regression models were used to estimate hazard ratios and 95% CIs.

*Results.*—Preterm birth was significantly associated with increased risk of psychiatric hospitalization in adulthood (defined as ≥16 years of age) in a monotonic manner across a range of psychiatric disorders. Compared with term births (37-41 weeks), those born at 32 to 36 weeks' gestation were 1.6 (95% CI, 1.1-2.3) times more likely to have nonaffective psychosis, 1.3 (95% CI, 1.1-1.7) times more likely to have depressive disorder, and 2.7 (95% CI, 1.6-4.5) times more likely to have bipolar affective disorder. Those born at less than 32 weeks' gestation were 2.5 (95% CI, 1.0-6.0) times more likely to have nonaffective psychosis, 2.9 (95% CI, 1.8-4.6) times more likely to have depressive disorder, and 7.4 (95% CI, 2.7-20.6) times more likely to have bipolar affective disorder.

*Conclusions.*—The vulnerability for hospitalization with a range of psychiatric diagnoses may increase with younger gestational age. Similar associations were not observed for nonoptimal fetal growth and low Apgar score.

▶ In Sweden, each episode of hospital care is entered into the Swedish National Hospital Discharge Register, a database that includes hospital discharges and discharge diagnoses. Because each episode of hospital care contains a unique personal identifier (a 10-digit National Registration Number), the investigators in this study were able to match individuals' hospital discharge diagnoses with information extracted from the Swedish Medical Birth Register, a database that contains prospectively collected information related to pregnancy, labor and delivery, and newborn characteristics.

The information presented would suggest that both preterm and late preterm birth are associated with an increased vulnerability for developing a wide spectrum of psychiatric disorders severe enough to warrant hospitalization. However, an important limitation of the study is that a psychiatric disorder listed as a discharge diagnosis was included in the analyses, even if the diagnosis was not the primary reason for the hospitalization. For example, an individual who was hospitalized for asthma and incidentally had a depressive disorder would be included in the data as being hospitalized for a psychiatric disorder. Individuals who are born preterm are known to interface with the medical system more frequently than their term counterparts. Thus, a plausible explanation for the apparent increased risk for psychiatric disorders is that the preterm population is overrepresented in the hospital data for reasons other than increased psychiatric disorders.

L. A. Papile, MD

## The effect of music-based listening interventions on the volume, fat content, and caloric content of breast milk-produced by mothers of premature and critically ill infants

Keith DR, Weaver BS, Vogel RL (Georgia College and State Univ, Milledgeville)
Adv Neonatal Care 12:112-119, 2012

*Purpose.*—Maternal breast milk is considered the nutritional "gold standard" for all infants, especially premature infants. However, preterm mothers are at risk of not producing adequate milk. Multiple factors affect the production of milk, including stress, fatigue, and the separation of the breastfeeding dyad-for example, when mother or infant is hospitalized. The purpose of this study was to examine the effects of listening and visual interventions on the quantity and quality of breast milk produced by mothers using a double electric breast pump.

*Subjects.*—Mothers of 162 preterm infants were randomly assigned to 1 of 4 groups.

*Methods.*—The control group received standard nursing care, whereas mothers in the 3 experimental groups additionally listened to a recording of 1 of 3 music-based listening interventions while using the pump.

*Results.*—Mothers in the experimental groups produced significantly more milk ($P < .0012$). Mothers in these groups also produced milk with significantly higher fat content during the first 6 days of the study.

▶ The provision of mother's milk is one of the most efficacious interventions for minimizing medical morbidity in patients in the neonatal intensive care unit. However, a mother's ability to provide adequate milk for her preterm or sick infant is limited by psychological as well as physiologic factors. Attempts to improve human milk production, including emotional support, instruction in the use of breast pumps, encouraging skin-to-skin contact (kangaroo care), and relaxation techniques have had varied success. In this study, women who wished to provide breast milk for their preterm infant were randomly assigned to a control group or an intervention that consisted of listening to a 12-minute recording of a progressive muscle relaxation protocol followed by guided imagery while using the breast pump. For some of the women in the intervention group, the relaxation section was accompanied by selections of lullabies for guitar; for others, images of their infants were added to the music. The volume of milk pumped by mothers in any of the 3 intervention groups was greater than that of the control group and by day 7 was approximately double the amount. From the data presented it would appear that listening to the 12-minute recording was sufficient. The most likely explanation for the beneficial effect is that the intervention reduced stress, leading to an increased quantity of milk.

**L. A. Papile, MD**

---

**The prognostic value of initial blood lactate concentration measurements in very low birthweight infants and their use in development of a new disease severity scoring system**
Phillips LA, Dewhurst CJ, Yoxall CW (Ysbyty Glan Clwyd, Rhyl, Denbighshire, UK; Liverpool Women's Hosp, Merseyside, UK)
*Arch Dis Child Fetal Neonatal Ed* 96:F275-F280, 2011

---

*Objectives.*—To investigate the predictive value of the Clinical Risk Index for Babies (CRIB) score in current practise, the predictive value of blood lactate concentrations ([L]) and to develop a new clinical scoring system for very low birthweight (VLBW) babies.

*Methods.*—The predictive ability of CRIB, [L] and the development of the new score was based on retrospective data collected from all inborn VLBW babies born between March 2001 and February 2004 in a tertiary neonatal unit. Predictive ability was determined from area under the receiver operator curve (AUC). A new score was developed and validated with a second cohort of VLBW babies.

*Results.*—408 babies were studied in the development cohort and 275 in the validation cohort. AUC for CRIB was 0.933 (95% CI 0.897—0.969). Initial [L] was significantly higher in babies who died than in those who survived (median (range) 9.2 (1.26—21.1) vs 3.64 (0.67—17.9) mmol/l, $p < 0.0001$) as was the highest [L] in the first 12 h (10.2 (3.37—26) vs 3.84 (1.05—20.7) mmol/l, $p < 0.0001$). A new score was developed using; highest [L], gestation and the presence of life-threatening malformation. AUC for the new score was 0.918 (95% CI 0.876—0.961) in the development cohort and 0.859 (95% CI 0.805—0.913) in the validation cohort.

*Conclusions.*—CRIB score retains its predictive ability for mortality in VLBW babies. Early hyperlactataemia is a predictor of death in VLBW

TABLE 4.—Components of the NIPI Score

| Variable | Score |
|---|---|
| Gestation | 8 |
| ≤24 | 4 |
| 25−26 | 1 |
| 27−29 | 0 |
| ≥30 | |
| Highest [L] | 0 |
| <3 | 2 |
| 3-6 | 4 |
| 7-9 | 6 |
| 10−14 | 8 |
| 15−19 | 10 |
| ≥ 20 | |
| Life threatening malformations* | 5 |
| Present | 0 |
| Absent | Out of 23 |
| Total score | |

[L] = blood lactate concentration.
*See text.

babies. The new score appears to perform as well as CRIB but requires fewer data items (Table 4).

▶ With the numerous quality improvement initiatives emerging in neonatal intensive care, it is critical to have information about risk status of populations to allow for meaningful comparisons of outcomes. Certain units may treat a large number of infants with good prognoses and others have a very high-risk population. To adequately compare outcomes among these units requires risk adjustment. This study reevaluates a commonly used 6-point indicator, the Clinical Risk Index for Babies (CRIB) score, developed 20 years ago, and finds that it remains a good indicator of predictive ability for death. The authors then used statistical methods to derive and develop a new score, the Neonatal Illness Prognosis Indicator, which uses 3 parameters (compared with 6 in the CRIB) that are highly objective (highest blood lactate, gestational age, and life-threatening malformations) and finds that these (Table 4) reach an area under the curve similar to that of the CRIB score. This score can be derived in the first hours after birth. The advantage of this newly developed score is that it does not contain components that may be affected by variation in clinical practice among units, and thus could be used for comparative purposes. It will be interesting to see if this gets adopted for quality improvement and comparative purposes.

**J. Neu, MD**

## The single-patient room in the NICU: maternal and family effects

Pineda RG, Stransky KE, Rogers C, et al (Washington Univ School of Medicine, St Louis, MO)

*J Perinatol* 32:1-7, 2011

*Objective.*—To explore differences in maternal factors, including visitation and holding, among premature infants cared for in single-patient rooms (SPR) compared with open-bay in the neonatal intensive care unit (NICU).

*Study Design.*—A total of 81 premature infants were assigned to a bed space in either the open-bay area or in a SPR upon NICU admission, based on bed space and staffing availability in each area. Parent visitation and holding were tracked through term equivalent, and parents completed a comprehensive questionnaire at discharge to describe maternal health. Additional maternal and medical factors were collected from the medical record. Differences in outcome variables were investigated using linear regression.

*Result.*—No significant differences in gestational age at birth, initial medical severity, hours of intubation or other factors that could affect the outcome were observed across room type. Significantly more hours of visitation were observed in the first 2 weeks of life ($P = 0.02$) and in weeks 3 and 4 ($P = 0.02$) among infants in the SPR. More NICU stress was reported by mothers in the SPR after controlling for social support ($P = 0.04$).

*Conclusion.*—Increased parent visitation is an important benefit of the SPR, however, mothers with infants in the SPR reported more stress.

▶ The latest trend in the design of neonatal intensive care units (NICUs) is single patient rooms rather than open-bay beds. The advantage of the single patient room is a reduction of noxious ambient stimuli for the medically fragile infant and provision of a private space for the family to engage in the care of their infant. The prospective benefits of single patient design in the NICU have been theoretically appreciated; however, the proven benefits are limited. Published studies have demonstrated increased satisfaction and decreased stress levels among nurses after transition to the single patient room design.[1] In addition, there are several studies that show reductions in the incidence of nosocomial infection, decreases in the length of hospital stay, and decreased use of supplemental oxygen.[2,3] However, there are few studies that have investigated the effect on the family and the mother.

This observational study took place in a NICU that had both single patient rooms and open-bay beds. Infants were assigned a bed space based on availability and remained in the assigned bed throughout their stay in the NICU. Although there was a wide range of parent visitation practices, overall, parents with infants in single patient rooms demonstrated more hours of visitation during their infant's NICU stay compared to parents with infants in the open-bay area. In spite of this, no differences were observed in the frequency of holding in general and skin-to-skin holding specifically. Additionally, the frequency of breast milk feeding at discharge was no different between the 2 cohorts. An interesting finding was the increase in reports of stress among mothers with infants in single patient rooms. It may be that mothers in single patient rooms feel isolated and miss the support of other mothers, or they may feel an increased obligation for the care of their medically fragile infants.

**L. A. Papile, MD**

*References*

1. Stevens DC, Helseth CC, Khan MA, Munson DP, Smith TJ. Neonatal intensive care nursery staff perceive enhanced workplace quality with the single-family room design. *J Perinatol.* 2010;30:352-358.
2. Domanico R, Davis DK, Coleman F, Davis BO. Documenting the NICU design dilemma: comparative patient progress in open-ward and single family room units. *J Perinatol.* 2011;31:281-288.
3. Ortenstrand A, Westruo B, Broström EB, et al. The Stockholm Neonatal Family Centered Care Study: effects on length of stay and infant morbidity. *Pediatrics.* 2010;125:e278-e285.

## When Bad Things Happen: Adverse Event Reporting and Disclosure as Patient Safety and Risk Management Tools in the Neonatal Intensive Care Unit

Donn SM, McDonnell WM (Univ of Michigan Health System, Ann Arbor; Univ of Utah Health Sciences Ctr, Salt Lake City)
*Am J Perinatol* 29:65-70, 2012

The Institute of Medicine has recommended a change in culture from "name and blame" to patient safety. This will require system redesign to identify and address errors, establish performance standards, and set safety expectations. This approach, however, is at odds with the present medical malpractice (tort) system. The current system is outcomes-based, meaning that health care providers and institutions are often sued despite providing appropriate care. Nevertheless, the focus should remain to provide the safest patient care. Effective peer review may be hindered by the present tort system. Reporting of medical errors is a key piece of peer review and education, and both anonymous reporting and confidential reporting of errors have potential disadvantages. Diagnostic and treatment errors continue to be the leading sources of allegations of malpractice in pediatrics, and the neonatal intensive care unit is uniquely vulnerable. Most errors result from systems failures rather than human error. Risk management can be an effective process to identify, evaluate, and address problems that may injure patients, lead to malpractice claims, and result in financial losses. Risk management identifies risk or potential risk, calculates the probability of an adverse event arising from a risk, estimates the impact of the adverse event, and attempts to control the risk. Implementation of a successful risk management program requires a positive attitude, sufficient knowledge base, and a commitment to improvement. Transparency in the disclosure of medical errors and a strategy of prospective risk management in dealing with medical errors may result in a substantial reduction in medical malpractice lawsuits, lower litigation costs, and a more safety-conscious environment.

▶ Few other fields in medicine have had the enormous successes that neonatology has seen in the past several decades. Infants who would have had little chance of survival are now routinely sent home and go on to lead full, productive lives. At the same time, few patients are more vulnerable and at risk of being harmed by the very system designed to save them than neonates. Long hospital stays, an inability to communicate, and multiple medications dosed based on weights that may triple during the hospitalization are just a few of the factors that place the tiniest patients at risk. Ensuring their safe care must be a priority for all. Unfortunately, there are some barriers in achieving this goal. An important one, as noted by these authors, is that a safety first approach is often "at odds with the present medical malpractice (tort) system."

Why might the medical malpractice system get in the way of improving safety? Fear plays a large role; clinicians fear that reporting information about an adverse event and disclosing that information to families will get them sued. Additionally, the legal system in the United States is an adversarial one, and clinicians are frequently specifically told not to talk with families after an adverse event. Besides litigation, clinicians also fear retaliation and punishment, which is reasonable in a culture of "name and blame." But what if this approach is completely backward?

In this article, the authors, both of whom are experienced with medicolegal issues in pediatrics, bring a more modern approach to patient safety in the neonatal intensive care unit. Since it is impossible to correct errors that are unknown, they discuss ways to improve error reporting. They review the different types of medical errors and the unique challenges of reducing medical errors in neonatology. Significantly, they advocate a different approach to error disclosure. There are ethical and legal reasons why open and honest disclosure of adverse events to families is the right thing to do. Surprisingly, when the University of Michigan (Donn's home institution) adopted a policy of full disclosure and fair compensation more than a decade ago, they also found that their legal liabilities actually decreased. This article provides brief advice on designing and implementing a disclosure program.

By changing the culture from one of blame to one of safety and being more open and honest with families, there is a much better chance to, as the article points out, "preserve the physician-patient relationship and increase patient satisfaction and trust." Just as important, it will allow caregivers to design the safest environment possible with the ultimate hope that there will be nothing disclosed because there truly is nothing to disclose.

**J. M. Fanaroff, MD, JD, FAAP, FCLM**

284 / Neonatal and Perinatal Medicine

Enrollment of Extremely Low Birth Weight Infants in a Clinical Research
Study May Not Be Representative

Rich W, for the SUPPORT and Generic Database Subcommittees of the *Eunice
Kennedy Shriver* National Institute of Child Health and Human Development
Neonatal Research Network (Univ of California at San Diego; et al)
*Pediatrics* 129:480-484, 2012

*Background and Objective.*—The Surfactant Positive Airway Pressure
and Pulse Oximetry Randomized Trial (SUPPORT) antenatal consent
study demonstrated that mothers of infants enrolled in the SUPPORT trial
had significantly different demographics and exposure to antenatal steroids
compared with mothers of eligible, but not enrolled infants. The objective of
this analysis was to compare the outcomes of bronchopulmonary dysplasia,
severe retinopathy of prematurity, severe intraventricular hemorrhage or
periventricular leukomalacia (IVH/PVL), death, and death/severe IVH/PVL
for infants enrolled in SUPPORT in comparison with eligible, but not
enrolled infants.

*Methods.*—Perinatal characteristics and neonatal outcomes were compared for enrolled and eligible but not enrolled infants in bivariate analyses. Models were created to test the effect of enrollment in SUPPORT
on outcomes, controlling for perinatal characteristics.

*Results.*—There were 1316 infants enrolled in SUPPORT; 3053 infants
were eligible, but not enrolled. In unadjusted analyses, enrolled infants had
significantly lower rates of death before discharge, severe IVH/PVL, death/
severe IVH/PVL (all <0.001), and bronchopulmonary dysplasia ($P = .003$)
in comparison with eligible, but not enrolled infants. The rate of severe retinopathy of prematurity was not significantly different. After adjustment for
perinatal factors, enrollment in the trial was not a significant predictor of any
of the tested clinical outcomes.

*Conclusions.*—The results of this analysis demonstrate significant outcome differences between enrolled and eligible but not enrolled infants in
a trial using antenatal consent, which were likely due to enrollment bias
resulting from the antenatal consent process. Additional research and regulatory review need to be conducted to ensure that large moderate-risk trials
that require antenatal consent can be conducted in such a way as to ensure
the generalizability of results.

▶ In this important article, the leaders of the National Institute of Child Health and
Human Development Neonatal Network—sponsored Surfactant Positive Airway
Pressure and Pulse Oximetry Randomized Trial (SUPPORT) provide a provocative
and thoughtful analysis of the challenges encountered in obtaining prior informed
consent for enrollment of newborn infants in randomized controlled trials. These
investigators previously reported that mothers who were approached for consent
for enrollment in SUPPORT were significantly more likely to be older, to have
completed high school, to have medical insurance, to have had at least 1 prenatal
care visit, and to be non-Hispanic white, as compared to mothers who were not
approached. Infants who were enrolled were more likely to have received

antenatal steroids, to have received intrapartum antibiotics, and were slightly (but statistically significantly) bigger and more mature. They were more likely to have Apgar scores greater than 3 at both 1 minute and 5 minutes of age and less likely to need resuscitation measures (intubation, surfactant, chest compressions, or epinephrine) in the delivery room. Unadjusted univariate analyses demonstrated that unenrolled infants had higher rates of death, oxygen use at 36 weeks' postmenstrual age, grade 3 or 4 intraventricular hemorrhage (IVH) or periventricular leukomalacia (PVL), and the combined outcomes of death or bronchopulmonary dysplasia (BPD) and death or IVH/PVL. Because of these differences in demographic characteristics and outcomes between enrolled and unenrolled subjects, the authors questioned the external validity of the SUPPORT results. In essence, they asked whether the main conclusions of the trial (substantial equivalence of early continuous positive airway pressure and intubation for early surfactant, higher mortality with lower oxygen saturation targets) are applicable to the less advantaged, sicker infants who were not enrolled in the trial. The primary conclusion of the article—that better strategies for more comprehensive enrollment of subjects in such trials of perinatal interventions are badly needed—should not obscure the implications of the logistic regression models developed to explore those concerns. After adjustment for gestational age, birth weight, gender, race, study center, and antenatal steroid exposure, there were no significant residual differences in rates of BPD, severe retinopathy of prematurity, death, severe IVH/PVL, or death/severe IVH/PVL. Although perhaps not definitive, those observations are actually reassuring in that they imply there were no major biological differences between enrolled and unenrolled subjects, so effects of the study interventions (similarly adjusted) are likely to be comparable as well. Methodological imperfections notwithstanding, we should not construe this study (or the intent of its authors) to suggest that the SUPPORT results should be discarded.

**W. E. Benitz, MD**

---

## Enrollment of Extremely Low Birth Weight Infants in a Clinical Research Study May Not Be Representative

Rich W, for the SUPPORT and Generic Database Subcommittees of the *Eunice Kennedy Shriver* National Institute of Child Health and Human Development Neonatal Research Network (Univ of California at San Diego; et al)
*Pediatrics* 129:480-484, 2012

---

*Background and Objective.*—The Surfactant Positive Airway Pressure and Pulse Oximetry Randomized Trial (SUPPORT) antenatal consent study demonstrated that mothers of infants enrolled in the SUPPORT trial had significantly different demographics and exposure to antenatal steroids compared with mothers of eligible, but not enrolled infants. The objective of this analysis was to compare the outcomes of bronchopulmonary dysplasia, severe retinopathy of prematurity, severe intraventricular hemorrhage or periventricular leukomalacia (IVH/PVL), death, and death/severe IVH/PVL for infants enrolled in SUPPORT in comparison with eligible, but not enrolled infants.

*Methods.*—Perinatal characteristics and neonatal outcomes were compared for enrolled and eligible but not enrolled infants in bivariate analyses. Models were created to test the effect of enrollment in SUPPORT on outcomes, controlling for perinatal characteristics.

*Results.*—There were 1316 infants enrolled in SUPPORT; 3053 infants were eligible, but not enrolled. In unadjusted analyses, enrolled infants had significantly lower rates of death before discharge, severe IVH/PVL, death/ severe IVH/PVL (all < 0.001), and bronchopulmonary dysplasia (P = .003) in comparison with eligible, but not enrolled infants. The rate of severe retinopathy of prematurity was not significantly different. After adjustment for perinatal factors, enrollment in the trial was not a significant predictor of any of the tested clinical outcomes.

*Conclusions.*—The results of this analysis demonstrate significant outcome differences between enrolled and eligible but not enrolled infants in a trial using antenatal consent, which were likely due to enrollment bias resulting from the antenatal consent process. Additional research and regulatory review need to be conducted to ensure that large moderate-risk trials that require antenatal consent can be conducted in such a way as to ensure the generalizability of results.

▶ This article and a previous publication from the National Institute of Child Health and Development's Neonatal Research Network analyze the process of prenatal consent for enrollment in the clinical Surfactant Positive Airway Pressure and Pulse Oximetry Randomized Trial. In the previous report,[1] the authors noted that mothers of infants enrolled in the trial were more likely to have a high school degree and private medical insurance compared with mothers of infants who were eligible but not enrolled. These mothers were also more likely to be non-Hispanic white and were 4 times more likely to have received antenatal steroids. The authors speculate that the selection bias most likely reflects a preponderance of mothers who were more likely to come to the hospital on an emergency basis to deliver their infants in the eligible but not enrolled cohort.

In this article, the authors compared demographics, delivery room data, and medical morbidity data for enrolled infants with data for eligible but not enrolled infants. Enrolled infants were significantly more mature and weighed more at birth. Eligible but not enrolled infants had significantly lower Apgar scores at 5 minutes and 10 minutes and a significantly greater need for delivery room intubation and cardiopulmonary resuscitation. An unadjusted analysis of mortality and medical morbidity showed a significantly higher frequency of mortality, bronchopulmonary dysplasia, and intraventricular hemorrhage (grades III and IV) for the cohort of eligible but not randomized infants. However, none of the differences in outcomes between the groups were significant after controlling for gestational age, birth weight, sex, race, center, and antenatal steroid exposure, indicating that birth characteristics rather than enrollment in the trial itself were likely responsible for the improved outcomes of enrolled infants.

These findings suggest that selection bias related to the consent process is an important issue when antenatal consent is needed to conduct a clinical trial involving neonates. This selection bias can create a threat to the external validity of a trial such that the results may not be generalizable to the sickest and most at-risk populations. The authors propose that a waiver or delay of parental consent be considered to promote generalizability of minimal-risk trials of interventions in the delivery room or shortly after birth.

**L. A. Papile, MD**

*Reference*

1. Rich WD, Auten KJ, Gantz MG, et al; National Institute of Child Health and Human Development Neonatal Research Network. Antenatal consent in the SUPPORT trial: challenges, costs, and representative enrollment. *Pediatrics*. 2010;126:e215-e221.

# 14 Pharmacology

**Are Proton Pump Inhibitors Safe during Pregnancy and Lactation?
Evidence to Date**
Majithia R, Johnson DA (Washington Hosp Ctr, DC; Eastern Virginia Med
School, Norfolk)
*Drugs* 72:171-179, 2012

Symptoms of gastro-oesophageal reflux disease (GORD or GERD) are estimated to occur in 30—50% of pregnancies, with the incidence approaching 80% in some populations. As with many other conditions in pregnancy, medical therapy with pharmaceutical agents is a concern, as the potential teratogenicity of medications is not well known. Although prevalence numbers are high, many patients have mild and infrequent symptoms, which often respond to lifestyle and dietary modifications. The exact mechanism and pathogenesis of GERD associated with pregnancy is likely multifactorial. Treatment strategies for patients not responding to conservative therapies include a step-up approach initially starting with antacids and alginates, and progressing to histamine $H_2$ receptor antagonists followed by proton pump inhibitor (PPI) therapy if indicated by symptoms. Although PPI therapy is the most effective treatment available for GERD, the data related to the safety for use during pregnancy and postpartum breastfeeding are mostly obtained from cohort analysis. Given the significant adverse impact of GERD on quality of life and functionality, the use of this class of medications should not be overly restricted based solely on the pregnancy. Based on the studies presented, exposure to PPI therapy during pregnancy seems to predispose the fetus to minimal risk and, overall, these medications should be discussed with the primary physician if symptomatically necessary in the pregnant patient. This evidence-based review will address the management and safety of PPI therapy during pregnancy and lactation, and briefly review the pathogenesis, clinical presentation and diagnosis of GERD in this population.

▶ Pregnancy category A adequate and well-controlled human studies have failed to demonstrate a risk to the fetus in the first trimester of pregnancy (and there is no evidence of risk in later trimesters).

Pregnancy category B animal reproduction studies have failed to demonstrate a risk to the fetus, and there are no adequate and well-controlled studies in pregnant women or animal studies that have shown an adverse effect, but adequate and well-controlled studies in pregnant women have failed to demonstrate a risk to the fetus in any trimester.

Pregnancy category C animal reproduction studies have shown an adverse effect on the fetus, and there are no adequate and well-controlled studies in humans, but potential benefits may warrant use of the drug in pregnant women despite potential risks.

In pregnancy category D studies, there is positive evidence of human fetal risk based on adverse reaction data from investigational or marketing experience or studies in humans, but potential benefits may warrant use of the drug in pregnant women despite potential risks.

Pregnancy category X studies in animals or humans have demonstrated fetal abnormalities or there is positive evidence of human fetal risk based on adverse reaction data from investigational or marketing experience, and the risks involved in use of the drug in pregnant women clearly outweigh potential benefits.

For pregnancy category N, the US Food and Drug Administration (FDA) has not classified this drug.

There is a constant concern regarding the balance between benefit and harm when prescribing drugs for pregnant women. The rule of thumb to avoid any potentially harmful agents before conception and during the period of organogenesis is sound in principle but not always easy to follow. Digestive disorders are extremely common in the first trimester, and the thalidomide story, familiar to all, serves to remind caretakers of the devastation that can be induced by pharmacologic agents during critical periods in organ formation. Heartburn occurs so frequently during pregnancy (in approximately two-thirds of pregnant patients), that it could be regarded as a normal occurrence. Most patients can be treated with the use of lifestyle modifications and antacids as the first line in therapy. Lifestyle modification, including smaller meals, not eating late at night, elevation of the head of the bed, and avoiding foods and medications causing heartburn, usually relieves the mild symptoms seen in early pregnancy. Abstinence from alcohol and tobacco are encouraged to reduce reflux symptoms and to avoid fetal exposure to these harmful substances.

Less than 1% of pregnant women will have proton pump inhibitors (PPIs) prescribed. They are reserved for women with severe and frequent symptoms of gastroesophageal reflux disease (GERD), which adversely impacts their quality of life.

Neonatal perinatal medicine specialists are often consulted regarding the safety of drugs during pregnancy and lactation. The meta-analysis by Gill,[1] the excellent article by Pasternak,[2] and this extensive review by Majithia and Johnson provide timely and up-to-date evidence on the effects of proton-pump inhibitors during pregnancy. In the meta-analysis conducted by Gill et al[1] the authors reviewed data from a total of 1530 patients exposed to PPIs in the first trimester or early pregnancy and 133 410 nonexposed controls. The odds ratio (OR) for the incidence of congenital malformations after in utero exposure to PPIs was 1.12 (95% confidence interval [CI], 0.86, 1.45). Their data suggest that PPIs may be used safely in the first trimester or in early pregnancy.

Pasternak and Hviid[2] conducted a cohort study to assess the association between exposure to PPIs during pregnancy and the risk of major birth defects among all infants born alive in Denmark between January 1996 and September 2008. Among 840 968 live births, 5082 involved exposure to PPIs between 4 weeks before conception and the end of the first trimester of pregnancy.

TABLE 1.—Summary of Proton Pump Inhibitor Safety Data After *In Utero* Exposure

| Study | Study Type | Exposed | Not Exposed | Odds Ratio for Fetal Malformations | 95% CI |
|---|---|---|---|---|---|
| Pasternak et al.,[18] 2010 | Prospective cohort | 3651 | 837 317 | 1.10 | 0.91, 1.34 |
| Gill et al.,[17] 2009 | Meta-analysis | 1530 | 133 410 | 1.12 | 0.86, 1.45 |
| Matok et al.,[33] 2005 | Retrospective cohort | 658 | 117 302 | 1.12 | 0.82, 1.54 |
| Diav-Citran et al.,[34] 2008 | Prospective cohort | 279 | 778 | 0.93 | 0.39, 2.21 |
| Nikfar et al.,[35] 2002 | Meta-analysis | 593 | | 1.18 | 0.72, 1.94 |
| Nielson et al.,[36] 1999 | Retrospective cohort | 38 | 13 327 | 1.55 | 0.48, 5.06 |
| Ruigomez et al.,[24] 1999 | Retrospective cohort | 139 | 1575 | 0.88 | 0.35, 2.22 |
| Lalkin et al.,[23] 1998 | Prospective cohort | 78 | 98 | 1.71 | 0.37, 7.88 |
| Kallen et al.,[21] 2001 | Prospective cohort | 275 | 255 | 1.17 | 0.45, 3.01 |

*Editor's Note:* Please refer to original journal article for full references

There were 174 major birth defects in infants whose mothers had been exposed to PPIs during this period (3.4%) compared with 21 811 in the group whose mothers had not been exposed (2.6%) (adjusted prevalence OR, 1.23; 95% CI, 1.05—1.44). In analyses limited to exposure during the first trimester, there were 118 major birth defects among 3651 infants exposed to PPIs (3.2%), and the adjusted prevalence OR was 1.10 (95% CI, 0.91—1.34). The risk of birth defects was not significantly increased in secondary analyses of exposure to individual PPIs during the first trimester or in analyses limited to the offspring of women who had filled PPI prescriptions and received enough doses to have a theoretical chance of first-trimester exposure. They concluded that in this large cohort, exposure to PPIs during the first trimester of pregnancy was not associated with a significantly increased risk of major birth defects.

Majithia and Johnson come to similar conclusions. However, it remains prudent and is safer to avoid these agents until after the first trimester.

Most PPIs are categorized as class B by the FDA for usage in pregnancy (Table 1). This means that although there are no adequate and well-controlled studies to evaluate safety, there have been no animal studies demonstrating potential fetal harm. The one exception is omeprazole, which is labeled as class C because of potential fetal toxicity evident from animal studies.

**A. A. Fanaroff, MBBCh, FRCPE**

*References*

1. Gill SK, O'Brien L, Einarson T, Koren G. The safety of proton pump inhibitors (PPIs) in pregnancy: a meta-analysis. *Am J Gastroenterol.* 2009;104:1541-1545.
2. Pasternak B, Hviid A. Use of proton-pump inhibitors in early pregnancy and the risk of birth defects. *N Engl J Med.* 2010;363:2114-2123.

**Medication Safety in Neonates**

Dabliz R, Levine S (Inst for Safe Medication Practices, Horsham, PA)
*Am J Perinatol* 29:49-56, 2012

Newborn intensive care units (NICUs) are high-risk areas of care, where complex medical interventions are performed, and are recognized as a resource for improved outcome in premature and low-birth-weight infants or those presenting with acute conditions. This critical environment, along with the vulnerable nature of the population it serves, places patients at risk for medication errors, which can result in permanent harm or death. Promoting safe medication practices requires participation of all individuals involved in the medication use process (e.g., physicians, nurses, nurse practitioners, physician assistants, pharmacists, respiratory therapists, pharmacy technicians). The following recommendations, organized in accordance with the Institute for Safe Medication Practices' Key Elements of the Medication Use System$^{TM}$, will focus on significant areas of concern within the NICU. All individuals caring for neonates, supported by administrators and organizational leaders, should recognize themselves as active partners responsible for the safety of this fragile patient population by participating in the design and sustainment of a safe and efficient medication use system.

▶ Medication errors continue to be a leading source of iatrogenic injury and frequently lead to malpractice litigation. In this article, the authors provide a thorough review of medication safety in the neonatal intensive care unit. One of the strengths of the article is the way in which they distinguish medication errors from adverse drug events (ADEs), and why the neonatal patient is so uniquely vulnerable for both medication errors and ADEs. Similar to most investigators in this field, the authors recognize the "systems failure" concept—that most errors result from a compendium of oversights and that system change is the key point to achieving quality improvement. In designing strategies to prevent medication errors, they present a 10-part process that encompasses both evidence-based and common-sense practices. Many of these focus on information, communication, and education, the triad of patient safety.

This article should be read by anyone even remotely connected to neonatal intensive care.

**S. M. Donn, MD**

---

**Ranitidine is Associated With Infections, Necrotizing Enterocolitis, and Fatal Outcome in Newborns**

Terrin G, Passariello A, De Curtis M, et al (Univ La Sapienza, Rome, Italy; Univ of Federico II, Naples, Italy; et al)
*Pediatrics* 129:e40-e45, 2012

---

*Background and Objectives.*—Gastric acidity is a major nonimmune defense mechanism against infections. The objective of this study was to investigate whether ranitidine treatment in very low birth weight (VLBW) infants is associated with an increased risk of infections, necrotizing enterocolitis (NEC), and fatal outcome.

*Methods.*—Newborns with birth weight between 401 and 1500 g or gestational age between 24 and 32 weeks, consecutively observed in neonatal intensive care units, were enrolled in a multicenter prospective observational study. The rates of infectious diseases, NEC, and death in enrolled subjects exposed or not to ranitidine were recorded.

*Results.*—We evaluated 274 VLBW infants: 91 had taken ranitidine and 183 had not. The main clinical and demographic characteristics did not differ between the 2 groups. Thirty-four (37.4%) of the 91 children exposed to ranitidine and 18 (9.8%) of the 183 not exposed to ranitidine had contracted infections (odds ratio 5.5, 95% confidence interval 2.9–10.4, $P < .001$). The risk of NEC was 6.6-fold higher in ranitidine-treated VLBW infants (95% confidence interval 1.7–25.0, $P = .003$) than in control subjects. Mortality rate was significantly higher in newborns receiving ranitidine (9.9% vs 1.6%, $P = .003$).

*Conclusions.*—Ranitidine therapy is associated with an increased risk of infections, NEC, and fatal outcome in VLBW infants. Caution is advocated in the use of this drug in neonatal age.

▶ Histamine-2 receptor (H2R) antagonists and proton pump inhibitors (PPI) have become very popular drugs in the neonatal intensive care unit. They are given for a variety of indications, including presumed gastroesophageal reflux disease, reflux-attributed apnea of prematurity, stress gastritis, and erythema or edema of the epiglottis and aryepiglottic folds. There is little evidence that these conditions are diseases in preterm infants and even less to support efficacy of suppression of gastric acid production in their management. The existence of infants whose clinical signs of severe postprandial discomfort are alleviated by antacid therapy makes it evident that some infants can be beneficiaries of that treatment, but it is likely that these agents are greatly overused in the neonatal population. Much of this can be attributed to the common perception that these drugs, which are safe enough to be available without prescription for adults, are similarly safe for neonates. This report suggests that this belief may be too sanguine. Although this study is observational, there were no substantial baseline differences between the infants who were or were not exposed to ranitidine. Prescription of ranitidine was not associated with gestational age, birth weight, gender, Apgar score of 1 at 5 minutes, Critical Risk Index for Babies score, central vascular access, or mechanical ventilation. Differences in rates of serious bacterial infection, necrotizing enterocolitis, and death were quite substantial, however (odds ratios of 5.5, 6.6, and 6.6, respectively, all significant at $P < .005$). Gram-negative bacilli (*Escherichia coli, Klebsiella pneumonia, Pseudomonas aeruginosa,* and *Serratia marcescens*) accounted for 74% of the infections in the ranitidine-exposed group, but only 22% of those in infants not exposed to ranitidine. The mean interval between initiation of ranitidine and onset of infection was 17.9 days. The authors posit that the risks of infection and necrotizing enterocolitis are increased by compromise of the gastric acid barrier to bacterial invasion. The causes of death are not specified in the report, but the higher mortality rate was presumably mediated by such infections. Although the evidence of a causal relationship between ranitidine and these outcomes is not definitive, the safety of this practice is certainly called into question. The authors suggest that ranitidine (and by implication other H2R blockers and PPI drugs) should be administered to preterm infants only after careful consideration of the risk/benefit ratio.

**W. E. Benitz, MD**

---

**Ranitidine is Associated With Infections, Necrotizing Enterocolitis, and Fatal Outcome in Newborns**

Terrin G, Passariello A, De Curtis M, et al (Univ La Sapienza, Rome, Italy; Univ Federico II, Naples, Italy; et al)

*Pediatrics* 129:e40-e45, 2012

---

*Background and Objectives.*—Gastric acidity is a major nonimmune defense mechanism against infections. The objective of this study was to investigate whether ranitidine treatment in very low birth weight (VLBW) infants is associated with an increased risk of infections, necrotizing enterocolitis (NEC), and fatal outcome.

*Methods.*—Newborns with birth weight between 401 and 1500 g or gestational age between 24 and 32 weeks, consecutively observed in neonatal intensive care units, were enrolled in a multicenter prospective observational study. The rates of infectious diseases, NEC, and death in enrolled subjects exposed or not to ranitidine were recorded.

*Results.*—We evaluated 274 VLBW infants: 91 had taken ranitidine and 183 had not. The main clinical and demographic characteristics did not differ between the 2 groups. Thirty-four (37.4%) of the 91 children exposed to ranitidine and 18 (9.8%) of the 183 not exposed to ranitidine had contracted infections (odds ratio 5.5, 95% confidence interval 2.9–10.4, $P < .001$). The risk of NEC was 6.6-fold higher in ranitidine-treated VLBW infants (95% confidence interval 1.7–25.0, $P = .003$) than in control subjects. Mortality rate was significantly higher in newborns receiving ranitidine (9.9% vs 1.6%, $P = .003$).

*Conclusions.*—Ranitidine therapy is associated with an increased risk of infections, NEC, and fatal outcome in VLBW infants. Caution is advocated in the use of this drug in neonatal age.

▶ H2 blockers have been commonly used in neonatal intensive care units. The rationale for their use spans a wide spectrum, including severe documented gastroesophageal acid reflux, surgical conditions such as PST congenital diaphragmatic hernia and tracheoesophageal fistula surgery to prophylaxis against stress, and as an adjunct to the use of glucocorticoids. In my experience, one of the most common uses has been in babies with apnea and bradycardia because of the putative association with gastroesophageal reflux. This has been common practice despite a lack of evidence that the H2 blockers provide any benefit.

Although a relationship between H2 blocker and critically ill patients has been recognized for quite some time, a retrospective analysis by Guillet et al[1] on babies in the National Institutes of Health Neonatal Network was one of the first to demonstrate a higher incidence of necrotizing enterocolitis (NEC) in babies who received H2 blocker prophylaxis. This study is very important in that in a prospective design, the authors demonstrate a more than 6-fold risk in NEC as well as an increase in death and late-onset sepsis in babies who receive ranitidine. One caveat is that even though the study was prospective, it is not totally clear what criteria the clinicians used to start the babies on this drug. Is it possible that this may have introduced some bias?

The mechanism of this effect is unclear. Preterm babies do have hypochlorhydria for a few weeks after birth, and further inhibition of the acid release may counteract one of our innate mechanisms to prevent pathogens from entering the gastrointestinal tract. It is of interest that the biggest difference between the treated and untreated groups was seen in *Escherichia coli, Klebsiella,* and *Pseudomonas,* microbes known to cause severe infections in these babies. Despite not yet understanding the mechanisms of this effect, it is clear that we need to be very selective in the use of these drugs in preterm infants.

**J. Neu, MD**

*Reference*

1. Guillet R, Stoll BJ, Cotten CM, et al. Association of H2-blocker therapy and higher incidence of necrotizing enterocolitis in very low birth weight infants. *Pediatrics.* 2006;117:e137-e142.

## Survival Without Disability to Age 5 Years After Neonatal Caffeine Therapy for Apnea of Prematurity

Schmidt B, for the Caffeine for Apnea of Prematurity (CAP) Trial Investigators (McMaster Univ, Hamilton, Ontario, Canada; et al)
*JAMA* 307:275-282, 2012

*Context.*—Very preterm infants are prone to apnea and have an increased risk of death or disability. Caffeine therapy for apnea of prematurity reduces the rates of cerebral palsy and cognitive delay at 18 months of age.

*Objective.*—To determine whether neonatal caffeine therapy has lasting benefits or newly apparent risks at early school age.

*Design, Setting, and Participants.*—Five-year follow-up from 2005 to 2011 in 31 of 35 academic hospitals in Canada, Australia, Europe, and Israel, where 1932 of 2006 participants (96.3%) had been enrolled in the randomized, placebo-controlled Caffeine for Apnea of Prematurity trial between 1999 and 2004. A total of 1640 children (84.9%) with birth weights of 500 to 1250 g had adequate data for the main outcome at 5 years.

*Main Outcome Measures.*—Combined outcome of death or survival to 5 years with 1 or more of motor impairment (defined as a Gross Motor Function Classification System level of 3 to 5), cognitive impairment (defined as a Full Scale IQ< 70), behavior problems, poor general health, deafness, and blindness.

*Results.*—The combined outcome of death or disability was not significantly different for the 833 children assigned to caffeine from that for the 807 children assigned to placebo (21.1% vs 24.8%; odds ratio adjusted for center, 0.82; 95% CI, 0.65-1.03; *P* = .09). The rates of death, motor impairment, behavior problems, poor general health, deafness, and blindness did not differ significantly between the 2 groups. The incidence of cognitive impairment was lower at 5 years than at 18 months and similar in the 2 groups (4.9% vs 5.1%; odds ratio adjusted for center, 0.97; 95% CI, 0.61-1.55; *P* = .89).

*Conclusion.*—Neonatal caffeine therapy was no longer associated with a significantly improved rate of survival without disability in children with very low birth weights who were assessed at 5 years.

▶ In 2006, the results of the Caffeine for Apnea of Prematurity (CAP) trial[1] were greeted with enthusiasm: At last, an effective strategy for reducing rates of bronchopulmonary dysplasia had been identified. Data demonstrating lower rates of death or neurodevelopmental impairment at 18 to 21 months of age soon followed.[2] Now we are presented with a longer-term follow-up that concludes that "Neonatal caffeine therapy was no longer associated with a significantly improved rate of survival without disability...at 5 years." In addition, doubts about external validity of the earlier results have been raised on the grounds that universal application in infants with birth weight less than 1250 g may be an inappropriate overgeneralization or that we cannot conclude that effects are beneficial when the original hypothesis was that caffeine is actually harmful. Was our enthusiasm for these findings misguided?

I do not think so. Criteria for enrollment in the CAP trial were birth weight of 500 to 1250 g and intent to use methylxanthine to prevent or treat apnea or to facilitate removal of an endotracheal tube during the first 10 days after birth. Of 5292 potential subjects, 977 were excluded by design, 681 were not approached, and the 1628 did not consent; the remaining 2006 infants were randomized. There is no apparent reason that this sample should not be representative of all eligible subjects, nor (given the very high prevalence of apnea of prematurity in infants less than 1250 g) is it likely that it differs substantially from the entire population of infants in that weight category. The finding that outcomes were better rather than worse (as hypothesized) in infants treated with caffeine is not less valid because it was unexpected. The null hypothesis was that the outcomes would differ, and that was demonstrated.

Does this article indicate that caffeine produces only transient effects and is therefore not valuable? Not necessarily. The CAP trial data still show several benefits. Infants treated with caffeine were substantially less likely to need supplemental oxygen at a postmenstrual age of 36 weeks (odds ratio [OR] 0.64; 95% confidence interval [CI], 0.52—0.78), to receive drugs to close a patent ductus arteriosus (PDA) (OR 0.67; 95% CI, 0.54—0.82), or to undergo ductal ligation (OR 0.29; 95% CI, 0.20—0.43), and they were extubated, weaned from positive airway pressure, and stopped using supplemental oxygen about 1 week earlier

($P$ < .001 for each comparison).[1] Long-term impacts remain to be determined but are likely to be favorable: Some infants clearly avoided vocal cord paresis from PDA ligation, for example, and late pulmonary morbidities of bronchopulmonary dysplasia will likely be ameliorated. Similarly, the neurodevelopmental effects seen at 18 to 21 months of age are genuine, even if not durable. Infants assigned to caffeine were less likely to die or survive with a neurodevelopmental disability (OR adjusted for gestational age, gender, maternal education, antenatal steroids, and multiple birth 0.79; 95% CI, 0.65—0.96), to have cerebral palsy (adjusted OR 0.59; 95% CI, 0.39—0.89), or to have severe cognitive impairment (Bayley MDI <70; unadjusted OR 0.70; 95% CI, 0.52—0.95).[2] Casual perusal of this article might suggest that these effects disappeared at age 5 years, but that is not correct. Although there were no differences in more global outcomes, caffeine was associated with lower (more favorable) scores on the Gross Motor Function Classification System (OR 0.66; 95% CI, 0.48—0.91) and better scores on tests of visual perception and motor coordination, so some differences did in fact persist. Infants with lower cognitive scores at 18 to 21 months had greater cognitive gains at 5 years of age; no analysis of the resources expended to achieve those gains is provided, but one might speculate that they were greater in the placebo group. It is reassuring that infants who did not receive caffeine are now approaching parity in outcomes with treated infants, but it would be premature to conclude that either pulmonary or neurodevelopmental outcomes, or the resources needed to achieve them, are truly equivalent. Until that is determined, caffeine should continue to have an important role in the care of infants who weigh 500 to 1250 g at birth.

**W. E. Benitz, MD**

*References*

1. Schmidt B, Roberts RS, Davis P, et al. Caffeine therapy for apnea of prematurity. *N Engl J Med.* 2006;354:2112-2121.
2. Schmidt B, Roberts RS, Davis P, et al. Long-term effects of caffeine therapy for apnea of prematurity. *N Engl J Med.* 2007;357:1893-1902.

# 15 Postnatal Growth and Development/ Follow-up

**Early Nutrition Mediates the Influence of Severity of Illness on Extremely LBW Infants**

Ehrenkranz RA, The Eunice Kennedy Shriver National Institute of Child Health and Human Development Neonatal Research Network (Yale Univ School of Medicine, New Haven, CT; et al)

*Pediatr Res* 69:522-529, 2011

To evaluate whether differences in early nutritional support provided to extremely premature infants mediate the effect of critical illness on later outcomes, we examined whether nutritional support provided to "more critically ill" infants differs from that provided to "less critically ill" infants during the initial weeks of life, and if, after controlling for critical illness, that difference is associated with growth and rates of adverse outcomes. One thousand three hundred sixty-six participants in the NICHD Neonatal Research Network parenteral glutamine supplementation randomized controlled trial who were alive on day of life 7 were stratified by whether they received mechanical ventilation for the first 7 d of life. Compared with more critically ill infants, less critically ill infants received significantly more total nutritional support during each of the first 3 wk of life, had significantly faster growth velocities, less moderate/severe bronchopulmonary dysplasia, less late-onset sepsis, less death, shorter hospital stays, and better neurodevelopmental outcomes at 18–22 mo corrected age. Rates of necrotizing enterocolitis were similar. Adjusted analyses using general linear and logistic regression modeling and a formal mediation framework demonstrated that the influence of critical illness on the risk of adverse outcomes was mediated by total daily energy intake during the first week of life.

▶ There are few areas in neonatal intensive care that are as controversial as (1) when to initiate components of parenteral nutrition, such as amino acids and lipids and (2) how rapidly to introduce enteral feedings. Although we still have a long way to go to find ideal parenteral or even enteral formulations for our critically ill babies, extremely slow initiation of enteral and parenteral feedings is

299

a hallmark of our intensive care practices. In this study from the National Institutes of Health Neonatal Network, enteral feedings were not initiated in less critically ill appropriate-for-gestational-age preterm infants until 5.4 days and more critically ill until 10.2 days. The age when enteral nutrition reached ≥110 kcal/kg/d in these babies was 24.9 and 35.1 days, respectively. This study took a very logical approach to evaluate the mediating effects of early nutrition on later morbidity in these infants. They evaluated 3 steps using logistic regressions and found the following: (1) Babies who are sicker to begin with have greater late morbidities. (2) Babies who are sicker to begin with are fed less. (3) Babies who are the sickest, but receive more nutrition in the first weeks after birth, have significantly lower odds of development of necrotizing enterocolitis (NEC), late-onset sepsis, bronchopulmonary dysplasia, and neurodevelopmental impairments. In fact, these morbidities decreased by approximately 2% for each 1 kcal/kg/d of total energy intake.

This is just 1 article among several recent studies that negates the message from Cochrane analyses that provide equivocal results[1] and may be interpreted as showing no benefits of early feeding. So why don't we start nutrition in these babies more rapidly, such as starting with some enteral feedings on day 0, providing 3 to 4 g/kg/d of amino acid and 3 g/kg/d of lipid starting on day 0? Studies in addition to the one reported here strongly support a strategy of providing more calories and protein to preterm babies in the first weeks after birth. One study showed marked improvement in neurodevelopment outcomes at 18 months[2] and actually quantified the increments of improvement that can be attained with different quantities of added amino acid and energy in the first week after birth. Furthermore, studies are now showing that NEC appears to be related to the lack of enteral feeding (overall risk, 2.41; 95% confidence interval, 1.08 to 5.52 if never enterally fed prior to diagnosis).[3]

So the data supporting the notion that we should provide more nutrition to these babies are rapidly emerging, and the basis for our excuses to not providing adequate early nutrition are rapidly declining. Let's stop starving these highly vulnerable babies.[4]

**J. Neu, MD**

*References*

1. Bombell S, McGuire W. Early trophic feeding for very low birth weight infants. *Cochrane Database Syst Rev.* 2009;(3):CD000504.
2. Stephens BE, Walden RV, Gargus RA, et al. First-week protein and energy intakes are associated with 18-month developmental outcomes in extremely low birth weight infants. *Pediatrics.* 2009;123:1337-1343.
3. Moss RL, Kalish LA, Duggan C, et al. Clinical parameters do not adequately predict outcome in necrotizing enterocolitis: a multi-institutional study. *J Perinatol.* 2008; 28:665-674.
4. Neu J. Is it time to stop starving premature infants? *J Perinatol.* 2009;29:399-400.

## Impact of Delivery Room Resuscitation on Outcomes up to 18 Months in Very Low Birth Weight Infants

DeMauro SB, for the Caffeine for Apnea of Prematurity Trial Investigators (Children's Hosp of Philadelphia and Univ of Pennsylvania; et al)
*J Pediatr* 159:546-550, 2011

*Objective.*—To examine the relationships between intensity of delivery room resuscitation and short- and long-term outcomes of very low birth weight infants enrolled in the Caffeine for Apnea of Prematurity (CAP) Trial. *Study Design.*—The CAP Trial enrolled 2006 infants with birthweights between 500 and 1250 g who were eligible for caffeine therapy. All levels of delivery room resuscitation were recorded in study participants. We divided infants in 4 groups of increasing intensity of resuscitation: minimal, n = 343; bag-mask ventilation, n = 372; endotracheal intubation, n = 1205; and cardiopulmonary resuscitation (chest compressions/epinephrine), n = 86. We used multivariable logistic regression models to compare outcomes across the 4 groups.

*Results.*—The observed rates of death or disability, death, cerebral palsy, cognitive deficit, and hearing loss at 18 months increased with higher levels of resuscitation. Risk of bronchopulmonary dysplasia, severe retinopathy of prematurity, and brain injury also increased with higher levels of resuscitation. Adjustment for prognostic variables reduced the differences between the groups for most outcomes. Only the adjusted rates of bronchopulmonary dysplasia and severe retinopathy remained significantly higher after more intense resuscitation.

*Conclusions.*—In CAP Trial participants, the risk of death or neurodevelopmental disability at 18 months did not increase substantially with increasing intensity of delivery room resuscitation.

▶ While the information in this study is interesting, it has limited usefulness in informing a clinician's decision whether to resuscitate an extremely low birth weight infant. The data set that was analyzed consisted of babies who were enrolled in the Caffeine for Apnea of Prematurity (CAP) trial. Thus, infants were included only if they survived delivery room resuscitation and the immediate postnatal period long enough to be considered eligible for the trial. In fact, the median age of enrollment in the CAP trial was 3 days. An additional limitation of the study is the inability to differentiate between infants who received delivery room resuscitation and infants who truly required resuscitation, especially for infants born at another facility and subsequently transferred to a study center. In fact, 24% of the infants in the cardiopulmonary resuscitation cohort were born outside a study center compared with 7% to 10% in the minimal and bag-mask ventilation cohorts. While this discrepancy may indicate that infants transferred to study centers were, on average, less stable than infants born at study centers, an alternative explanation is that these infants inappropriately received aggressive delivery room resuscitation.

**L. A. Papile, MD**

### Intraventricular Hemorrhage and Developmental Outcomes at 24 Months of Age in Extremely Preterm Infants
O'Shea TM, for the ELGAN Study Investigators (Wake Forest School of Medicine, Winston-Salem, NC; et al)
*J Child Neurol* 27:22-29, 2012

Whether intraventricular hemorrhage increases the risk of adverse developmental outcome among premature infants is controversial. Using brain ultrasound, we identified intraventricular hemorrhage and white matter abnormalities among 1064 infants born before 28 weeks' gestation. We identified adverse developmental outcomes at 24 months of age using a standardized neurologic examination and the Bayley Scales of Infant Development Mental and Motor Scales. In logistic regression models that adjusted for gestational age, sex, and public insurance, isolated intraventricular hemorrhage was associated with visual fixation difficulty but no other adverse outcome. Infants who had a white matter lesion unaccompanied by intraventricular hemorrhage were at increased risk of cerebral palsy, low Mental and Motor Scores, and visual and hearing impairments. Except when accompanied or followed by a white matter lesion, intraventricular hemorrhage is associated with no more than a modest increase (and possibly no increase) in the risk of adverse developmental outcome during infancy.

▶ As is intimated in the first sentence of this abstract, there are conflicting data concerning the negative impact of isolated intraventricular hemorrhage (IVH) on developmental outcome. Unfortunately, this article on a subset of infants enrolled in the Extremely Low Gestational Age Newborn Study (ELGANS) adds to the controversy.

The study sample includes 80% of surviving infants enrolled in ELGANS and was limited to infants who had both an early (between 1 and 4 days of age) and a "late" (between 15 days and 40 weeks of age) cranial ultrasound (CUS), and had 1 of more of the following evaluations available at 24 months of corrected age: neurologic examination, Bayley assessment, head circumference measurement, information about visual dysfunction. White matter injury (WMI) was defined as the presence of a parenchymal hyperechoic or hypoechoic lesion or ventriculomegaly on the late cranial ultrasound. Infants were allocated to 1 of 4 groups based on CUS findings: no WMI or IVH; WMI alone; IVH alone; WMI and IVH. Thus, the no WMI or IVH group encompassed both infants with grade I periventricular, intraventricular hemorrhage (PIVH), as well as infants with no PIVH, and the WMI and IVH group included infants with grade III PIVH as well as those with grade IV PIVH.

The conclusion that an isolated IVH is associated with no more than a modest increase in the risk for adverse developmental outcome during infancy needs to be qualified. Because the number of infants with cerebral palsy who had an isolated IVH was relatively small (n = 11), the confidence intervals are wide and imprecise. Also, although the data were adjusted for gestational age, sex, and public insurance, medical conditions known to adversely impact developmental outcome, such as chronic lung disease, were not accounted for.

**L. A. Papile, MD**

---

**Early postnatal hypotension and developmental delay at 24 months of age among extremely low gestational age newborns**
Logan JW, for the ELGAN Study Investigators (New Hanover Regional Med Ctr, Wilmington, NC; et al)
*Arch Dis Child Fetal Neonatal Ed* 96:F321-F328, 2011

---

*Objectives.*—To evaluate in extremely low gestational age newborns, relationships between indicators of hypotension during the first 24 postnatal hours and developmental delay at 24 months of age.

*Methods.*—The 945 infants in this prospective study were born at < 28 weeks, were assessed for three indicators of hypotension in the first 24 postnatal hours, and were evaluated with the Bayley Mental Development Index (MDI) and Psychomotor Development Index (PDI) at 24 months corrected age. Indicators of hypotension included: (1) mean arterial pressure in the lowest quartile for gestational age; (2) treatment with a vasopressor; and (3) blood pressure lability, defined as the upper quartile for the difference between the lowest and highest mean arterial pressure. Logistic regression was used to evaluate relationships between hypotension and developmental outcomes, adjusting for potential confounders.

*Results.*—78% of infants in this cohort received volume expansion or vasopressor; all who received a vasopressor were treated with volume expansion. 26% had an MDI < 70 and 32% had a PDI < 70. Low MDI and PDI were associated with low gestational age, which in turn, was associated with receipt of vasopressor treatment. Blood pressure in the lowest quartile for gestational age was associated with vasopressor treatment and labile blood pressure. After adjusting for potential confounders, none of the indicators of hypotension were associated with MDI < 70 or PDI < 70.

*Conclusions.*—In this large cohort of extremely low gestational age newborns, we found little evidence that early postnatal hypotension indicators are associated with developmental delay at 24 months corrected gestational age.

▶ The Extremely Low Gestational Age Newborn (ELGAN) study was designed to identify characteristics and exposures that increase the risk of structural and functional neurological disorders in extremely low gestational age newborns. This report is a post hoc analysis of blood pressure parameters measured in the first 24 hours after birth as they relate to developmental delay.

Because no single definition of hypotension in extremely low gestational age infants is widely accepted, the investigators examined 3 separate indicators of hypotension. The rate of hypotension defined as the lowest quartile for gestational age was 25%; 64% of the infants had hypotension defined as a mean arterial blood pressure less than gestational age; and hypotension defined as labile blood pressure was noted in 24%. In contrast, 75% of the study cohort received volume expansion and 26% received 1 or more vasopressor. The proportion of infants treated for hypotension varied greatly among the 14 study centers, with the most important determinant being the identity of the unit in which the infant was treated and not the degree of illness or hypotension.

The finding of no correlation between blood pressure and developmental delay in this article suggests that early postnatal hypotension might not be a reliable indicator of cerebral perfusion that is sufficiently compromised to result in brain injury. However, the study has several limitations that temper this proposal. Many of the infants had intermittent measurement of blood pressure, so periods of hypotension may have been missed. In addition, the duration of low blood pressure, which may be a more important factor than hypotension for brain injury, was not analyzed. Nevertheless, the results of this study challenge the long-held assumption that treatment of hypotension in the extremely preterm infant decreases the risk of brain injury.

**L. A. Papile, MD**

---

**Early term and late preterm birth are associated with poorer school performance at age 5 years: a cohort study**
Quigley MA, Poulsen G, Boyle E, et al (Univ of Oxford, UK; Univ of Leicester, UK; et al)
*Arch Dis Child Fetal Neonatal Ed* 97:F167-F173, 2012

---

*Objective.*—To compare school performance at age 5 years in children born at full term (39–41 weeks gestation) with those born at early term (37–38 weeks gestation), late preterm (34–36 weeks gestation), moderately preterm (32–33 weeks gestation) and very preterm (< 32 weeks gestation).

*Design.*—Population-based cohort (UK Millennium Cohort Study).

*Participants.*—Seven thousand six hundred and fifty children born in 2000–2001 and attending school in England in 2006.

*Methods.*—School performance was measured using the foundation stage profile (FSP), a statutory assessment by teachers at the end of the child's first school year. The FSP comprises 13 assessment scales (scored from 1 to 9). Children who achieve an average of 6 points per scale and at least 6 in certain scales are classified as 'reaching a good level of overall achievement'.

*Results.*—Fifty-one per cent of full term children had not reached a good level of overall achievement; this proportion increased with prematurity (55% in early term, 59% in late preterm, 63% in moderately preterm and 66% in very preterm children). Compared with full term children, an elevated risk remained after adjustment, even in early term (adjusted RR 1.05, 95% 1.00 to 1.11) and late preterm children (adjusted RR 1.12, 95% CI 1.04 to 1.22). Similar effects were noted for 'not working securely' in mathematical development, physical development and creative development. The effects of late preterm and early term birth were small in comparison with other risk factors.

*Conclusions.*—Late preterm and early term birth are associated with an increased risk of poorer educational achievement at age 5 years.

▶ The source population for this analysis is the Millennium Cohort Study (MCS), a nationally representative UK longitudinal study of 18 818 infants born in the United Kingdom (England and Wales) between September 2000 and August 2001. This article showed the likelihood of failing to achieve a good level of school performance progressively increased with advancing prematurity. Not only extremely or very preterm infants, but also late preterm (34 to 36 weeks' gestational age) and early term (37 to 38 weeks' gestational age) infants were found to be at increased risk of school underachievement, compared with the term cohort, in domains that most often included mathematical, physical, or creative development. There was a 5% risk of poorer performance in early term and a 12% increase in poorer performance at age 5 years among late preterm infants. Although the measure of effects for early term and late preterm contributions to underachievement was not as great as were sociodemographic risk factors, the association persisted after adjustment in multivariate analyses for these and other risk factors. Although the late preterm and early term infants in this study were more likely to be born in the context of multiple gestation and by cesarean section, the findings are consistent with results of prior studies. Marlow's[1] accompanying editorial titled "Full Term; an Artificial Concept" says it all: We must fully explore and establish the likely contributions of late preterm, early term, and post-term gestation and do all we can to minimize iatrogenic contributions, including gestational age, to adverse outcomes.

**L. J. Van Marter, MD, MPH**

*Reference*

1. Marlow N. Full term; an artificial concept. *Arch Dis Child Fetal Neonatal Ed.* 2012;97:F158-F159.

---

**Prediction of outcome at 5 years from assessments at 2 years among extremely preterm children: A Norwegian national cohort study**
Leversen KT, Sommerfelt K, Elgen IB, et al (Univ of Bergen, Norway; et al)
*Acta Paediatr* 101:264-270, 2012

---

*Aim.*—To examine the predictive value of early assessments on developmental outcome at 5 years in children born extremely preterm.
*Methods.*—This is a prospective observational study of all infants born in Norway in 1999—2000 with gestational age (GA) < 28 weeks or birth weight (BW) < 1000 g. At 2 years of age, paediatricians assessed mental and motor development from milestones. At 5 years, parents completed questionnaires on development and professional support before cognitive function was assessed with Wechsler Preschool and Primary Scale of Intelligence-Revised (WPPSI-R) and motor function with the Movement Assessment Battery for children (ABC test).

*Results.*—Twenty-six of 373 (7%) children had cerebral palsy at 2 and 29 of 306 (9%) children at 5 years. Of children without major impairments, 51% (95% CI 35—67) of those with and 22% (95% CI 16-28) without mental delay at 2 years had IQ < 85 at 5 years, and 36% (95% CI 20—53 with and 16% (95% CI 11—21) without motor delay at 2 years had an ABC score > 95th percentile (poor function). Approximately half of those without major impairments but IQ < 85 or ABC score > 95th percentile had received support or follow-up beyond routine primary care.

*Conclusion.*—Previous assessments had limited value in predicting cognitive and motor function at 5 years in these extremely preterm children without major impairments.

▶ "Only time will tell" and "the proof is in the pudding" are the take-home messages delivered in this Norwegian report comparing 2-year outcomes of extremely preterm children to early school age assessments. The robust national registry of Norway allows the authors to evaluate a large cohort of children born in the modern era with gestational age less than 28 weeks or birth weight less than 1000 g and followed up 5 years. Although the majority survived without major neurodevelopmental impairment, early school age cognitive and motor problems were prevalent. Pediatric assessments at 2 years were poorly predictive of cognitive and motor function at 5 years. Furthermore, despite being children at known high risk for developmental delay and living in a society in which virtually all children are followed regularly through preschool age according to a national protocol to identify special needs, only half of the children with IQ less than 85 were receiving educational support at school entry. These findings will affect the future planning of long-term educational resources and policies aimed at enhancing early intervention. They emphasize the importance of school age follow-up and continued interventions at school entry for high-risk children.

Although this study lends more support to the long-abiding theme that when it comes to long-term outcomes of preterm infants, there are a slew of cognitive and motor problems, all should not be doom and gloom. Half of those children with subnormal IQ at 2 years outgrew this delay by school age. The task for the future will be to determine which interventions will best minimize morbidity and enhance the ability to outgrow the long-term sequelae of prematurity.

**D. Wilson-Costello, MD**

---

### Stability of Cognitive Outcome From 2 to 5 Years of Age in Very Low Birth Weight Children

Munck P, the PIPARI Study Group (Turku Univ Hosp, Finland; et al)
*Pediatrics* 129:503-508, 2012

---

*Objective.*—This study assessed the stability of cognitive outcomes of premature, very low birth weight (VLBW; ≤1500 g) children.

*Methods.*—A regional cohort of 120 VLBW children born between 2001 and 2004 was followed up by using the Bayley Scales of Infant Development, Second Edition, at 2 years of corrected age and the Wechsler

Preschool and Primary Scale of Intelligence–Revised at the age of 5 years. The Mental Development Index (MDI) and the full-scale IQ (FSIQ) were measured, respectively. A total of 168 randomly selected healthy term control children born in the same hospital were assessed for MDI and FSIQ.
  *Results.*—In the VLBW group, mean ± SD MDI was 101.2 ± 16.3 (range: 50–128), mean FSIQ was 99.3 ± 17.7 (range: 39–132), and the correlation between MDI and FSIQ was 0.563 ($P < .0001$). In the term group, mean MDI was 109.83 ± 11.7 (range: 54–128), mean FSIQ was 111.73 ± 14.5 (range: 73–150), and the correlation between MDI and FSIQ was 0.400 ($P < .0001$). Overall, 83% of those VLBW children who had significant delay (−2 SD or less) according to MDI had it also in FSIQ. Similarly, 87% of those children who were in the average range in MDI were within the average range in FSIQ as well.
  *Conclusions.*—Good stability of cognitive development over time was found in VLBW children and in term children between the ages of 2 and 5 years. This conclusion stresses the value and clinical significance of early assessment at 2 years of corrected age. However, we also emphasize the importance of a long-term follow-up covering a detailed neuropsychological profile of these at-risk children.

▶ In contrast to the marked improvement in cognitive scores between 18 months and 5 years of age observed in both the caffeine-treated and control cohorts enrolled in the Caffeine for Apnea of Prematurity (CAP) trial,[1] the authors of this observational study report stable cognitive scores between 2 and 5 years of age in a regional cohort of very low birth weight infants born in Finland. The assessment tools used in the 2 studies were the same, and in both studies the level of education achieved by the parents was high. However, the study population in the CAP trial was younger and lighter weight than the Finnish group (mean birth weight and gestational age was 960 g and 27.4 weeks vs 1061 g and 28.7 weeks), and the initial developmental assessments were done at a younger age than those in the Finnish study (18 months vs 24 months). Twenty-four months is a critical transition period in cognitive development during which skills in symbolic function, language development, and early concept formation emerge. This suggests that the predictors of developmental outcomes of children are more robust the older the child is at the time of testing, and this may help to explain the discrepancy between the 2 studies.

**L. A. Papile, MD**

*Reference*

1. Schmidt B, Roberts RS, Davis P, et al. Caffeine for Apnea of Prematurity Trial Group. Long-term effects of caffeine therapy for apnea of prematurity. *N Engl J Med.* 2007;357:1893-1902.

## High Blood Pressure in 2.5-Year-Old Children Born Extremely Preterm

Edstedt Bonamy A-K, Källén K, Norman M (Karolinska Institutet, Stockholm, Sweden; Univ of Lund, Sweden)

*Pediatrics* 129:e1199-e1204, 2012

*Objective.*—Adolescents and young adults born preterm have elevated blood pressure (BP). The objective of this study was to investigate if BP is elevated at 2.5 years of age after an extremely preterm birth (EXPT).

*Methods.*—In a regional subset of the national population-based cohort Extremely Preterm Infants in Sweden Study, BP at 2.5 years of age was studied in 68 survivors of EXPT (gestational age: 23.6−26.9 weeks; mean ± SD birth weight: 810 ± 164 g), and 65 matched controls born at term.

*Results.*—At follow-up at 2.5 years of corrected age, EXPT children had significantly higher systolic blood pressure (SBP) and diastolic blood pressure (DBP) $z$ scores than controls born at term, according to pediatric BP nomograms by age, gender, and height. The proportion of SBP $\geq$ 90th percentile was 44% (30 of 68) in EXPT children and 23% (15 of 65) in controls ($P = .01$). In logistic regression analyses stratified according to gender, EXPT was associated with an odds ratio for a SBP $\geq$ 90th percentile of 3.32 (95% confidence interval: 1.25−8.81) among boys. The corresponding odds ratio among EXPT girls was 2.18 (95% confidence interval: 0.62−7.61). In EXPT children, SBP and DBP $z$ scores were inversely correlated to catch-up growth from 36 weeks' postmenstrual age to follow-up at 2.5 years of age.

*Conclusions.*—Children born extremely preterm have elevated office SBP and DBP at a corrected age of 2.5 years. This finding might have implications for their cardiovascular health later in life.

▶ In a follow-up comparison of 68 extremely preterm infants at 2.5 years of age with 65 term controls, differences in blood pressure were seen. Although several previous studies have reported higher blood pressures when preterm infants reach adolescence, this study evaluated children at a younger age to determine if early signs of hypertension might be detectable at 2.5 years. Here, extremely preterm infants had a higher blood pressure at 2.5 years of age. The effect on systolic blood pressure was confined to boys, whereas higher diastolic blood pressures were seen in both boys and girls. Higher blood pressures associated with extreme prematurity were related to slower growth between the neonatal period and follow-up at 2.5 years of corrected age.

These findings and previous studies referred to in this article support the likelihood that preterms have a propensity to higher blood pressures than babies born at term. Furthermore, although the differences were statistically significant, does a mean diastolic blood pressure that is higher by 4 mm Hg really matter in terms of overall health and later outcomes? The fact that boys seemed to be more susceptible is of interest, but as with the rest of this association, there was no solid evidence to implicate any particular mechanism. If these differences actually matter, the mechanism needs to be found to intervene early. If the differences are genetic and related to what caused the preterm birth in the first place, or maternal factors such as preeclampsia, this may not be easy to address. However, if it is related to a discrete factor such as type of feeding (maternal milk vs formula) or other nutritional factor, this could be addressed in preventative approaches.

So, as stated by the authors, these infants who were preterm should have their blood pressures followed as they grow older, but it also behooves us as neonatologists to find the cause of this and, if possible, prevent it.

**J. Neu, MD**

---

## Outcome of Extremely Low Birth Weight Infants Who Received Delivery Room Cardiopulmonary Resuscitation

Wyckoff MH, for the National Institute of Child Health and Human Development Neonatal Research Network (Univ of Texas Southwestern Med Ctr, Dallas; et al)
*J Pediatr* 160:239-244, 2012

---

*Objective.*—To determine whether delivery room cardiopulmonary resuscitation (DR-CPR) independently predicts morbidities and neurodevelopmental impairment (NDI) in extremely low birth weight infants.

*Study Design.*—We conducted a cohort study of infants born with birth weight of 401 to 1000 g and gestational age of 23 to 30 weeks. DR-CPR was defined as chest compressions, medications, or both. Logistic regression was used to determine associations among DR-CPR and morbidities, mortality, and NDI at 18 to 24 months of age (Bayley II mental or psychomotor index <70, cerebral palsy, blindness, or deafness). Data are adjusted ORs with 95% CIs.

*Results.*—Of 8685 infants, 1333 (15%) received DR-CPR. Infants who received DR-CPR had lower birth weight (708 ± 141 g versus 764 ± 146g, $P < .0001$) and gestational age (25 ± 2 weeks versus 26 ± 2 weeks, $P < .0001$). Infants who received DR-CPR had more pneumothoraces (OR, 1.28; 95% CI, 1.48-2.99), grade 3 to 4 intraventricular hemorrhage (OR, 1.47; 95% CI, 1.23-1.74), bronchopulmonary dysplasia (OR, 1.34; 95% CI, 1.13-1.59), death by 12 hours (OR, 3.69; 95% CI, 2.98-4.57), and death by 120 days after birth (OR, 2.22; 95% CI, 1.93-2.57). Rates of NDI in survivors (OR, 1.23; 95% CI, 1.02-1.49) and death or NDI (OR, 1.70; 95% CI, 1.46-1.99) were higher for DR-CPR infants. Only 14% of DR-CPR recipients with 5-minute Apgar score < 2 survived without NDI.

*Conclusions.*—DR-CPR is a prognostic marker for higher rates of mortality and NDI for extremely low birth weight infants. New DR-CPR strategies are needed for this population.

---

▶ A recent meta-analysis of published studies of very low birth weight (VLBW) infants who received delivery room cardiopulmonary resuscitation (CPR) found an increased risk for mortality and brain injury.[1] Although an increased risk for neurodevelopmental impairment was not noted, the number of infants included was small and the confidence intervals were wide.

The data for this article were abstracted from the National Institute of Child Health and Development's Neonatal Research Network generic database from 1996 through 2002. Infants were excluded from the analysis if they were outborn, had major congenital anomalies, or were not considered candidates for CPR and mechanical ventilation. The percentage of infants needing delivery room CPR (15%) is 2.5-fold higher than that reported previously from the Vermont Oxford Network.[2]

Maternal characteristics that increased the likelihood of delivery room CPR were antepartum hemorrhage and vaginal breech delivery; infant characteristics included younger gestational age, lower birth weight, and male sex. Death during the initial hospitalization occurred in 42% of resuscitated infants, with the majority of deaths occurring by 72 hours of age. At 18 to 22 months corrected age, 44% of resuscitated infants had died compared with 24% of similar infants who did not require delivery room resuscitation. The combined rate of death or neurodevelopmental impairment at 18 to 22 months corrected age was 72% for the resuscitated cohort compared with 54% of those who did not require delivery room CPR. This report suggests that the need for delivery room CPR can be used to counsel parents regarding the death and neurodevelopmental outcome in early childhood of VLBW infants.

**L. A. Papile, MD**

*References*

1. Shah PS. Extensive cardiopulmonary resuscitation for VLBW and ELBW infants: a systematic review and meta-analyses. *J Perinatol.* 2009;29:655-661.
2. Finer NN, Horbar JD, Carpenter JH. Cardiopulmonary resuscitation in the very low birth weight infant: the Vermont Oxford Network Experience. *Pediatrics.* 1999;104:428-434.

---

**Outcome of Extremely Preterm Infants (<1,000 g) With Congenital Heart Defects From the National Institute of Child Health and Human Development Neonatal Research Network**
Pappas A, Shankaran S, Hansen NI, et al (Wayne State Univ, Beaubien, Detroit, MI; Statistics and Epidemiology Unit, NC; et al)
*Pediatr Cardiol* 2012 [Epub ahead of print]

---

Little is known about the outcomes of extremely low birth weight (ELBW) preterm infants with congenital heart defects (CHDs). The aim of this study was to assess the mortality, morbidity, and early childhood outcomes of ELBW infants with isolated CHD compared with infants with no congenital defects. Participants were 401–1,000 g infants cared for at National Institute of Child Health and Human Development Neonatal Research Network centers between January 1, 1998, and December 31, 2005. Neonatal morbidities and 18–22 months' corrected age outcomes were assessed. Neurodevelopmental impairment (NDI) was defined as moderate to severe cerebral palsy, Bayley II mental or psychomotor developmental index < 70, bilateral blindness, or hearing impairment requiring aids. Poisson regression models were used to estimate relative risks for outcomes while adjusting for gestational age, small-for-gestational-age status, and other variables. Of 14,457 ELBW infants, 110 (0.8%) had isolated CHD, and 13,887 (96%) had no major birth defect. The most common CHD were septal defects, tetralogy of Fallot, pulmonary valve stenosis, and coarctation of the aorta. Infants with CHD experienced increased mortality (48% compared with 35% for infants with no birth defect) and poorer growth. Surprisingly, the adjusted risks of other short-term neonatal morbidities associated with prematurity were not significantly different. Fifty-seven (52%) infants with CHD survived to 18—22 months' corrected age, and 49 (86%) infants completed follow-up. A higher proportion of surviving infants with CHD were impaired compared with those without birth defects (57 vs. 38%, $p = 0.004$). Risk of death or NDI was greater for ELBW infants with CHD, although 20% of infants survived without NDI.

▶ This article is a retrospective analysis of the National Institute of Child Health and Human Development's Neonatal Research Network center's generic database for infants who were born between January 1, 1998, and December 31, 2005, and weighed less than 1001 g at birth. Although the database is selective, there are several findings that most likely are applicable to all US neonatal intensive care units that care for extremely low birth weight infants (ELBW) with congenital heart disease (CHD).

Compromised intrauterine growth was significantly greater among ELBW infants with CHD compared to that of the ELBW cohort without CHD (27% vs 15%) and head circumference at birth was on average 1 cm less. At 36 weeks, postmenstrual age weight gain and head growth among the CHD cohort were markedly less than that of the cohort without CHD. These differences persisted, and by 18 to 22 months, corrected age recumbent height was also adversely affected.

Predictably, CHD was associated with a 2-fold increase in the risk of dying, but the proportion of infants who survived to 18 to 22 months corrected age varied by the type of CHD. None of the infants with hypoplastic left heart syndrome or hypoplastic right heart syndrome survived. Likewise, survival rates were poor for transposition of the great vessels (20%), tetralogy of Fallot (33%), pulmonary atresia (33%), total anomalous venous return (33%), complete atrioventricular canal (33%), double outlet right ventricle (40%), and coarctation of the aorta (44%). Surprisingly, the rates of medical major morbidities, including severe intraventricular hemorrhage, necrotizing enterocolitis, and chronic lung disease, were not higher in the CHD cohort.

The risk of neurodevelopmental impairment in early childhood was approximately 1.5 times greater if CHD was present and was related primarily to poor performance on the Mental Developmental Index test of the Bayley Scales of Infant Development-II test. Although there was no difference in the frequency of retinopathy of prematurity between the groups, infants with CHD had a 7-fold increase in the risk of bilateral blindness in early childhood, suggesting that a central lesion was the cause.

**L. A. Papile, MD**

## Outcomes at 7 years for babies who developed neonatal necrotising enterocolitis: the ORACLE Children Study

Pike K, Brocklehurst P, Jones D, et al (Univ of Bristol, UK; Univ College London, UK; Univ of Leicester, UK; et al)
*Arch Dis Child Fetal Neonatal Ed* 2012 [Epub ahead of print]

*Background.*—Within the ORACLE Children Study Cohort, the authors have evaluated long-term consequences of the diagnosis of confirmed or suspected neonatal necrotising enterocolitis (NEC) at age of 7 years.

*Methods.*—Outcomes were assessed using a parental questionnaire, including the Health Utilities Index (HUI-3) to assess functional impairment, and specific medical and behavioural outcomes. Educational outcomes for children in England were explored using national standardised tests. Multiple logistic regression was used to explore independent associates of NEC within the cohort.

*Results.*—The authors obtained data for 119 (77%) of 157 children following proven or suspected NEC and compared their outcomes with those of the remaining 6496 children. NEC was associated with an increase in risk of neonatal death (OR 14.6 (95% CI 10.4 to 20.6)). At 7 years, NEC conferred an increased risk of all grades of impairment. Adjusting for confounders, risks persisted for any HUI-3 defined functional impairment (adjusted OR 1.55 (1.05, 2.29)), particularly mild impairment (adjusted OR 1.61 (1.03, 2.53)) both in all NEC children and in those with proven NEC, which appeared to be independent. No behavioural or educational associations were confirmed. Following NEC, children were more likely to suffer bowel problems than non-NEC children (adjusted OR 3.96 (2.06, 7.61)).

*Conclusions.*—The ORACLE Children Study provided opportunity for the largest evaluation of school age outcome following neonatal NEC and demonstrates significant long-term consequences of both gut function (presence of stoma, admission for bowel problems and continuing medical care for gut-related problems) and motor, sensory and cognitive outcomes as measured using HUI-3.

▶ The ORACLE trial evaluated the effects of broad-spectrum antibiotic therapy for women with either preterm rupture of the membranes (PROM) or spontaneous preterm labor with intact membranes and no infection. The composite primary outcome of neonatal death, the need for supplemental oxygen at 36 weeks' corrected age, or major cerebral abnormality on head ultrasound was essentially the same for infants born to women allocated to antibiotic therapy and those whose mothers received placebo therapy.

This investigation is a secondary study focusing on the outcome of 209 study infants who were diagnosed with proven or suspected necrotizing enterocolitis (NEC). Of these, 52 died before hospital discharge and 3 after discharge. Information on outcome was available for 119 (77%) of eligible children. Study data were obtained through parent questionnaires that gathered information related to functional impairment and behavior (Health Utilities Index, Strengths and Difficulties

Questionnaire), and a query of the national curriculum test, given to children in England at 7 years of age to assess children's educational attainment. Functional impairment included difficulty with speech, vision, ambulation, dexterity, emotion, cognition, or pain. Children with NEC or suspected NEC were noted to have a greater frequency of mild functional impairment that was not associated with any educational or behavioral concerns. Additionally, children with NEC or suspected NEC were more likely to have bowel problems, particularly hospital admissions for diarrhea and constipation who still have a bowel stoma.

Although the number of children in the NEC cohort who still had a bowel stoma at 7 years of age was small (5%), it is noteworthy because typically a bowel stoma after operative treatment of NEC is a temporizing measure, even with a significant loss of bowel. Additionally, the persistence of other bowel problems that occurred in 10% of this cohort is a reminder that neonatal disease may affect well-being far beyond infancy.

**L. A. Papile, MD**

---

## Survival Without Disability to Age 5 Years After Neonatal Caffeine Therapy for Apnea of Prematurity

Schmidt B, for the Caffeine for Apnea of Prematurity (CAP) Trial Investigators (McMaster Univ, Hamilton, Canada; et al)
*JAMA* 307:275-282, 2012

---

*Context.*—Very preterm infants are prone to apnea and have an increased risk of death or disability. Caffeine therapy for apnea of prematurity reduces the rates of cerebral palsy and cognitive delay at 18 months of age.

*Objective.*—To determine whether neonatal caffeine therapy has lasting benefits or newly apparent risks at early school age.

*Design, Setting, and Participants.*—Five-year follow-up from 2005 to 2011 in 31 of 35 academic hospitals in Canada, Australia, Europe, and Israel, where 1932 of 2006 participants (96.3%) had been enrolled in the randomized, placebo-controlled Caffeine for Apnea of Prematurity trial between 1999 and 2004. A total of 1640 children (84.9%) with birth weights of 500 to 1250 g had adequate data for the main outcome at 5 years.

*Main Outcome Measures.*—Combined outcome of death or survival to 5 years with 1 or more of motor impairment (defined as a Gross Motor Function Classification System level of 3 to 5), cognitive impairment (defined as a Full Scale IQ < 70), behavior problems, poor general health, deafness, and blindness.

*Results.*—The combined outcome of death or disability was not significantly different for the 833 children assigned to caffeine from that for the 807 children assigned to placebo (21.1% vs 24.8%; odds ratio adjusted for center, 0.82; 95% CI, 0.65-1.03; P =.09). The rates of death, motor impairment, behavior problems, poor general health, deafness, and blindness did not differ significantly between the 2 groups. The incidence of cognitive impairment was lower at 5 years than at 18 months and similar in the 2 groups (4.9% vs 5.1%; odds ratio adjusted for center, 0.97; 95% CI, 0.61-1.55; $P = .89$).

*Conclusion.*—Neonatal caffeine therapy was no longer associated with a significantly improved rate of survival without disability in children with very low birth weights who were assessed at 5 years.

▶ The impetus behind the Caffeine for Apnea of Prematurity (CAP) trial was concern that neonatal caffeine therapy may cause long-term harm. But the CAP trial showed that caffeine therapy not only improves the rate of survival without neurodevelopmental impairment in early childhood, it also reduces the rates of neonatal medical morbidities, such as bronchopulmonary dysplasia and retinopathy of prematurity.[1,2]

In this observational study, the investigators report the outcome at 5 years of age for 84.9% of the original CAP cohort. Unlike the results in early childhood, the rates of motor impairment and an IQ less than 70 (2 standard deviations below the mean) were essentially the same in both groups. Caffeine therapy was associated with better mean scores on tests of manual dexterity, visual perception and motor coordination, and gross motor function; however, the differences did not reach statistical significance.

Perhaps the most noteworthy observation is that rates of cognitive impairment were much lower at 5 years than at 18 months for both treated and untreated infants. Only 18.5% of the children with a Bayley Scales of Infant Development II (BSID II) Mental Developmental Index (MDI) less that 70 at 18 months of age had a Wechsler Preschool and Primary Scale of Intelligence (WPPSI) III Full Scale IQ less that 70 at 5 years. A linear regression model of the difference in cognitive scores between 18 months and 5 years suggested that, on average, a child with MDI of 70 at 18 months had a WPPSI full scale IQ that was almost 20 points higher at 5 years.

The higher rates of cognitive impairment noted on the BSID compared with later cognitive testing have been reported by others[3,4] and have important implications for outcome studies after extremely preterm birth, especially those evaluating the long-term effects of common neonatal therapies.

**L. A. Papile, MD**

*References*

1. Schmidt B, Roberts RS, Davis P, et al. Caffeine for Apnea of Prematurity Trial Group. Caffeine therapy for apnea of prematurity. *N Engl J Med.* 2006;354: 2112-2121.
2. Schmidt B, Roberts RS, Davis P, et al. Caffeine for Apnea of Prematurity Trial Group. Long-term effects of caffeine therapy for apnea of prematurity. *N Engl J Med.* 2007;357:1893-1902.
3. Hack M, Taylor HG, Drotar D, et al. Poor predictive validity of the Bayley Scales of Infant Development for cognitive function of extremely low birth weight children at school age. *Pediatrics.* 2005;116:333-341.
4. Roberts G, Anderson PJ, Doyle LW; Victorian Infant Collaborative Study Group. The stability of the diagnosis of developmental disability between ages 2 and 8 in a geographic cohort of very preterm children born in 1997. *Arch Dis Child.* 2010; 95:786-790.

## Breastfeeding, Long-Chain Polyunsaturated Fatty Acids in Colostrum, and Infant Mental Development

Guxens M, Mendez MA, Moltó-Puigmartí C, et al (Ctr for Res in Environmental Epidemiology, Barcelona, Spain; CIBER Epidemiologia y Salud Pública, Barcelona, Spain; et al)

*Pediatrics* 128:e880-e889, 2011

---

*Background.*—Breastfeeding has been associated with improved neurodevelopment in children. However, it remains unknown to what extent nutritional advantages of breast milk may explain this relationship.

*Objective.*—We assessed the role of parental psychosocial factors and colostrum long-chain polyunsaturated fatty acid (LC-PUFA) levels in the relationship between breastfeeding and children's neurodevelopment.

*Methods.*—A population-based birth cohort was established in the city of Sabadell (Catalonia, Spain) as part of the INMA-INfancia y Medio Ambiente Project. A total of 657 women were recruited during the first trimester of pregnancy. Information about parental characteristics and breastfeeding was obtained by using a questionnaire, and trained psychologists assessed mental and psychomotor development by using the Bayley Scales of Infant Development in 504 children at 14 months of age.

*Results.*—A high percentage of breastfeeds among all milk feeds accumulated during the first 14 months was positively related with child mental development (0.37 points per month of full breastfeeding [95% confidence interval: 0.06–0.67]). Maternal education, social class, and intelligence quotient only partly explained this association. Children with a longer duration of breastfeeding also exposed to higher ratios between $n$-3 and $n$-6 PUFAs in colostrum had significantly higher mental scores than children with low breastfeeding duration exposed to low levels.

*Conclusions.*—Greater levels of accumulated breastfeeding during the first year of life were related to higher mental development at 14 months, largely independently from a wide range of parental psychosocial factors. LC-PUFA levels seem to play a beneficial role in children's mental development when breastfeeding levels are high (Fig 2).

▶ Convincing evidence exists that breastfeeding is associated with improved cognitive development. Whether the composition of lipids in breast milk underlies these conferred advantages has been postulated. As referred to in this article, several studies of supplementation of formulas with long-chain polyunsaturated fatty acids (LC-PUFAs) have not found any clear effects. This study assessed the association between LC-PUFA levels in colostrum and children's mental development in a large population-based study. The combination of length of breastfeeding and LC-PUFA levels in colostrums appeared to have a beneficial effect on neurodevelopment at 14 months. As shown in the figure (Fig 2), the "high" tertile of cumulative intensity of breastfeeding along with milk with high m-3/n-6 PUFA ratio showed the highest mental development scores. They also found that the neurodevelopmental increment was largely independent from

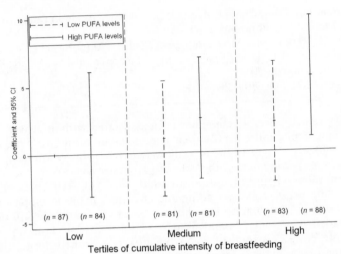

**FIGURE 2.**—Association between PUFA levels (total $n$-3/$n$-6 PUFAs ratio), tertiles of cumulative intensity of breastfeeding, and infant mental development score.[1] The reference group was subjects with low tertile of cumulative breastfeeding and low PUFA levels. $\beta$ coefficients were adjusted for psychologist, child's age in days, quality of the neuropsychological test, parental education, social class, attachment to the child, IQ, and mental health, maternal age, maternal alcohol use during pregnancy, use of a gas stove at home during pregnancy, and child's age of food introduction. *Editor's Note:* Please refer to original journal article for full references. (Reproduced with permission from Pediatrics, Guxens M, Mendez MA, Moltó-Puigmartí C, et al. Breastfeeding, long-chain polyunsaturated fatty acids in colostrum, and infant mental development. *Pediatrics.* 2011;128:e880-e889. Copyright © 2011 by the American Academy of Pediatrics.)

a wide range of parental psychosocial factors. Although this study makes sense from a physiologic perspective, it is not clear how the higher concentrations of lipids within the matrix of breast milk confer a benefit whereas the benefit was not seen in the studies of LC-PUFA supplementation of formulas. There are several caveats here. This study was only done at 14 months, so the long-term effects, when they really matter, such as at school age, were not seen. Furthermore, the fatty acid analysis was only done on colostrum and not more mature milk, so it is not clear how much and for how long these infants were actually receiving higher levels of LC-PUFAs. However, if in fact additional studies by this group in this cohort of patients continue to show this effect as the babies get older, what is the chemical component in the matrix of human milk that is different from formula that makes the LC-PUFA more bioactive in terms of neurodevelopment?

**J. Neu, MD**

## Does maternal depression predict developmental outcome in 18 month old infants?

Piteo AM, Yelland LN, Makrides M (Women's and Children's Hosp, Adelaide, Australia; Univ of Adelaide, Australia)
*Early Hum Dev* 2012 [Epub ahead of print]

*Aim.*—Our aim was to examine the associations between maternal depression in the first 6 months postpartum, home environment and cognitive, language and motor development in infants at 18 months of age.

*Study Design and Methods.*—This article reports results from the control group ($n = 312$ full term; $n = 48$ preterm) of the prospective Docosahexaenoic acid (DHA) to Optimise Maternal Infant Outcome (DOMInO) Randomised Controlled Trial. Mothers in South Australia completed the Edinburgh Postnatal Depression Scale (EPDS) at 6 weeks and 6 months postpartum. Infant development was assessed when children were 18 months old with the Bayley Scales of Infant and Toddler Development Version III and mothers completed the Home Screening Questionnaire at this assessment.

*Results.*—There were no significant associations between maternal depression in the first 6 months postpartum and cognitive, language or motor development after controlling for infant prematurity, breastfeeding status and socio-economic level. Home environment remained a significant predictor of development after controlling for potential confounding variables. Using mediation models, we did not find an association between maternal depression and developmental outcome through home environment.

*Conclusions.*—Maternal depression in the first 6 months postpartum was not associated with infant development at 18 months of age. Further studies should focus on women with chronic depression.

▶ It is uncertain if the impact of maternal depression on the subsequent developmental outcome of an infant is direct or mediated through indirect paths such as a poor home environment. In this study, the authors used standardized questionnaires to measure maternal depression at both 6 weeks and 6 months postpartum and quality of the home environment when the infant was 18 months of age. The results of these assessments were compared with scores on the Bayley Scales of Infant and Toddler Development Edition III that was done at 18 months of age.

Overall, maternal depression was noted in 7% at 6 weeks postpartum and 8% at 6 months postpartum. Only 3% showed symptoms of depression at both time points. Among the women with postpartum depression, only 16% of those who manifested postpartum depression were depressed at both 6 weeks and 6 months. Maternal depression did not have a negative effect on developmental outcome. The quality of the home environment was an independent predictor of infant development; however, maternal depression did not influence the quality of the home environment. Although maternal occupation, maternal education, breastfeeding at 6 months, and home environment were significant predictors of cognitive development, when the model was adjusted for potential confounders, only maternal education was significant.

As the authors acknowledge, there are several limitations to the study. Because depression was not assessed beyond 6 months postpartum, it does not address the effect of chronic depression on infant development. In addition, the cohort was not at high risk for lack of infant stimulation in the home environment; the socioeconomic status of the women was high, with 70% completing further studies beyond high school. It may be that the longer the duration of maternal depression, the more likely it is to be associated with a poor home environment, which, in turn, leads to less-than-optimal development for children, especially in more disadvantaged families.

**L. A. Papile, MD**

---

## The effects of giving pacifiers to premature infants and making them listen to lullabies on their transition period for total oral feeding and sucking success

Yildiz A, Arikan D (Abant Izzet Baysal Univ, Bolu, Turkey; Atatürk Univ, Erzurum, Turkey)

*J Clin Nurs* 21:644-656, 2012

---

*Aim and Objective.*—This research aimed to assess the effect of giving pacifiers to premature infants and making them listen to lullabies on the transition period to total oral feeding, their sucking success and their vital signs (peak heart rate, respiration rate and oxygen saturation).

*Background.*—It is very important that preterm infants start oral feeding as soon as possible to survive and get healthy quickly. Previous studies have shown that by using some external stimuli, premature babies can move to oral feeding at an earlier period than 34th gestational week, have increased daily weight gain and be discharged from hospital earlier.

*Design.*—In this quasi-experimental and prospective study, 90 premature infants were studied with 30 premature infants allocated to each of pacifier, lullaby and control groups.

*Method.*—The research was conducted at a neonatal intensive care clinic and premature unit of a university hospital in the east of Turkey between December 2007—January 2009. The data were collected through demographic information form for premature infants, the LATCH Breastfeeding Charting System and patient monitoring.

*Results.*—We found that the group who proceeded to the oral feeding in the shortest period was the pacifier group ($p < 0.05$), followed by the lullaby group and the control group, respectively ($p > 0.05$). We also found that the highest sucking success was achieved by infants in the pacifier group ($p < 0.05$) followed by the lullaby group ($p > 0.05$).

*Conclusion.*—These results demonstrate that giving pacifiers to premature infants and making them listen to lullabies has a positive effect on their transition period to oral feeding, their sucking success and vital signs (peak heart rate and oxygen saturation).

▶ The use of various stimuli, including pacifier, music, breast milk smell, and kangaroo care, has been associated with a reduction in the transition period from gavage to full oral feeding and duration of hospital stay. In this study, the investigators compared the efficacy of pacifier use with that of listening to a lullaby during gavage feeding.

Study infants were on average greater than 31 weeks of gestational age and weighed more than 1400 g at birth. Infants were included in the study only if they were medically stable from birth and were breastfed. Control and study infants were gavage fed their mother's own breast milk. Infants in the pacifier cohort were given a pacifier at the beginning of a gavage feeding that was removed when the feeding was completed. For the lullaby group, a speaker system was placed at the foot of the infants in the incubator and connected to a CD player. The music was played when the gavage feeding was started and was terminated at the end of the feeding. The intervention was carried out daily for 3 feedings until the infant graduated to oral feeding. All infants transitioned from gavage feeding directly to breastfeeding. To evaluate sucking behavior, the LATCH Breastfeeding Charting System form was completed when full oral feeding was established.

The average time to full oral feeding was 11.7 days for the control group compared with 7.7 days and 10.1 days for the pacifier and lullaby groups, respectively. On average, the hospital stay for infants in the pacifier group was 15.4 days compared with 21.7 days and 20.7 days for the control and lullaby groups, respectively. The pacifier group also had the highest sucking success as measure by the LATCH score.

As the authors note, their results are in accordance with a recent meta-analysis that found nonnutritive sucking significantly decreases the length of hospital stay in preterm infants and is associated with positive clinical outcome including transition from tube to full oral feedings and better feeding performance.[1] Although a positive trend in the transition period to oral feeding and sucking success was documented with listening to lullabies, the lack of statistical difference between this intervention and usual care contradicts the authors' conclusion that making preterm infants listen to lullabies is an effective strategy.

**L. A. Papile, MD**

*Reference*

1. Pinelli J, Symington AJ. Non-nutritive sucking for promoting physiologic stability and nutrition in preterm infants. *Cochrane Database Syst Rev.* 2005;(4):CD001071.

---

### Changing long-term outcomes for infants 500–999 g birth weight in Victoria, 1979–2005

Doyle LW, the Victorian Infant Collaborative Study Group (Royal Women's Hosp, Parkville, Victoria, Australia; et al)
*Arch Dis Child Fetal Neonatal Ed* 96:F443-F447, 2011

---

*Objective.*—To determine the survival and neurological outcome at 2 years of age of extremely low birthweight (ELBW, birth weight 500–999 g) infants born in the state of Victoria compared with term controls, and contrasted with ELBW cohorts from previous eras.

*Design and Setting.*—A population-based cohort study of consecutive ELBW infants born during 2005 in the state of Victoria, and also in 1979–1980, 1985–1987, 1991–1992 and 1997.

*Participants.*—All 257 live births free of lethal malformations weighing 500–999 g in 2005, 220 randomly selected term, normal birthweight (birth weight > 2499 g) controls, and equivalent cohorts born in earlier eras.

*Main Outcome Measures.*—Survival rates and quality-adjusted survival rates at 2 years of age, contrasted between cohorts.

*Results.*—Of 257 ELBW live births in 2005, 66.9% survived to 2 years of age, significantly lower than the survival rate of 75.2% for 1997 (odds ratio (OR) 0.67, 95% CI 0.45 to 0.99, $p = 0.046$), but not after adjustment for confounders of birth weight, gestational age and gender (adjusted OR 0.73, 95% CI 0.46 to 1.16, $p = 0.18$). This was a reversal of the steady increase in survival rates up to 1997. Rates of blindness, severe developmental delay and severe disability were significantly lower in 2005 than in ELBW survivors from previous eras. Consequently the difference in the quality-adjusted survival rates between 2005 and 1997 was only −3.8% (95% CI −11.4% to 3.7%, $p = 0.32$).

*Conclusions.*—Regional survival rates for ELBW infants have plateaued since the late 1990s, but the neurosensory outcome in survivors has improved in 2005.

▶ "It's not the quantity but the quality that counts." Although this statement is a familiar one in the world of industry, it has not traditionally been used as a measure of outcome in the world of medicine. However, in the modern period, where the vast majority of extremely preterm infants survive, the next challenge will be to design and implement interventions to minimize morbidity. The findings of these authors are reassuring, that despite a continuation in the outstanding survival rates of extremely low birth weight infants in Australia, the neurodevelopmental outcomes of these infants born since 2000 have not deteriorated. In fact, they report that the quality-adjusted survival rates reflecting intact survival without major disability have improved in the most recent period. This is exciting and encouraging news in an era where trepidation about the long-term impact of recently lowered rates of viability in neonatal intensive care units around the globe has shrouded the achievements made in survival. Unfortunately, although rates of major morbidity have not increased, the developmental outcomes of the extremely preterm children still reveal high rates of cognitive and motor delays, with 86% having developmental quotients greater than 1 standard deviation below the mean. These minor delays discovered at 2 years may translate into many more not so minor cognitive, motor, and behavioral problems with a variety of functional limitations at school age. These authors are among the first to report 2-year outcomes using the Bayley-III Developmental Assessment, which has demonstrated higher scores than the previous edition of the test. We know that developmental outcomes previously reported according to Bayley-II standards show lower scores at 2 years than those seen at school age, suggesting the Bayley-II overestimates delays. Whether the new Bayley-III tool will underestimate rates of school-age delay or better predict school age outcomes is yet to be determined. Nonetheless, the cup measuring these most recent 2-year outcomes remains both half empty and half full, with low rates of major impairment and high rates of minor delays. One more sobering fact to consider: outcome statistics are reported for populations, not individuals. Although the reported overall rates of impairment are low, they are 100% for those affected. Thus, the ultimate impact of prematurity on each individual cup remains uncertain. Only time will tell on an individual basis whether each cup will runneth over with joy or hardship as each of these children matures into adulthood.

Since neonatal risk factors have been the most consistent predictors of neurodevelopmental outcomes, future efforts must concentrate on minimizing the neurologic and pulmonary sequelae of prematurity, an undertaking that has traditionally been much easier said than done!

**D. E. Wilson-Costello, MD**

---

## Changing long-term outcomes for infants 500–999 g birth weight in Victoria, 1979–2005

Doyle LW, the Victorian Infant Collaborative Study Group (Royal Women's Hosp, Parkville, Victoria, Australia; et al)
*Arch Dis Child Fetal Neonatal Ed* 96:F443-F447, 2011

---

*Objective.*—To determine the survival and neurological outcome at 2 years of age of extremely low birthweight (ELBW, birth weight 500–999 g) infants born in the state of Victoria compared with term controls, and contrasted with ELBW cohorts from previous eras.

*Design and Setting.*—A population-based cohort study of consecutive ELBW infants born during 2005 in the state of Victoria, and also in 1979–1980, 1985–1987, 1991–1992 and 1997.

*Participants.*—All 257 live births free of lethal malformations weighing 500–999 g in 2005, 220 randomly selected term, normal birthweight (birth weight > 2499 g) controls, and equivalent cohorts born in earlier eras.

*Main Outcome Measures.*—Survival rates and quality adjusted survival rates at 2 years of age, contrasted between cohorts.

*Results.*—Of 257 ELBW live births in 2005, 66.9% survived to 2 years of age, significantly lower than the survival rate of 75.2% for 1997 (odds ratio (OR) 0.67, 95% CI 0.45 to 0.99, $p = 0.046$), but not after adjustment for confounders of birth weight, gestational age and gender (adjusted OR 0.73, 95% CI 0.46 to 1.16, $p = 0.18$). This was a reversal of the steady increase in survival rates up to 1997. Rates of blindness, severe developmental delay and severe disability were significantly lower in 2005 than in ELBW survivors from previous eras. Consequently the difference in the quality-adjusted survival rates between 2005 and 1997 was only −3.8% (95% CI −11.4% to 3.7%, $p = 0.32$).

*Conclusions.*—Regional survival rates for ELBW infants have plateaued since the late 1990s, but the neurosensory outcome in survivors has improved in 2005.

▶ Steadily increasing survival rates for extremely low birth weight (ELBW) (<1000 g) infants from the 1970s though the 1990s were not accompanied by declining rates of neurodevelopmental or neurosensory impairment among survivors, raising concerns that the successes of neonatal-perinatal medicine in this high-risk population might be mixed victories. This population-based report from Australia provides some much needed reassurance. Using methods that enabled comprehensive ascertainment of cases and a very high follow-up rate, these authors found that survival rates plateaued between 1997 and 2005; the survival rate for infants born at 750 g to 999 g remained steady (86% and 90%, respectively; odds ratio [OR] 1.42; 95% confidence interval [CI], 0.66–3.07), while that for infants with birth weights of 500 g to 749 g decreased from 63% to 45% (OR 0.48; 95% CI, 0.29–0.82). After adjustment for gender, gestational age, and birth weight, that decrease was no longer statistically significant, however. Rates of severe developmental delay and severe neurodevelopmental impairment were significantly lower in 2005 (OR 0.24; 95% CI, 0.09–0.60 for both outcomes). In 2005, intensive care was not initiated for a larger proportion of infants over 750 g (25% vs 16%; OR 1.74; 95% CI, 0.91–3.34), so it may be that more infants died who otherwise would have had adverse neurological outcomes. The authors also speculate that improved outcomes may be a consequence of widespread adoption of early caffeine use between 1997 and 2005. These data suggest that changes in care may be producing better long-term results in ELBW infants. On the other hand, recent reports[1] describing increasing survival rates after 2000 among infants at the very margins of viability once again heighten concern that these "better" statistics may come with an upward trend in rates of neurodevelopmental and neurosensory impairments.

**W. E. Benitz, MD**

*Reference*

1. Fischer N, Steurer MA, Adams M, Berger TM. Survival rates of extremely preterm infants (gestational age <26 weeks) in Switzerland: impact of the Swiss guidelines for the care of infants born at the limit of viability. *Arch Dis Child Fetal Neonatal Ed.* 2009;94:F407-F413.

**Aberrant Adiposity and Ectopic Lipid Deposition Characterize the Adult Phenotype of the Preterm Infant**
Thomas EL, Parkinson JR, Hyde MJ, et al (Imperial College London, UK; et al)
*Pediatr Res* 70:507-512, 2011

Our investigation addresses the hypothesis that disruption of third trimester development by preterm birth alters multiple biological pathways affecting metabolic health in adult life. We compared healthy adult volunteers aged 18–27 y born at ≤ 33 wk gestation or at term. We used whole-body MRI, $^1$H magnetic resonance spectroscopy (MRS) of liver and muscle, metabonomic profiling of blood and urine, and anthropometric and blood pressure measurements. Preterm subjects had greater (mean difference (95% CI)) total [2.21 L (0.3, 4.1), $p = 0.03$] and abdominal adipose tissue [internal 0.51 (0.1, 0.9), $p = 0.007$]; blood pressure [systolic 6.5 mm Hg (2.2, 10.8), $p = 0.004$; diastolic 5.9 (1.8, 10.1), $p = 0.006$]; and ectopic lipid (ratio (95% CI)), intrahepatocellular lipid (IHCL) 3.01 (1.78, 5.28) $p < 0.001$, and tibialis-intramyocellular lipid (T-IMCL) [1.31 (1.02, 1.69) $p = 0.04$]. In preterm, compared with term men, there was greater internal adipose tissue [mean (SD); men: preterm 4.0 (1.6), term 2.7 (1.1) liters; women: preterm 2.6 (0.9); term 2.6 (0.5); gender-gestation interaction $p = 0.048$] and significant differences in the urinary metabolome (elevated methylamines and acetyl-glycoproteins, lower hippurate). We have identified multiple premorbid biomarkers in ex-preterm young adults, which are most marked in men and indicative of risks to later wellbeing. These data offer insight into biological trajectories affected by preterm birth and/or neonatal care.

▶ This is an interesting extension of a previous study[1] reported by this group in 2004 that compared body fat of preterm infants with that of term infants. In that study, the authors showed that babies born at term had greater subcutaneous fat, but preterm babies had more intra-abdominal visceral body fat. Of interest was the fact that the visceral intra-abdominal fat correlated with level of intensity of care to which the preterm babies were exposed. In the more recent study, the authors evaluated young men and women who were ex-preterms versus ex-term controls. Again, they found differences in body composition with the ex-preterm men showing a greater degree of difference, especially in both the internal adipose tissue compartments and in various metabolic markers. The significance of the metabolic markers and how they might be traced to being born prematurely or at term and having been exposed to neonatal intensive care certainly would be highly speculative, but is of interest and requires additional scrutiny. Overall, this study underlines the fact that prematurity does have long-term metabolic consequences that could be reflected in metabolic syndrome in adulthood. However, these individuals may still have been too young to analyze for full-blown metabolic consequences of their having been born preterm. Whether these findings can be causally linked to early nutrition, medication use, high levels of stress, and endogenous (or perhaps exogenous) glucocorticoid responses raises some interesting questions than could be addressed for determining potential prevention. As stated by the authors, these findings add to the growing justification to monitor the health of preterm men and women beyond infancy and childhood.

**J. Neu, MD**

*Reference*

1. Uthaya S, Thomas EL, Hamilton G, Doré CJ, Bell J, Modi N. Altered adiposity after extremely preterm birth. *Pediatr Res.* 2005;57:211-215.

# 16 Ethics

**The ethics of obtaining consent in labour for research**
Reid R, Susic D, Pathirana S, et al (Royal Hosp for Women, Randwick, New South Wales, Australia; Univ of New South Wales, Randwick, Australia; Univ of Newcastle, UK)
*Aust N Z J Obstet Gynaecol* 51:485-492, 2011

*Background.*—It is widely acknowledged that the pregnant population is a vulnerable and potentially disadvantaged one with regard to research. We sought to evaluate compliance with this concept by examining current Australian practices of obtaining consent for research during labour through the published literature and from Australian Human Research Ethics Committees (HRECs) as well as reviewing the relevant literature.

*Methods.*—We surveyed Australian HRECs requesting information about their opinions and/or practices surrounding the ethics of research consent during labour or birth. In addition, a literature search was performed to find randomised controlled trials (RCTs) involving interventions during labour in Australia in the last five years.

*Results.*—Of the HREC respondents, 75% believed it to be ethical to obtain consent for research in labour, 87% would require additional expert assistance to approve, 57% felt the partner should be involved and all proposed research scenarios were thought to require protocol changes. Recent local RCTs reflected a variety of consent strategies, each having their limitations.

*Conclusions.*—An under-used but potentially useful strategy may be staged recruitment and consent. Despite the evidence supporting labour as a time requiring increased acuity for informed consent, there is little to suggest that this knowledge is being applied to current Australian HREC and RCT practices. We suggest that further practical guidelines be devised to aid researchers and human ethics committees.

▶ Research involving pregnant women is important for several reasons, but an article in *Nature*, titled "Pregnant women deserve better," provides a concise explanation: "Pregnant women get sick, and sick women get pregnant. Patients who happen to be pregnant are as entitled as anyone else to safe and effective treatments, yet they are denied this and will be for as long as pregnant women are excluded from clinical studies."[1]

While studies involving pregnant women are needed, they are considered a vulnerable population and subject to additional research protections in the United States under the regulations of the National Institutes of Health. In this study, a group of Australian researchers focus on ethical issues surrounding the process of obtaining consent for research studies while the woman is in labor. This is an important issue, because the studies may involve the pregnant woman, her as yet unborn child, or both. Labor, of course, is a particularly difficult time to obtain consent from a pregnant woman. There is pain, sometimes alleviated with narcotics. There is often anxiety. The labor and delivery environment itself may be noisy and unfamiliar. And of course, as the study notes, there is an understandable "preferential focus of attention and energy on the anticipated delivery."

The study thoughtfully approaches the issue from 2 perspectives. First via a survey of Australian Human Research Ethics Committees (HRECs) and, second, via a literature search looking at randomized, controlled trials performed in Australia over a 5-year period that involved interventions during labor. The survey had a reasonable 46% response rate. Unfortunately, only 9 of the 64 respondents went beyond the initial survey question. Among that group, a majority (75%) felt that it could ever be ethical to ask for consent in labor. None of the committees had a formal policy or guideline relating to obtaining consent in labor. Interestingly, 100% felt that partners should have a role in providing consent to participate in labor, even in cases in which the baby would not be involved in the research.

The literature search found 8 studies involving interventions during labor, but only 2 of the studies were published, with the rest being registered trials. In contrast to the survey results, none of these studies required consent from the partner. Timing of consent was inconsistent. Under ideal circumstances, consent would be obtained prior to labor or in early labor and prior to any narcotics. In the reviewed studies, 3 obtained consent prior to labor, 3 during active labor, and 2 unstated.

The 20th century saw tremendous advances in both obstetric and neonatal care. To continue these advances, it has been argued that "it is not only permissible but also imperative that pregnant women be judiciously included in research."[2] Inevitably, some of that research will involve laboring women. It is incumbent on all involved to ensure that true informed consent is obtained in a sensitive and respectful manner.

**J. Fanaroff, MD**

*References*

1. Baylis F. Pregnant women deserve better. *Nature*. 2010;465:689-690.
2. Goldkind SF, Sahin L, Gallauresi B. Enrolling pregnant women in research—lessons from the H1N1 influenza pandemic. *N Engl J Med*. 2010;362:2241-2243.

---

**The Prediction and Cost of Futility in the NICU**
Meadow W, Cohen-Cutler S, Spelke B, et al (The Univ of Chicago, IL; et al)
*Acta Paediatr* 101:397-402, 2012

---

*Aim.*—To quantify the cost and prediction of futile care in the Neonatal Intensive Care Unit (NICU).

*Methods.*—We observed 1813 infants on 100 000 NICU bed days between 1999 and 2008 at the University of Chicago. We determined costs and assessed predictions of futility for each day the infant required mechanical ventilation.

*Results.*—Only 6% of NICU expenses were spent on nonsurvivors, and in this sense, they were futile. If only money spent *after* predictions of death is considered, futile expenses fell to 4.5%. NICU care was preferentially directed to survivors for even the smallest infants, at the highest risk to die. Over 75% of ventilated NICU infants were correctly predicted to survive on every day of ventilation by every caretaker. However, predictions of 'die before discharge' were wrong more than one time in three. Attendings and neonatology fellows tended to be optimistic, while nurses and neonatal nurse practitioners tended to be pessimistic.

*Conclusions.*—Criticisms of the expense of NICU care find little support in these data. Rather, NICU care is remarkably well targeted to patients who will survive, particularly when contrasted with care in adult ICUs. We continue to search for better prognostic tools for individual infants.

▶ This article sets out to respond to a perceived criticism of the expense of neonatal intensive care unit (NICU) care that at times overtreats infants "who are doomed to die." In the study, futile care was interpreted as providing care for nonsurviving infants. Two distinct definitions of futile care were assessed: the number of bed days of infants who died before discharge, and the number of bed days occupied by nonsurvivors after they had been predicted to die. Over a 10-year period in the NICU at the University of Chicago, the caregivers of ventilated premature infants were asked whether they thought the baby would survive to be discharged; they were also asked to rate their confidence level in that prediction. Attempts were made to obtain 3 predictions for each baby on each day. No explanation or reasoning was required for these instinctive responses. The length of stay for 92% of infants over this time period was determined and the per diem costs calculated.

The key finding was that NICU care is well targeted to those who will survive. Over 90% of NICU bed days were occupied by infants who survived to be discharged home, and only 7% of overall NICU expenses were spent on nonsurvivors. Although the prediction of futility was fairly accurate in that more than 75% of infants were consistently predicted to survive and did so, the authors certainly are not advocating the predictive capability as a guide. There was sufficient inaccuracy and caregiver variation, and the predictions to die before discharge for even the most accurate caretaker group were wrong more than 1 time in 3, all of which would be evidence that daily predictions cannot solely be used to target resources. One small quibble, however: the authors tried to quantify professional intuition or judgment about prognosis. The question asked of caregivers was will the baby live or die, not should the baby live or die and not what will the prognosis be. So, before lamenting the inaccuracy of clinical judgment, we need to make sure we ask the right question.

The sound justification of this study for providing neonatal intensive care to these infants does come with at least two caveats. What if there were more deaths, say a 10% nonsurvival rate. Would that justification still hold and is there a tipping point? But the bigger issue really is the morbidity in survivors.

What if the quality of that survival is not "good enough"? There are no data on postdischarge deaths or neurodevelopmental outcomes, making this unknowable. But the question must be raised, for if we looked at mortality as well as other outcomes, we might come to a different conclusion. What if 15% of infants have cerebral palsy or blindness—would the argument still hold?

Certainly the authors are to be commended for showing the real costs for such NICU care. The authors justifiably refute any notion that this care is less cost-effective than adult medical intensive care unit care: NICU costs are roughly one-fifth that of many interventions accepted for adult patients, and if end-of-life care cost savings for society as a whole are desired, it is not the NICU that should be the site of cost reduction. Despite this spirited defense of NICU care and the favorable comparisons with adult care, it is certainly sobering to see that the overall cost per surviving early low birth weight infant to discharge was approximately $226 000.

Extrapolation and generalization of the findings may, however, be limited. First, the authors describe the demographics of their parent population as "poor, inner city, black, religious, distrustful of medical authority and believing in miracles," suggesting that decision making is largely a reflection of this culture and that the frequency of "negotiated deaths" in their NICU is extremely low. Second, the definition of futility in this study is solely in economic terms, excluding other consideration such as the views of parents or nursing staff, who might have described their experience as more or less rewarding or futile in ways other than economic.

**J. Hellmann, MBBCh, FCP(SA), FRCPC, MHSc**

---

## How Infants Die in the Neonatal Intensive Care Unit: Trends From 1999 Through 2008

Weiner J, Sharma J, Lantos J, et al (Univ of Missouri, Kansas City)
*Arch Pediatr Adolesc Med* 165:630-634, 2011

---

*Objective.*—To determine whether trends toward decreasing use of cardiopulmonary resuscitation at the time of death and increasing frequency of forgoing life-sustaining treatment had continued, as few studies quantifying mode of death for hospitalized infants have been conducted in the last 10 years.

*Design.*—Retrospective descriptive study.

*Setting.*—Regional referral neonatal intensive care unit.

*Participants.*—Infants who died from January 1, 1999, to December 31, 2008. Infants were categorized into following categories: (1) very preterm (≤ 32 weeks' gestation); (2) congenital anomaly; and (3) other.

*Main Outcome Measures.*—The primary outcome was level of clinical service provided at the end of life (care withheld, care withdrawn, or full resuscitation).

*Results.*—For 10 years, 414 neonatal patients died. Of these, 61.6% had care withdrawn, 20.8% had care withheld, and 17.6% received cardiopulmonary resuscitation. The percentage of deaths that followed withholding of treatment rose by 1% per year ($P = .01$). Most of this change was accounted for by withholding of therapy in the very premature group.

*Conclusion.*—During the 10-year period, the primary mode of death in this regional referral neonatal intensive care unit was withdrawal of life-sustaining support. When death is imminent or medical care is considered futile, the approach is thought to provide a peaceful, controlled setting. Significant increase in withholding of care suggests improved recognition of medical futility and desire to provide a peaceful death.

▶ This retrospective descriptive study examined the methods of death of infants in a single-center neonatal intensive care unit over a 10-year period (1999–2008). Examination of more than 400 neonatal deaths found that more than 80% were associated with either withdrawal or noninitiation of support. Withdrawal of support was the most frequent mode of death irrespective of diagnostic category. The authors also looked at the mode of death for very preterm infants (defined as ≤ 32 weeks' gestation) over this time period in 2-year epochs. Both withdrawing and withholding care showed increasing trends beginning in 2001, whereas death following cardiopulmonary resuscitation showed a declining trend over the same time period.

I found 2 important messages in this study. First, it may represent a real change in both physician and parental acceptance of futility of care and input in decision making. Second, it should force us, as clinical investigators, to reconsider death as a primary outcome measure in clinical trials, and if this parameter is chosen, it should be obligatory that we disclose the causes of death or at least the percentage of deaths attributed to withdrawal or noninitiation of support. It would also be of interest to know if these results are representative of national practices. I suspect they are.

**S. M. Donn, MD**

---

**Evidence to Inform Decisions About Maternal–Fetal Surgery: Technical Brief**

Hartmann KE, McPheeters ML, Chescheir NC, et al (Vanderbilt Med Ctr, Nashville, TN; Univ of North Carolina, Chapel Hill)
*Obstet Gynecol* 117:1191-1204, 2011

---

*Objective.*—To summarize the state of research in maternal–fetal surgery regarding the surgical repair of abnormalities in fetuses in the womb.

*Data Sources.*—We searched MEDLINE from 1980 to 2010 for studies of maternal–fetal surgery for the following conditions: twin–twin transfusion syndrome, obstructive uropathy, congenital diaphragmatic hernia, myelomeningocele, thoracic lesions, cardiac malformations, and sacrococcygeal teratoma.

*Methods of Study Selection.*—We used pilot-tested data collection forms to screen publications for inclusion and to extract data. We compiled information about how fetal diagnoses were defined, maternal inclusion criteria, type of surgery, study design, country, setting, comparators used, length of follow-up, outcomes measured, and adverse events.

*Tabulation, Integration, and Results.*—Two reviewers independently extracted data and discordance was resolved by a third party. Of 1,341 articles located, we retained 258 (comprising 166 unique study populations). Three studies were randomized controlled trials; the majority of the evidence was observational (116 case series [70%], 36 retrospective [22%], and 11 prospective [7%] cohorts). Twin—twin transfusion is the most studied condition, with 84 studies including 2,532 pregnancies. Fewer than 500 pregnancies are represented in the literature for each of the other conditions except congenital diaphragmatic hernia (n = 503). Inclusion criteria were poorly specified. Outcomes typically measured were survival to birth, preterm birth, and neonatal death. Longer-term outcomes were sparse but included pulmonary, renal, and neurologic status and developmental milestones. Maternal outcome data were rare.

*Conclusion.*—Although developing rapidly, maternal—fetal surgery research has yet to achieve the typical quality of studies and aggregate strength of evidence needed to optimally inform care.

▶ In their review, Hartmann et al provide a highly practical review of the existing evidence about available in utero interventions for a number of fetal problems, model a methodologically sound example of systematic literature review, and highlight the poignant problems that families and perinatal care providers face when it comes to deciding about fetal intervention. The broad scope and thorough nature of this review are reasons enough to include this work on one's highlight reel for 2011, and this article will no doubt be quite useful to practitioners new and old who are not intimately familiar with the evidence in support of these high-risk high-stakes procedures. It is regrettable that this article was written before the results of the Management of Myelomeningocele study (Adzick et al, 2011) were published,[1] as discussion of that study no doubt would have enriched this work even more.

This article brings to the foreground several ethically difficult questions for the many stakeholders in the evolving field of fetal intervention for congenital anomalies and twin-twin transfusion syndrome. First, it reminds us that for women and families considering these interventions, decisions remain highly sensitive to specific contextual features of each case and in many cases are appropriately value driven. Clearly the adverse health outcomes associated with the conditions themselves and with the interventions (both before and after birth) require careful weighing of risks and benefits for both the fetus and the expectant mother. This is complicated, of course, by the paucity of gold standard evidence to inform the risk-benefit calculus. How informed can consent possibly be while we remain so uncertain of the likely outcomes associated with these procedures? For those who counsel women about pregnancy termination, in utero intervention, and postnatal care, how can we appropriately provide support for this kind of decision making, knowing that for most of fetal interventions, few or no data from randomized control trials are available? What is the obligation to explain this academic reality to patients? Good ethics start with good facts, but the facts remain elusive.

Beyond the strengths of this article as a scholarly endeavor in systematic literature review, the authors provide an articulate and balanced discussion, pointing out both the need for more data to support decisions about fetal intervention and the realities that complicate the conduct of large multicenter randomized control trials in this field. Their optimism is not misplaced—this look back at the evolution of in utero fetal intervention does suggest that things are moving in the right direction, but it seems that after 50 years, the need remains for robust prospective research on short- and long-term outcomes using mutually agreed-upon, relevant end points.

N. T. Laventhal, MD

Reference

1. Danzer E, Adzick NS. Fetal Surgery for myelomeningocele: patient selection, perioperative management and outcomes. <i>Fetal Diagn Ther.</i> 2011;30:163-173.

# Article Index

## Chapter 1: The Fetus

## Chapter 2: Epidemiology and Pregnancy Complications

## Chapter 3: Genetics and Teratology

## Chapter 4: Labor and Delivery

## Chapter 5: Infectious Disease and Immunology

## Chapter 6: Cardiovascular System

## Chapter 7: Respiratory Disorders

## Chapter 8: Central Nervous System and Special Senses

## Chapter 9: Behavior and Pain

## Chapter 10: Gastrointestinal Health and Nutrition

## Chapter 11: Hematology and Bilirubin

## Chapter 12: Renal, Metabolism, and Endocrine Disorders

## Chapter 15: Postnatal Growth and Development/Follow-up

## Chapter 16: Ethics

# Author Index